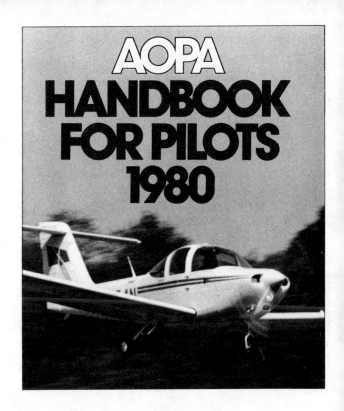

Published by
Aircraft Owners and Pilots Association
7315 Wisconsin Avenue
Washington, D.C. 20014
Phone (301) 654-0500

Price: $6 to AOPA members; $10 to nonmembers.

FOREWORD

The *AOPA Handbook for Pilots* is a quick and easy source of aviation information for pilots. And this year the information contained in the publication has been reorganized to make it easier to locate.

The contents have been updated and revised and the eight sections found in past editions have been condensed into six. A more detailed table of contents and revised index makes the information in the book easier to locate.

Added features in the 1980 edition include a list of the major air shows and aviation conventions in the U.S.; new customs regulations; an extensively updated list of FSS numbers, which for the first time includes the Pacific region; a Pilot's Checklist; and a Flight Plan checklist. Also, we have indicated new additions to the FARs with brackets, to enable the busy pilot to locate important changes quickly.

Other information contained in this edition which the user may find particularly helpful are aircraft performance charts and conversion tables; weather information (including an aviation weather key); the complete pilot/controller glossary; emergency survival procedures; names and addresses of key aviation agencies and organizations; plus much more.

Keep in mind, though, that the Handbook should be used as a supplement of, not a substitute for, the many specialized publications used for flight planning—for example, the Airman's Information Manual and aeronautical charts.

The contents have been thoroughly revised and updated to reflect the most current and accurate information available at the time of publication. However, we acknowledge that some information may change during the year; any comments, suggestions, and/or corrections to the material you may wish to send to us are most appreciated.

TABLE OF CONTENTS

Section 2 Weather

Section 3 In Flight

Section 4 Emergency Procedures

Section 5 Addresses and Services

Section 6   Federal Aviation Regulations

General Aviation at a Glance

Active Civil Aircraft (as of Dec. 31, 1978)

General Aviation	198,800
Piston	184,700
Turbine	5,500
Rotorcraft	5,000
Other	3,600

Active Airman Certificates (as of Dec. 31, 1978)

TOTAL	798,833
Student	204,874
Private	337,644
Commercial	185,833
ATP	55,881
Helicopter (only)	4,874
Glider and Lighter than Air	9,727

General Aviation Totals (1978)

Hours flown	33,600,000 (84.4%)
Miles flown	4,519,900,000 (61.8%)
Aircraft Operations	51,664,261 (75.6%)
Instrument Operations	16,780,693 (49.0%)

U.S. General Aviation Aircraft Production (1978)

Single engine	13,650
Ag Planes	784
Multi-engine	2,634
Turboprop	548
Turbojet	231
Helicopters	904

U.S. Civil Aircraft Landing Facilities (as of Dec. 31, 1978)

Airports	12,006
Heliports	1,986
Seaplane bases	436

1980 Air Shows and Aviation Conventions

Following is a listing of major air shows and aviation conventions around the country for 1980. This is not a complete listing. Check the **AOPA Pilot** "Calendar" section for additional information.

Abbotsford International Airshow Canada, Abbotsford, B.C., Canada, August 8–10

Aircraft Electronics Association Convention, Kansas City, MO, April 21–23

Aircraft Owners and Pilots Association Convention and Industry Exhibit, San Diego, CA, October 28–November 2

American Association of Airport Executives, Dallas, TX, May 18–22

American Bonanza Society, Nashville, TN, July 16–20

Aviation/Space Writers Association Annual News Conference, Toronto, Canada, May 18–23

Confederate Air Force, Harlingen, TX; Wintersho'—February 16; Airsho'—October 2–5

Experimental Aircraft Association Convention, Oshkosh, WI, August 2–9

Flying Dentists Association, San Antonio, TX, June 29–July 3

Flying Farmers Annual Conference, San Diego, CA, August 3–8

Flying Physicians Association, Monterey, CA, July 20–24

Helicopter Association of America, Las Vegas, NV, February 10–13

Lawyer-Pilots Bar Association, Marco Island, FL, February 6–10; Vancouver, B.C., Canada, August 6–10

National Agricultural Aviation Association, Las Vegas, NV, December 1–4

National Air Transportation Association, Las Vegas, NV, March 23–26

National Association of Flight Instructors Annual Meeting, San Diego, CA (at the AOPA Convention), October 29–30

National Business Aircraft Association, Kansas City, MO, September 23–25

National Intercollegiate Flying Association National Air Meet, University of North Dakota, Grand Forks, ND, May 15–18

The Ninety-Nines Annual Convention, Vail, CO, July 23–27

Reading Air Show, Reading Municipal Airport, Reading, PA, June 10–13

Reno Air Races, Reno/Stead Airport, Reno, NV, September 12–14

World Aerobatic Contest, Oshkosh, WI, August 17–30

SECTION 1
Flight Preparation

Aeronautical Charts

Any National Ocean Survey aeronautical chart may be ordered from AOPA, individually or in any quantity, at standard list prices plus first class postage.

Jeppesen Airway Manual Service subscriptions are also available through AOPA. Address information queries and orders to Listing, Title Search and Chart Department. For Foreign Trip Kits contact the AOPA Chart Department. For Domestic Trip Kits write Jeppesen & Co., 8025 E. 40th Ave., Denver, CO, 80207.

AOPA maintains a chart subscription service for members to all U.S. sectional, WAC, and TCA charts plus Alaskan and Hawaiian WAC charts. Subscriptions to other types of National Ocean Survey aeronautical charts are available directly from AOPA and the National Ocean Survey, Distribution Division, Washington, DC, 20235. Proper order forms for all NOS subscriptions are available upon request to the AOPA Chart Dept., P.O. Box 5800, Washington, DC, 20014.

Subscriptions available from the National Ocean Survey include:

Instrument Navigation Charts

(All charts are replaced every 56 days.)

En Route Low Altitude Charts (data required for instrument flight below 18,000 ft. in the 48 states and at all altitudes in the Caribbean).

En Route Alaska and Hawaii Charts (data required for instrument flight at all altitudes in Alaska and Hawaii).

En Route High Altitude Charts (data required for instrument flight above 18,000 ft. in the 48 states).

Area Charts (data required to safely execute arrivals and departures in high density terminal areas).

Standard Instrument Departures (SIDs). (Data depicting preferential departure routing from high density terminal areas.)

Standard Terminal Arrival Routes (STARs). (Data depicting preplanned air traffic control IFR arrival clearance routings.)

Note: All subscriptions include special notices and revisions for one year. En Route Low Altitude subscriptions also include Area Charts. SIDs, under separate subscription, are furnished in a bound booklet, revised every 56 days.

Instrument Approach Procedure Charts

The 15 bound volumes provide complete conterminous (48 states) U.S. coverage, including Puerto Rico and the Virgin Islands but excluding Alaska and Hawaii. Each volume completely replaces the former looseleaf format. Each successive volume also totally supercedes its predecessor.

Changes to procedures between publication dates are reflected in a single Change Notice volume, covering the entire U.S. (48 states).

Bound volumes may be ordered as a set, individually or in any combination or number to meet individual needs.

Subscriptions are broken down as follows:

Northeast, books 1, 2, 3—ME, NH, VT, MA, CT, RI, NY, PA, NJ, DE, MD, VA, WV, DC

Southeast, books 1, 2, 3—KY, TN, AL, MS, NC, SC, GA, FL, PR, VI

East Central, books 1, 2, 3—MI, IN, OH, WI, IL

North Central, books 1, 2—ND, SD, MN, IA, NE, KS, MO

South Central, books 1, 2—OK, AR, LA, TX, NM

Northwest, book 1—WA, OR, ID, MT, WY

Southwest, book 1—NV, UT, CO, AZ, CA

Change Notice—full conterminous U.S. (48 states)

Jet Navigation Charts

JN series charts are suitable for long-range, high-altitude, high-speed navigation. Four charts provide complete coverage of the United States, much of northern Mexico and most of southern Canada. JN coverage is available for most of the northern hemisphere.

Aircraft Radio Station Licenses

Both a station license and an operator license must be obtained from the Federal Communications Commission for operation of an aircraft radio station. The radio station license must be posted in a prominent place in the aircraft or kept with the aircraft registration certificate.

Before making application, the applicant should refer to Part 87 of the FCC Rules Governing Aviation Services. Copies are available through the Government Printing Office, Washington, DC, 20402. Subscription cost is $15.00 for domestic subscriptions (including U.S. Territories, Canada and Mexico) and $18.75 for foreign subscriptions. The subscription request should be for Volume V, which contains Parts 87, 90 and 94. Make check or money order payable to the Superintendent of Documents.

Use FCC Form 404 to make application for a new aircraft radio station license or for the modification of such license. Application for renewal without modification should be made on FCC Form 405-B. Renewal applications should be filed within 90 days of, and not less than 30 days prior to, the license expiration. The application should be completed and sent to the Federal Communications Commission, P.O. Box 1030, Gettysburg, PA, 17325.

The Federal Communications Commission suspended all fee collections effective January 1, 1977. Until a new fee schedule is adopted, applications for aircraft radio station licenses should *not* include any remittance or filing fee. If application for renewal is filed prior to expiration of the station license, operation may continue until the renewal application is acted upon by the commission.

In the purchase and sale of used private aircraft, the seller's license (if valid at time of sale) serves as evidence of 60-day interim authority for the benefit of the buyer, in accordance with authority on the face of the license document. Persons buying a new aircraft are also afforded a 60-day interim authority to operate radio equipment installed in the aircraft at the aircraft factory. This is accomplished through aircraft manufacturers, distributors and dealers using FCC Form 453-B. A person who owns an aircraft or is having the initial installation of radio equipment installed by an avionics manufacturer, dealer or distributor may also be afforded a 60-day interim authority to operate the radio equipment. This is accomplished through the avionics manufacturer, dealer or distributor using FCC Form 453-B. In these instances the interim authority is valid only if application for a regular aircraft radio station license is made by the buyer at the time of the sale. Radio station licenses are not transferable between aircraft.

Aircraft Radio Operator's License

The radio transmitter must be operated by or under the direct supervision of a licensed radio operator. The license normally held by persons operating aircraft radios is the Restricted Radiotelephone Operators Permit (RRTOP). To obtain the permit, complete FCC Form 753 and mail to the FCC at P.O. Box 1050, Gettysburg, PA, 17325. No oral or written examination is required. Field offices will accept applications for the permit if the applicant makes a satisfactory showing, in writing, of immediate need for safety, and if the application is presented in person by the applicant or his agent. This permit does not authorize the holder to make transmitter adjustments that may affect the proper operation of the station. Any adjustments must be made by the holder of a first- or second-class radiotelegraph or radiotelephone license. Alien pilots applying for permits should submit the application, FCC Form 755, to the FCC's Washington, DC, office. (To expedite handling, also send a copy of U.S. pilot certificate.) The alien permit is good for five years.

Effective January 1, 1977, the Federal Communications Commission suspended all fee collections relating to obtaining an aircraft radio operator's permit. Until a new fee schedule is adopted by the FCC, applications for Restricted Radiotelephone Operator Permits should *not* include remittance. (See Section 5 for FCC Field Operating Offices.)

Notams

FAA Notices to Airmen (NOTAMS) are used to provide information over weather teletypes that is not known sufficiently in advance to be publicized by any other means. The NOTAM is generally unrelated to weather, but instead concerns establishment, condition, or changes in facilities and procedures in the airspace system. Specific hazards may also be noted. NOTAMS will be found listed at the end of hourly sequence reports for each region of the country and may also be broadcast on VOR voice frequencies.

Air Navigation Formulas

true course $\pm$ wind correction angle = true heading
   (Add wind corr. angle right; subtract wind corr. angle left.)

true heading $\pm$ variation = magnetic heading

magnetic heading $\pm$ deviation = compass heading
   $TC \pm WCA = TH \pm Var = MH \pm Dev = CH$

true course $\pm$ variation = magnetic course
   $TC \pm Var = MC$

$$time = \frac{distance}{groundspeed} \qquad\qquad distance = groundspeed \times time$$

$$groundspeed = \frac{distance}{time}$$

Converting minutes to tenths of an hour, 6 minutes = 0.1 hour.

Air Navigation Definitions

Calibrated Airspeed (CAS)—Airspeed after corrections made for manufacturer and installation errors.

Compass Heading (CH)—Heading flown by reference to the magnetic compass. Magnetic heading corrected for compass deviation is compass heading.

Deviation—Compass instrument error caused by magnetic attractions from parts of the aircraft. Deviated amount usually recorded in cockpit near magnetic compass.

Groundspeed (GS)—Actual speed of aircraft over the ground.

Indicated Airspeed (IAS)—Airspeed read directly from the airspeed indicator.

Magnetic Course (MC)—Proposed flight-path direction relative to magnetic north. (Victor airways are plotted on aeronautical charts as magnetic courses.)

Magnetic Heading (MH)—Actual heading of the aircraft in flight relative to magnetic north.

Track—Actual path over the earth's surface.

True Airspeed (TAS)—Indicated airspeed corrected for instrument error, altitude and temperature.

True Course (TC)—Proposed flight-path direction relative to true north.

True Heading (TH)—Actual aircraft heading in flight relative to true north. TH is the TC plus or minus WCA.

Variation—The difference in degrees, plus or minus between true north and magnetic north at any given point on the earth's surface. East variation is subtracted and west variation is added to true course to obtain magnetic course.

Wind Correction Angle (WCA)—Correction angle needed to make the aircraft's track and course the same.

Wind Direction—The *true* direction *from* which the wind is blowing. (FSS and airport towers report winds from a *magnetic* direction when queried by radio.)

Windspeed—Rate of movement of an air mass over the ground, reported in knots.

Weight and Balance

Each pilot is responsible for ensuring that the weight and balance of his aircraft is within prescribed limits prior to flight.

Typical loading for a small airplane—L indicates the distance of each load item from a reference, datum, line. From this example you can make your own weight and balance format, inserting the correct **L** numbers applicable to your own airplane.

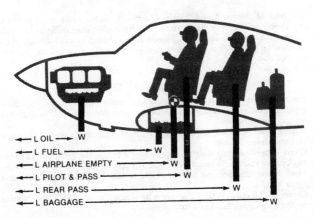

ITEM	LENGTH-INCHES (ARM)	×	WEIGHT-LBS.	=	MOMENT IN.-LBS.
Oil	_____	×	_____	=	_____
Fuel	_____	×	_____	=	_____
Airplane Basic Weight Empty	_____	×	_____	=	_____
Pilot	_____	×	_____	=	_____
Front Passenger	_____	×	_____	=	_____
Rear Passengers	_____	×	_____	=	_____
Baggage	_____	×	_____	=	_____
TOTAL	_____		_____		_____

TOTAL MOMENT DIVIDED BY THE TOTAL WEIGHT EQUALS THE CENTER OF GRAVITY (CG) LOCATION IN INCHES FROM DATUM LINE.

	FORWARD	AFT
APPROVED CG LIMITS FOR AIRCRAFT		
MAXIMUM ALLOWABLE GROSS WEIGHT	_____	_____
	INCHES FROM DATUM	

WARNING: If the CG does not fall between the forward and aft limits, the load must be rearranged prior to takeoff. If the weight exceeds the maximum allowable, the load must be reduced prior to takeoff.

(Percent of Mean Aerodynamic Chord—% MAC. This is a different reference used to locate the center of gravity. Rather than using inches from an imaginary datum line, the CG limits are computed as a percentage of the mean wing chord. This method is used primarily for large or long aircraft.)

Weight and Balance Definitions

Empty Weight—The weight of the basic airplane—the structure, the powerplant, fixed equipment, all fixed ballast, and unusable fuel, undrainable oil and hydraulic fluid.

Useful Load (payload)—The weight of pilot, passengers, baggage, usable fuel and drainable oil.

Gross Weight—Empty weight plus the useful load is the gross weight of the airplane at takeoff. When an airplane is carrying the maximum load for which it is certificated, the takeoff weight is called the **maximum allowable gross weight.**

Center of Gravity (CG)—The point at which the aircraft would balance perfectly if suspended from that point.

Datum—The location along the aircraft's longitudinal axis from which all horizontal measurements are taken.

Arm—The distance between an object in the aircraft and the datum.

Moment—The weight of an object in the aircraft multiplied by the arm.

• Since in most modern aircraft the pilot has a loading option, he must carefully consider all factors that might possibly have an adverse effect on flight safety. Any condition that will affect takeoff and climb performance must be considered. Of prime importance are high elevations, high temperatures and high humidity, all of which decrease performance. Other factors include runway length, runway surface, winds and obstacle-clearance margins.

• When loading the aircraft one must keep the center of gravity (CG) within prescribed limits so that the aircraft will properly "balance." In most aircraft this can be done by using common sense and distributing the load by following placards located in the aircraft. Refer to the weight and balance data in the airplane flight manual if any question exists about whether the aircraft is loaded within acceptable tolerances of balance.

• Pilots of aircraft loaded with an improper forward center of gravity can expect: excessive nosewheel loads, or tendency to nose over in tailwheel airplanes; decreased performance; higher stalling speeds; higher stick forces.

• Pilots of aircraft loaded with an improper aft center of gravity can expect: decreased static and dynamic longitudinal stability (under some conditions it may be uncontrollable); violent stall characteristics; very light stick forces.

Standard figures used in weight and balance computations:

    Fuel—6 pounds per gallon (varies from 5.85 to 6.4)

    Oil—7.5 pounds per gallon

    Passengers—170 pounds average

Special VFR Clearances

A Special VFR clearance allows a pilot to fly inside a control zone in lower weather minimums than normally permitted. An ATC clearance MUST be obtained prior to initiating a Special VFR operation. Within most control zones, a VFR pilot may request and be given a clearance to conduct special VFR flight to, from, or within the control zone providing the flight will not delay IFR operations.

While flying under an SVFR clearance, visibility requirements for fixed-wing aircraft are 1 mile flight visibility, and 1 mile ground visibility if taking off or landing. All special VFR flights must remain clear of the clouds.

When a control zone tower is located within the control zone, requests for clearances should be to the tower. If no tower is located within the control zone, a clearance may be obtained from the nearest tower, flight service station, or center.

In some control zones special VFR operations are prohibited due to the volume of IFR traffic. A list of these zones is in FAR 93.113, which is included in Section 6 of this Handbook.

In addition, special VFR operations by fixed-wing aircraft are prohibited between sunset and sunrise unless the pilot is instrument rated and his aircraft is equipped for IFR flight.

High Density Traffic Airports

FAA has designated John F. Kennedy International, LaGuardia, Washington National, and O'Hare as "high-density traffic airports." At all, IFR reservations are required for general aviation aircraft except those on medical emergency flights. The reservations system applies at LaGuardia and Washington National between the hours of 6 a.m. and midnight; at JFK International and O'Hare, between 3 p.m. and 8 p.m.

Reservations are allocated hourly, All VFR arrivals must obtain a reservation granted by ATC and have an alternate airport planned for use if necessary. A reservation does not preclude traffic delays.

To obtain an IFR reservation, contact the nearest FSS, or call the Airport Reservation Office at the following locations: New York—(212) 632-7806, Chicago—(312) 263-2575, Washington, DC—(202) 488-1491. Requests for a reservation will be accepted any time after 6 a.m. local time on the day which is 48 hours in advance of the proposed operation.

Flight Plan

Federal Aviation Regulations do not require that a VFR flight plan be filed except as specified for flight in a coastal or domestic ADIZ or DEWIZ. Flight plans can be submitted to the nearest Flight Service Station (FSS) in person or by telephone. They may be filed by radio if no other means are available.

VFR flight plans are transmitted only to the FSS with which the pilot has stated his arrival report will be filed. If the flight plan is not closed within ½ hour after the estimated time of arrival (ETA), search and rescue operations are started.

When a flight is terminated before the destination specified in the flight plan is reached, the pilot should contact the nearest FSS and request that an arrival report be transmitted to the FSS at the specified destination. The importance of closing the flight plan cannot be overemphasized. The pilot who forgets to do so may incur civil penalties.

Pilots operating on VFR flight plans and desiring to make flight progress reports should include in the report the phrase: "VFR from (blank) to (blank)," along with aircraft identification, position, time and altitude.

The use of the term "VFR" instead of an actual altitude indicates that the pilot intends to fly in accordance with visual flight rules. Aircraft may be operated VFR above a well-defined cloud or other formation, provided climb to and descent from such "on top" flight can also be made in VFR conditions.

A DVFR (Defense Visual Flight Rules) flight plan is mandatory for VFR flight within an ADIZ except as specified in Part 99 of the FARs.

For IFR flight (Instrument Flight Rules) the pilot must have an instrument rating and the aircraft must be properly equipped. The required equipment includes a properly functioning two-way radio.

For details see Part 91 of the FARs in Section 6 of this Handbook.

For filing flight plans, 14 equipment suffixes are used along with aircraft type. These are:

X—no transponder

T—transponder with no altitude encoding capability

U—transponder with altitude encoding capability

D—DME, no transponder

B—DME, transponder with no altitude encoding capability

A—DME, transponder with altitude encoding capability

M—TACAN only, no transponder

N—TACAN only, transponder with no altitude encoding capability

P—TACAN only, transponder with altitude encoding capability

C—RNAV, transponder with no altitude encoding capability

F—RNAV, transponder with altitude encoding capability

W—RNAV, no transponder

Examples: BE-50/B, PA-30/D, C-152/U

Close Flight Plan Upon Arrival

This format is used by the FAA on Flight Plan forms. Complete each item as necessary when filing.

1. Type: ☐VFR ☐IFR ☐DVFR

2. Aircraft Identification:

3. Aircraft Type/Special Equipment:

4. True Airspeed: _____ Kts.

5. Departure Point:

6. Departure Time: _____ Proposed
   (Zulu)
   _____ Actual

7. Cruising Altitude:

8. Route of Flight:

9. Destination (Name of Airport and City):

10. Estimated Time Enroute:

    _____ Hrs. _____ Mins.

11. Remarks:

12. Fuel on Board:

    _____ Hrs. _____ Mins.

13. Alternate Airport(s):

14. Pilot's Name, Address, Telephone Number, and Aircraft Home Base:

15. Number Aboard:

16. Color Aircraft:

Great Circle Distances Between U.S. Cities

(statute miles) (Source: U.S. National Ocean Survey)

	Atlanta	Baltimore	Boston	Buffalo	Chicago	Cincinnati	Cleveland	Dallas	Denver	Detroit	Great Falls	Houston	Indianapolis	Jacksonville	Kansas City, Mo.	Little Rock	Los Angeles	Louisville
Atlanta	•	577	937	697	587	369	554	721	1212	596	1689	701	426	285	676	456	1936	319
Baltimore	577	•	360	274	606	424	308	1212	1510	397	1818	1251	511	681	963	920	2320	499
Boston	937	360	•	400	851	740	551	1551	1769	613	1983	1605	807	1017	1251	1259	2596	826
Buffalo	697	274	400	•	454	393	173	1198	1370	216	1603	1286	435	879	861	913	2198	483
Chicago	587	606	851	454	•	252	308	803	920	238	1223	940	165	863	414	552	1745	269
Cincinnati	369	424	740	393	252	•	222	814	1094	235	1460	892	100	626	541	524	1897	90
Cleveland	554	308	551	173	308	222	•	1025	1227	90	1510	1114	263	770	700	740	2049	311
Dallas	721	1212	1551	1198	803	814	1025	•	663	999	1268	225	763	908	451	293	1240	726
Denver	1212	1510	1769	1370	920	1094	1227	663	•	1156	621	879	1000	1467	558	780	831	1038
Detroit	596	397	613	216	238	235	90	999	1156	•	1423	1105	240	831	645	723	1983	316
Great Falls	1689	1818	1983	1603	1223	1460	1510	1268	621	1423	•	1490	1361	1968	1020	1320	995	1436
Houston	701	1251	1605	1286	940	892	1114	225	879	1105	1490	•	865	821	644	388	1374	803
Indianapolis	426	511	807	435	165	100	263	763	1000	240	1361	865	•	699	453	483	1809	107
Jacksonville	285	681	1017	879	863	626	770	908	1467	831	1968	821	699	•	950	690	2147	594

Kansas City, Mo.	676	963	1251	861	414	541	700	451	558	645	1020	644	453	950	•	325	1356	480
Little Rock	456	920	1259	913	552	524	740	293	780	723	1320	388	483	690	325	•	1480	435
Los Angeles	1936	2320	2596	2198	1745	1897	2049	1240	831	1983	995	1374	1809	2147	1356	1480	•	1829
Louisville	319	499	826	483	269	90	311	726	1038	316	1436	803	107	594	480	435	1829	•
Memphis	337	793	1137	803	482	410	630	420	879	623	1388	484	384	590	369	129	1603	320
Miami	604	954	1255	1181	1188	952	1087	1111	1726	1152	2260	968	1024	326	1241	949	2339	919
Minneapolis	907	939	1123	731	355	605	630	862	700	543	880	1056	511	1191	413	708	1524	605
New Orleans	424	999	1359	1086	833	706	924	443	1082	939	1657	318	712	504	680	355	1673	623
New York City	748	172	188	292	713	570	405	1374	1631	482	1893	1420	646	838	1097	1081	2451	652
Oklahoma City	757	1177	1495	1120	692	758	951	190	505	910	1092	413	689	986	296	301	1181	678
Omaha	817	1028	1282	883	432	622	739	586	488	669	872	794	525	1098	166	492	1315	580
Philadelphia	666	90	271	279	666	503	360	1299	1579	443	1864	1341	585	758	1038	1007	2394	582
Phoenix	1592	2005	2300	1906	1453	1581	1749	887	586	1690	970	1017	1499	1794	1049	1137	357	1508
Pittsburgh	521	197	483	178	410	257	115	1070	1320	205	1622	1137	330	703	781	779	2136	344
Portland, Ore.	2172	2361	2540	2156	1758	1985	2055	1633	982	1969	559	1836	1885	2439	1497	1759	825	1950
St. Louis	467	733	1038	662	262	309	492	547	796	455	1225	679	231	751	238	291	1589	242
Salt Lake City	1583	1861	2099	1699	1260	1453	1568	999	371	1492	466	1200	1356	1837	925	1148	579	1402
San Francisco	2139	2457	2699	2300	1858	2043	2166	1483	949	2091	876	1645	1949	2374	1506	1688	347	1986
Seattle	2182	2334	2493	2117	1737	1972	2026	1681	1021	1938	515	1891	1872	2455	1506	1785	959	1943
Tulsa	678	1081	1398	1023	598	661	853	236	550	813	1108	442	591	921	216	231	1266	582
Washington, D.C.	543	35	393	292	597	404	306	1185	1494	396	1814	1220	494	647	945	892	2300	476
Wichita	776	1126	1424	1036	591	702	873	340	437	821	980	559	620	1031	177	348	1197	633

Great Circle Distances Between U.S. Cities

(statute miles)

	Memphis	Miami	Minneapolis	New Orleans	New York City	Oklahoma City	Omaha	Philadelphia	Phoenix	Pittsburgh	Portland, Ore.	St. Louis	Salt Lake City	San Francisco	Seattle	Tulsa	Washington, D.C.	Wichita
Atlanta	337	604	907	424	748	757	817	666	1592	521	2172	467	1583	2139	2182	678	543	776
Baltimore	793	954	939	999	172	1177	1028	90	2005	197	2361	733	1861	2457	2334	1081	35	1126
Boston	1137	1255	1123	1359	188	1495	1282	271	2300	483	2540	1038	2099	2699	2493	1398	393	1424
Buffalo	803	1181	731	1086	292	1120	883	279	1906	178	2156	662	1699	2300	2117	1023	292	1036
Chicago	482	1188	355	833	713	692	432	666	1453	410	1758	262	1260	1858	1737	598	597	591
Cincinnati	410	952	605	706	570	758	622	503	1581	257	1985	309	1453	2043	1972	661	404	702
Cleveland	630	1087	630	924	405	951	739	360	1749	115	2055	492	1568	2166	2026	853	306	873
Dallas	420	1111	862	443	1374	190	586	1299	887	1070	1633	547	999	1483	1681	236	1185	340
Denver	879	1726	700	1082	1631	505	488	1579	586	1320	982	796	371	949	1021	550	1494	437
Detroit	623	1152	543	939	482	910	669	443	1690	205	1969	455	1492	2091	1938	813	396	821
Great Falls	1388	2260	880	1657	1893	1092	872	1864	970	1622	559	1225	466	876	515	1108	1814	980
Houston	484	968	1056	318	1420	413	794	1341	1017	1137	1836	679	1200	1645	1891	442	1220	559
Indianapolis	384	1024	511	712	646	689	525	585	1499	330	1885	231	1356	1949	1872	591	494	620
Jacksonville	590	326	1191	504	838	986	1098	758	1794	703	2439	751	1837	2374	2455	921	647	1031

22

City	Memphis	Miami	Minneapolis	New Orleans	New York	Oklahoma City	Omaha	Philadelphia	Phoenix	Pittsburgh	Portland, Ore.	St. Louis	Salt Lake City	San Francisco	Seattle	Tulsa	Washington, D.C.	Wichita
Kansas City, Mo.	369	1241	413	680	1097	296	166	1038	1049	781	1497	238	925	1506	1506	216	945	177
Little Rock	129	949	708	355	1081	301	492	1007	1137	779	1759	291	1148	1688	1785	231	892	348
Los Angeles	1603	2339	1524	1673	2451	1181	1315	2394	357	2136	825	1589	579	347	959	1266	2300	1197
Louisville	320	919	605	623	652	678	580	582	1508	344	1950	242	1402	1986	1943	582	476	633
Memphis	•	872	699	358	957	422	529	881	1263	660	1849	240	1250	1802	1867	341	765	442
Miami	872	•	1511	669	1092	1226	1397	1019	1982	1010	2708	1061	2089	2594	2734	1176	923	1297
Minneapolis	699	1511	•	1051	1018	693	290	985	1280	743	1427	466	987	1584	1395	626	934	546
New Orleans	358	669	1051	•	1171	577	847	1089	1316	919	2063	598	1434	1926	2101	548	966	677
New York	957	1092	1018	1171	•	1328	1144	83	2145	317	2445	875	1972	2571	2408	1231	205	1266
Oklahoma City	422	1226	693	577	1328	•	408	1260	842	1014	1486	459	862	1388	1524	98	1153	153
Omaha	529	1397	290	847	1144	408	•	1094	1036	836	1371	354	833	1429	1369	352	1014	257
Philadelphia	881	1019	985	1089	83	1260	1094	•	2083	259	2412	811	1925	2523	2380	1163	123	1204
Phoenix	1263	1982	1280	1316	2145	842	1036	2083	•	1828	1005	1272	504	653	1114	932	1983	879
Pittsburgh	660	1010	743	919	317	1014	836	259	1828	•	2165	559	1668	2264	2138	917	192	950
Portland, Ore.	1849	2708	1427	2063	2445	1486	1371	2412	1005	2165	•	1723	636	534	145	1531	2354	1411
St. Louis	240	1061	466	598	875	459	354	811	1272	559	1723	•	1162	1744	1560	361	917	394
Salt Lake City	1250	2089	987	1434	1972	862	833	1925	504	1668	636	1162	•	600	701	917	712	808
San Francisco	1802	2594	1584	1926	2571	1388	1429	2523	653	2264	534	1744	600	•	678	1461	1848	1369
Seattle	1867	2734	1395	2101	2408	1524	1369	2380	1114	2138	145	1560	701	678	•	1369	2442	1437
Tulsa	341	1176	626	548	1231	98	352	1163	932	917	1531	361	917	1461	1369	•	1058	130
Washington, D.C.	765	923	934	966	205	1153	1014	123	1983	192	2354	917	712	1848	2442	1058	•	1106
Wichita	442	1297	546	677	1266	153	257	1204	879	950	1411	394	808	1369	1437	130	1106	•

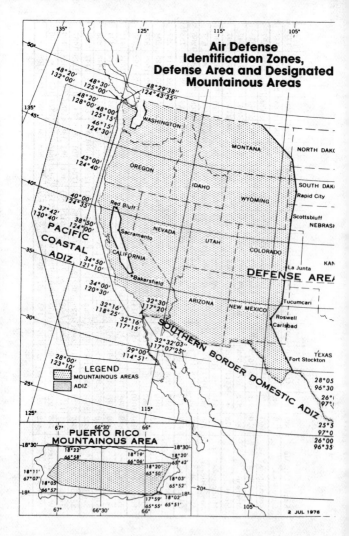

Air Defense Identification Zones, Defense Area and Designated Mountainous Areas

PACIFIC COASTAL ADIZ

SOUTHERN BORDER DOMESTIC ADIZ

DEFENSE AREA

LEGEND
MOUNTAINOUS AREAS
ADIZ

PUERTO RICO MOUNTAINOUS AREA

2 JUL 1976

24

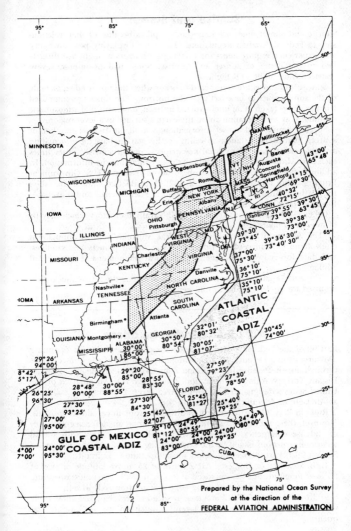

Sunrise and Sunset

Sunrise and sunset times are important to pilots because of their relationship to Federal Aviation Regulations. Times for displaying position lights, and experience requirements for carrying passengers at night are directly tied to the hours of sunset and sunrise. Some nations impose severe restrictions on night VFR flight.

Sunrise and sunset are considered to occur when the upper edge, or limb, of the sun appears to be exactly on the horizon. The times are computed from readings taken of an unobstructed horizon, under normal atmospheric conditions, at zero elevation above the earth's surface in a level region.

Specific sunrise and sunset information is available from a number of sources. Flight Service stations as well as weather stations have the information available on request. Many local newspapers contain sunrise/sunset times each day. Also many almanacs publish tables containing the information. In addition, sunrise/sunset tables can be ordered from the U.S. Government Printing Office (Washington, D.C. 20402). A booklet containing the tables for northern latitudes is called "Astronomical Phenomena," and is available for $2.40 (1980 edition).

Other GPO publications from the U.S. Naval Observatory which may be of interest to pilots are:

"The American Ephemeris and Nautical Almanac." Issued annually in one volume. Contains ephemerides of the sun, moon, planets, and satellites, and data for eclipses and other astronomical phenomena. $11.25 (1980 edition).

"The Air Almanac." Issued twice a year. Contains the astronomical data required for air navigation. $11.00 per volume.

ADIZ Rules and Regulations

Part 99 of the Federal Aviation Regulations prescribes rules for operating civil aircraft in a Defense Area, or within, into, or out of the United States through an Air Defense Identification Zone (ADIZ), including the Alaskan Distant Early Warning Identification Zone (DEWIZ). All airspace of the United States is designated as a Defense Area except that airspace designated as Air Defense Identification Zones.

Rules in Part 99 for the control of air traffic contain certain exemptions. However, these exemptions do not apply during an air defense emergency or defense emergency, when all civil aircraft must comply with special security instructions issued by the FAA. During normal periods, except for Section 99.7, Part 99 does not apply to the operation of aircraft:

1. In a Coastal or Domestic ADIZ north of 25° north latitude or west of 85° west longitude at a true airspeed of less than 180 knots, unless operating on a flight between Mexico and the United States (see FAR 91.84);

2. In the Alaskan DEWIZ at a true airspeed of less than 180 knots while the pilot maintains a continuous listening watch on the appropriate frequency;

3. Within the Continental United States, or within the state of Alaska, and remaining within 10 nautical miles of the point of departure; or

4. Over any island, or within three nautical miles of the coastline of any island, in the Hawaiian ADIZ.

An aircraft without two-way radio may penetrate or operate within an ADIZ if:

1. The flight is exempt from filing a DVFR flight plan by the exceptions listed above; or

2. The pilot adheres to the filed DVFR flight plan, which includes the point of penetration, and if the departure is made within five minutes of estimated time of departure.

Other operations may be exempted by an FAA ARTCC on a local basis only, with the concurrence of the military commanders concerned, provided they are conducted wholly within the boundaries of an ADIZ and are not currently significant to the air defense system. Civil aircraft may operate within the Panama Canal Zone Domestic ADIZ only under a flight plan that has been approved by appropriate military authority acting through an FAA air traffic control facility.

For operations not covered by the foregoing exemptions, a pilot must file a Defense Visual Flight Rules (DVFR) flight plan prior to operating VFR within or penetrating an ADIZ or DEWIZ. The flight plan must contain the information basic to a standard VFR flight plan and, in the case of DEWIZ operations, must include the estimated time and point of DEWIZ penetration (ETDP). Before penetrating an ADIZ, the pilot must report the time, position, and altitude of passing an appropriate reporting point and estimate time of arrival over the next appropriate reporting point along the route of flight. If there is no appropriate reporting point, the pilot must give an estimated time, position and altitude for penetrating an ADIZ to the appropriate facility at least 15 minutes before penetration.

The Air Defense Command has advised that an air-filed flight plan makes the aircraft subject to interception for positive identification. Interception can be avoided if a flight plan is filed prior to takeoff.

Aircraft complying with instrument flight rules within controlled airspace will automatically conform to the requirements of Part 99. In uncontrolled airspace, the same position reports are required for IFR and DVFR flights.

In an emergency that requires immediate decision and action, a pilot may deviate from the rules of Part 99 to the extent required by the emergency. He shall, however, report deviations and reasons for them as soon as possible to the appropriate facility where flight plans or position reports are normally filed.

Questions regarding local application of these regulations should be referred to the nearest FAA Flight Service Station or ATC facility.

ATC Clearance Shorthand

Climb and maintain .... ↑   Out of control zone .... ♂

Descend and maintain .... ↓   Through control zone .... ⊖•

Cruise	→	Before	>
At	@	After	<
Cross	X	Below	⊥
Maintain	⋈	Above	⊤
Cross airways	≠	Until	/
Join or intercept airways, track or course	⇌	Alternate instructions	( )
While on airways	=	Takeoff (direction, if specified)	T→N
While in control area	△		
While in control zone	O	Restriction (remain at or below)	50̅
Enter control area	◿	Restriction (remain at or above)	20̲
Out of control area	◺		
Enter control zone	◒	Clearance void after	V<
Hold (direction)	H-S	Shuttle climb	$
Report leaving	RL	Shuttle descent	$
Report passing	RP	Special VFR	SVFR
Report reaching	RR	Expect further clearance	EFC
Radar vector	RV		
Contact (name, freq.)	119.1	Altitude, 5,000-15,000 etc.	50-150

Phonetic Alphabet and Morse Code

(International—ICAO)

A—Alfa ·–	M—Mike ––	Y—Yankee –·––
B—Bravo –···	N—November –·	Z—Zulu ––··
C—Charlie –·–·	O—Oscar –––	0—Zero –––––
D—Delta –··	P—Papa ·––·	1—Wun ·––––
E—Echo ·	Q—Quebec ––·–	2—Too ··–––
F—Foxtrot ··–·	R—Romeo ·–·	3—Tree ···––
G—Golf ––·	S—Sierra ···	4—Fow-er ····–
H—Hotel ····	T—Tango –	5—Fife ·····
I—India ··	U—Uniform ··–	6—Six –····
J—Juliett ·–––	V—Victor ···–	7—Sev-en ––···
K—Kilo –·–	W—Whiskey ·––	8—Ait –––··
L—Lima ·–··	X—Xray –··–	9—Nin-er ––––·

28

Omni Test Signal Stations

Note: VOR limitations for IFR flight are outlined in FAR 91.25.

Akron, OH—Akron-Canton 110.6
Albany, NY—Albany County 109.0
Albuquerque, NM—Albuquerque International-Sunport 111.0
Anchorage, AK—Anchorage 111.0
Atlanta, GA—Atlanta Municipal 111.0
Bakersfield, CA—Bakersfield 111.2
Bedford, MA—L.G. Hanscom Field 110.0
Birmingham, AL—Birmingham Municipal 110.0
Boston, MA—Logan International 111.0
Buffalo, NY—Greater Buffalo International 109.0
Burlington, VT—Burlington International 109.0
Camp Springs, MD—Andrews AFB 109.6
Charleston, WV—Kanawha 108.8
Charlotte, NC—Charlotte 112.0
Chicago, IL—Midway 111.0
            O'Hare International 112.0
Cincinnati, OH—Cincinnati Municipal-Lunken 108.4
Cleveland, OH—Cleveland-Hopkins International 110.4
Columbus, OH—Port Columbus International 111.0
Dallas, TX—Love Field 113.8
Dayton, OH—J.M. Cox–Dayton Municipal 111.0
Denver, CO—Stapleton International 110.0
Detroit, MI—Detroit City 111.6
            Detroit Metropolitan-Wayne County 109.8
El Paso, TX—El Paso International 111.0
Fort Belvoir, VA—Davidson 109.4
Fort Worth, TX—Meacham 108.2
Ft. Wayne, IN—Baer 111.0
Honolulu, HI—Honolulu 111.0
Houston, TX—Houston–W. P. Hobby 111.6
Indianapolis, IN—Indianapolis Municipal 109.0
Jacksonville, FL—Jacksonville International 111.0
Kansas City, MO—Kansas City Municipal 108.6
Knoxville, TN—McGhee Tyson Municipal 112.0
Long Beach, CA—Long Beach Daugherty 109.0
Los Angeles, CA—San Pedro Hill 113.9
Louisville, KY—Standiford Field 111.0
Memphis, TN—Memphis Metropolitan 111.0
Miami, FL—Miami 112.0
Milwaukee, WI—Milwaukee 109.0
Minneapolis, MN—Minneapolis-St. Paul International 111.0
Nashville, TN—Nashville Metropolitan 112.0
New Orleans, LA—New Orleans Lakefront 111.0
New York, NY—J.F. Kennedy 115.1
            La Guardia 109.0

Newark, NJ—Newark Municipal 110.0
Oklahoma City, OK—Will Rogers 108.8
Philadelphia, PA—Philadelphia International 109.8
Phoenix, AZ—Phoenix Sky Harbor 109.0
Pittsburgh, PA—Greater Pittsburgh 111.0
Portland, OR—Portland International 111.0
Richmond, VA—E. Byrd Field 110.8
Saint Louis, MO—Lambert Field 111.0
Salt Lake City, UT—Salt Lake City Municipal 111.0
San Antonio, TX—San Antonio International 110.4
San Diego, CA—Lindbergh 109.8
San Francisco, CA—San Francisco International 111.0
Santa Monica, CA—Santa Monica Municipal 110.2
Savannah, GA—Travis Field 111.0
Seattle, WA—Boeing Field 108.6
Spokane, WA—Spokane International 109.6
Tallahassee, FL—Tallahassee Municipal 111.0
Tampa, FL—Tampa International 111.0
Tulsa, OK—Tulsa International 109.0
Van Nuys, CA—Van Nuys 109.0
Washington, DC—National 108.2
West Palm Beach, FL—Palm Beach 109.0

Preventive Maintenance

Part 43 of the FARs allows the holder of a pilot certificate to perform preventive maintenance on any aircraft owned or operated by him. Some examples of work typical of preventive maintenance are:

1. Removal, installation, and repair of landing-gear tires.
2. Servicing landing-gear shock struts by adding oil, air, or both.
3. Servicing landing-gear wheel bearings e.g., cleaning and greasing.
4. Lubrication not requiring disassembly other than removal of non-structural items such as coverplates, cowlings, and fairings.
5. Making simple fabric patches not requiring rib stitching or the removal of structural parts or control surfaces.
6. Replenishing hydraulic fluid in the hydraulic reservoir.
7. Making small, simple repairs to fairings, nonstructural cover plates, cowlings, and small patches and reinforcements, but not changing the contour so as to interfere with proper air flow.
8. Replacing safety belts.
9. Replacing seats or seat parts with replacement parts approved for the aircraft, not involving disassembly of any primary structure or operating system.

10. Trouble-shooting and repairing broken circuits in landing-light wiring circuits.
11. Replacing bulbs, reflectors, and lenses of position and landing lights.
12. Replacing wheels and skis where no weight and balance computation is involved.
13. Replacing or cleaning spark plugs and setting spark-plug gap clearance.
14. Replacing any hose connection except hydraulic connections.
15. Cleaning fuel and oil strainers.
16. Replacing batteries and checking fluid level and specific gravity.

In addition to preventive maintenance, a pilot can perform other maintenance if he works under the direct supervision of a properly certificated mechanic.

For more complete information on owner maintenance, obtain the *Aircraft Inspection for the General Aviation Aircraft Owner* (April 1978, AC 20-106, $2.75) from the Superintendent of Documents, U.S. Government Printing Office, Washington, DC 20402.

Aircraft Fuel and Oil

Fuel. Normal engine operation depends on use of the proper fuel grade. Follow airplane manual recommendations. If the proper grade of fuel is not available, it is sometimes permissible to burn the next higher grade of fuel, but check with the aircraft operating manual. Never allow a grade lower than that specified for normal operation to be used. To do so may cause extensive heat damage to the engine. Automotive fuel may NOT be used in aircraft engines. Know the color of the proper fuel for your aircraft and check it on every flight.

Octane	Color Code
80/87	Red
100LL	Blue
100/130	Green
115/145	Purple
Jet A	Clear or straw-colored

In recent years, the availability of 80/87 grade (red) fuel has diminished. Instead, fuel suppliers have been providing 100LL grade for use in all light piston-engine airplanes. Some engines designed for 80/87 require modifications for continuous use of the higher grade fuel. Additionally, maintenance problems in some engines—primarily exhaust valve erosion and spark plug fouling—have been attributed to the higher leaded fuel. Engine manufacturers advise strict adherence to their latest recommended operating procedures to help assure proper operation of the affected engines.

Oil. Two basic types of oil are used in general aviation aircraft piston engines: straight mineral and ashless dispersant (AD). Most engines use straight mineral oil for break-in purposes with new, remanufactured, or overhauled engines. After break-in, AD oil is used in the engine. There are exceptions to this procedure, however.

Clean engine oil is essential to long engine life. Oil filter elements, if installed, should be replaced after each 50 hours of engine operation. However, operation in dusty areas, cold climates, and where the engine is used infrequently may require more frequent oil changes, despite use of an oil filter.

Pilots and mechanics should know the weight, type and brand of oil used at each oil change. This information should be recorded in the engine logbook. Mixing of oil may create high oil consumption, or clogged oil control rings and oil screens. Manufacturers do not generally recommend use of either fuel or oil additives.

Ground Radio Procedures

- Pilots of departing aircraft should communicate with the control tower on the appropriate ground control frequency for taxi and clearance information and, unless otherwise advised, should remain on that frequency until they are ready to request takeoff clearance. If there is a designated clearance delivery frequency, it should be contacted before contacting ground control.

- Airport ground control frequencies are provided in the 121.6–121.9 MHz band to eliminate frequency congestion, thus providing a clear VFR channel for aircraft movements and airport utility vehicle operations on the airfield. Ground control frequencies are used for issuance of taxi information, clearances, and other necessary contacts between the tower and aircraft or other vehicles operated on the airport. Normally, only one of these ground control frequencies is assigned for use at an airport; however, at locations where the amount of traffic warrants, additional frequencies may be assigned, with one designated as a clearance delivery frequency.

- When the appropriate ground control frequency is not available or out of service (tower or aircraft) the tower normally will transmit to aircraft over an appropriate ground-to-air frequency.

- Pilots of aircraft not equipped to transmit on a ground control frequency should transmit on the tower frequency and tune their receivers to the appropriate ground control frequency in accordance with the above.

- At non-tower airports, the frequencies to use to advise others of your location and intentions (flight or ground) are: 123.6 MHz at airports with an FSS; on the Unicom frequency specified on the sectional chart; and on 122.9 MHz at airports with neither FSS nor Unicom.

Ground Handling an Airplane

- When taxiing in tight quarters, don't stand on one brake, blast the throttle and pivot—you'll cause unnecessary wear on tires and brakes. Instead, while holding modest rpm, try a series of quick little jabs on the brake pedal. If quarters are too tight, shut down the engine and get out and move the plane bodily.

• When moving the plane into a parking space or tiedown spot, it's okay to push it back a few feet providing the nosewheel remains straight. If it is cocked, or the distance is too great, apply muscle power at the tail end of the aircraft.

• To move a plane at the tail, face rearward and push gently, but firmly, against the leading edges of the horizontal and vertical stabilizers. Hands should be as close to the fuselage as possible. Never push or pull on trailing edges of the wings or tail surfaces.

• If you must push or pull on a propeller, use both hands, placing one on either side of the hub or spinner, as close to the hub as possible. In pulling, use only as much of your fingers as needed—preferably not more than the first joint curled around the edge of the prop blade. In pushing, use only the "flat" of the hand. This technique equalizes the force on the crankshaft and prop, and safeguards you should the prop turn out to be "hot." USE A TOW BAR IF YOU HAVE ONE.

• Use caution when pulling or pushing a plane by its wing struts. You can pull on them, providing you pull as close to either end as possible. Again, use gentle force. Some struts are sturdier than others. Be careful, and don't stand on struts to check fuel or the top of the wings.

Model Check List

The model check list that follows contains some items that are not applicable to all lightplanes, while some other items may be omitted that the individual pilot may feel are equally important. This list is intended merely as a guide from which the individual may draw up a check list more suitable to the airplane he flies.

The Walk-Around

A. Make sure both magnetos are off and landing gear is locked down. Remove control locks.

B. During walk-around, check all openings in engine compartment, fuselage and empennage for bird nests.

C. Wings:
    1. Check tips, leading/trailing edges and surfaces for damage.
    2. Check struts for damage and proper safetying.
    3. Check ailerons and flaps for cracks in hinges, safetying; control-cable attachment and tension.
    4. Remove frost, snow or ice.

D. Fuselage:
    1. Check for skin damage.
    2. Check to insure inspection plates are in place.
    3. Check static ports for obstructions.

E. Empennage:
   1. Check for skin damage.
   2. Check brace wires for tension, wear and safetying.
   3. Check control surface hinges for cracks, safetying; control-cable attachment and tension.
   4. Remove frost, snow or ice.

F. Undercarriage:
   1. Check tires for wear and proper inflation.
   2. Check struts for damage and proper inflation.
   3. Check visible nuts and bolts for safetying.
   4. Check brake lines for damage, attachment and signs of leaks.
   5. Check for obstructions (mud, ice, etc.) to proper operation.

G. Fuel system:
   1. Visual check of fuel for contamination and quantity.
   2. Replace gas caps properly and check breather hole.
   3. Drain fuel lines and tanks of water and sediment.

H. Propeller:
   1. Check blades for damage.
   2. Check hub for proper safetying of nuts and bolts.
   3. Check spinner for cracks.

I. Engine:
   1. Check mounts, battery, wiring and all visible items for cracks, security, safetying.
   2. Check exhaust manifold for cracks and leakage.
   3. Check oil level, insure dip stick is replaced and filler cap secure.
   4. Check cowl to insure it is closed properly and securely.

J. Turn on master switch and check all lights.

K. Remove chocks and untie tiedown ropes.

Starting (Starting procedures vary so much depending on the aircraft, engine and operating conditions, that no attempt has been made to give a detailed check list. As a general rule of thumb, the following items are common to most starting procedures.)

A. Brakes set.

B. Fuel selector on.

C. Electrical equipment off.

D. Cowl flaps open.

E. Clear area around. Sound off, "Clear!"

F. Master switch on.

G. Manufacturer's recommended starting procedure.

H. After engine starts, check oil and fuel pressure. (Oil pressure gauge should begin to show pressure in 30 seconds in summer, 60 seconds in winter. If it does not, shut off engine.)

Pre-Takeoff

A. Warm up at recommended r.p.m. (usually one-third power).

B. Check instruments:
   1. Altimeter to field elevation or reported altimeter setting, if available.
   2. Directional gyro set to magnetic compass or runway heading.
   3. Other instruments for proper readings.

C. Check magnetos singly and set on "both."

D. Exercise propeller.

E. Check carburetor heat.

F. Check controls for freedom of movement and proper rigging (including flaps).

G. Check trim tabs for proper settings.

H. Check fuel selector for proper setting.

I. Check radio equipment.

J. Check that seat belts are in use and properly fastened.

K. Check that doors are locked.

L. Check for aircraft in the pattern and on crossing runways.

M. Electric fuel pumps on. (If required by manufacturer's specifications.)

N. Uncage directional gyro on takeoff roll (if vacuum operated).

In Flight

A. Maintain continual lookout for other traffic.

B. Be aware of changing weather conditions ahead, behind and on both sides.

C. Check directional gyro against magnetic compass.

D. Check periodically for carburetor icing.

Pre-Landing

A. Carburetor heat on.

B. Cowl flaps properly positioned.

C. Fuel selector on proper tank.

D. Gear down and locked.

E. Mixture rich.

F. Propeller to low pitch (high rpm).

G. Electric fuel pumps on. (If required by manufacturer's specifications).

H. Seat belts securely fastened.

I. Check surface wind direction.

J. Check for other traffic in the air and on the ground.

Postflight

A. Tune to 121.5 and check for inadvertent ELT activation.

B. Engine shut down.

C. All switches off.

D. Aircraft properly tied down.

E. Fuel tanks topped off.

F. Doors closed and locked.

G. Pitot tube covered.

H. Close flight plan.

Pilot's Checklist

Preflight Action:

The FAA requires that before any flight the pilot familiarize his or herself with all available information concerning the flight. For both VFR and IFR flights, this should include:

1. Current weather reports and forecasts.

2. General fuel requirements:
   IFR—enough fuel must be on board to complete the flight to the first airport of intended landing, plus enough to fly from there to an alternate airport, and then 45 minutes beyond at cruise;
   VFR—enough fuel must be on board to fly to destination airport and 30 minutes beyond during the day, and 45 minutes beyond during night.

3. Alternate airport(s).

4. Known traffic delays.

5. Runway lengths at destination airport(s).

6. Takeoff and landing data for the aircraft being flown.

Certificates Required:

In the aircraft:

1. Aircraft Airworthiness Certificate
2. Aircraft Registration Certificate
3. FCC Radio Station Permit
4. Operating manual (including weight and balance information)

On the pilot's person:

1. Appropriate category pilot's license with ratings held
2. Current medical
3. FCC Radio Operators Permit

International Travel

For the pilot who is visiting other countries, the first landing must be made at a designated airport for Customs, Immigration and Health inspections. Upon return to the United States he must also report for the same inspections.

Certain procedures must be followed to meet Customs and Immigration requirements. Knowledge of the services available will promote a safer, more enjoyable and more economical flight. Useful flight suggestions and precautions, plus detailed information on the Customs and Immigration requirements of many countries, are published by the Aircraft Owners and Pilots Association. These "Flight Reports" are available to AOPA members at no charge through the AOPA Flight Operations Department.

Currently available AOPA Flight Reports include:

    U.S. Customs
    Alaska Flight Report
    Bahamas Flight Report
    Bermuda Flight Report
    Canada Flight Report
    Central America Flight Report
    Latin American Flight Guide
    Mexico Flight Report
    Routes for Latin America Flight Report
    The West Indies Flight Report
    Trans-Atlantic and Europe Flight Report

Special guidance is available to AOPA members, through the AOPA Flight Operations Department, for flights anywhere in the world. Members should contact the Flight Operations Department as early as possible, when planning an international flight, to realize the benefits of professional flight-planning assistance and sound guidance regarding accommodations, airport facilities, fuel, repairs, insurance, currency, credit cards, car rentals, survival gear, personal and aircraft documents, and immunizations required. These considerations are necessary to the conduct of a pleasant and safe flight. Pilots operating corporate jet aircraft should contact the Flight Operations Department for special services available for their particular international flight requirements.

Documents

Documents required to be in your possession for international travel may include the following:

> Passport
> Visa or Tourist Card
> Birth Certificate or U.S. Citizen ID card
> Pilot Identification (License and Medical Certificate)
> International Driver's License
> International Certificate of Vaccination

Aircraft documents should include:

> Certificate of Registration
> Certificate of Airworthiness
> License for Temporary Export (required for any modified type of military aircraft)
> Bill of Sale for Aircraft
> Export License (if required)
> Flight Permits (if required)
> General Declaration Forms
> Copies of Advance Notice (if required)

Passports

Obtaining a passport—An application for a passport must be personally presented to and executed by (1) a passport agent; (2) a clerk of any Federal court; (3) a clerk of any State court of record or a judge or clerk of any probate court; or (4) a postal clerk designed by the Postmaster General. (Postal clerks have been designated only in certain areas.)

Under certain circumstances, a person holding an expired passport issued within the last eight years, can submit the expired passport with his application, by mail.

Location of passport agencies:

Boston, Massachusetts 02203: John F. Kennedy Bldg., Room E123 Government Center; 617-223-2946

Chicago, Illinois 60604: Everett M. Dirksen Bldg., Room 244A, 219 S Dearborn Street; 312-353-5426

Honolulu, Hawaii 96813: 335 Merchant Street, Federal Bldg.; 808-546-2130

Los Angeles, California 90261: Hawthorne Federal Bldg., Room 2W16, 15000 Aviation Blvd., Lawndale; 213-536-6500

Miami, Florida 33130: Federal Office Bldg., 51 S.W. First Avenue; 305-350-5395

New Orleans, Louisiana 70130: Room 400 International Trade Mart, 2 Canal St.; 504-589-6161

New York, New York 10020: Rockefeller Center, 630 Fifth Avenue; 212-541-7700

Philadelphia, Pennsylvania 19106: Federal Building, 600 Arch St.; 217-597-7480

San Francisco, California 94102: Room 1405, Federal Bldg., 450 Golden Gate Avenue; 415-556-4516

Seattle, Washington 98101: Room 906, Federal Bldg., 500 2nd Street; 206-442-7945

Washington, D.C. 20524: Passport Office, 1425 K Street, N.W.; local: 783-8200, long distance: 202-783-8170

Mutilation or loss of passports—Passports which are mutilated or altered shall not be used for travel. Such passports shall be turned in to passport agents, clerks of courts or other officials of the U.S. Government. Any new passport issued to replace a lost valid passport will be limited to three months.

The address and notification data appearing on the inside front cover of the passport may be changed by the passport bearer. The passport need not be submitted to a Government official for such changes. All other entries or changes, however, must be made by an authorized official.

The loss of a valid passport is a serious matter and should be reported in writing immediately to the Passport Office, Department of State, Washington, D.C. 20524, or to the nearest consular office of the U.S. when abroad.

Applicants should allow at least two weeks for the receipt of their passports after application is made.

Visas

A visa is a permit to enter and leave the country to be visited. It is a stamp of endorsement placed in a passport by a consular official of the country to which entry is requested. Nearly all countries require visitors from other nations to have in their possession a valid visa obtained before departing from their home country. A visa may be obtained from foreign embassies or consulates located in the U.S. (visas are not always obtainable at the airport of entry of the foreign location and verification of visa issuance must be made in advance of departure). Various types of visas are issued depending upon the nature of the visit and the intended length of stay. A VALID PASSPORT MUST BE SUBMITTED WHEN APPLYING FOR A VISA OF ANY TYPE.

Several countries do not require U.S. citizens to obtain passports and visas for certain types of travel, mostly tourist. Instead they issue a simple tourist card which can be obtained from the nearest consulate of the country in question (presentation of a birth certificate or similar documentary proof of citizenship may be required). In some countries, the transportation company is authorized to grant tourist cards.

The photographs required in submitting visa applications should be full view and should not be larger than 3 × 3 inches nor smaller than 2½ × 2½ inches on white background.

Innoculations

Contact your local or state health department or the AOPA Flight Operations Department for information.

U.S. Customs Requirements

The following is a brief resumé of U.S. Customs requirements for departure from and entry into the United States. Only the major requirements are listed, and this is not intended as a substitute for the detailed information available to AOPA members through the AOPA Flight Operations Department.

Outbound

Private Tourist Flight—No requirement to clear with Customs.

Aliens Aboard—You must assure that they check with U.S. Immigration officials.

Carrying Items of Foreign Manufacture—Since time and place of acquisition may be asked for by Customs upon your reentry, you should report to a Customs officer and ask to fill out Customs Form 4457, "Certificate of Registration for Personal Effects Taken Abroad."

Inbound

Arrival Examination—Pilot and passengers will be examined. All must declare any articles acquired abroad. If you are carrying passengers for hire, or merchandise, a general declaration form must be filed. Baggage declarations may be made orally.

What To Declare—ALL articles acquired abroad and in your possession at the time of your return. Declaration must include:

a. Items brought home for another person.
b. Any article intended for sale or use in business.
c. Alterations or repairs made to articles abroad.
d. Gifts received while abroad—even though you may be wearing them.

Duty Free Exemptions—There are certain exceptions from paying duty on items obtained while abroad:

a. **$300 Exemption**—Articles totaling $300 (based on the *fair retail value* of each item in the country where acquired) may be entered free of duty, subject to the limitations on liquors, cigars and cigarettes, *if*:

- Articles were acquired as an incident of your trip for your personal or household use.
- You bring the articles with you at the time of your return to the United States and they are properly declared to Customs. Articles purchased and left for alterations or other reasons cannot be applied to your $300 exemption when shipped to follow at a later date.
- You are returning from a stay abroad of at least 48 hours. Example: A resident who leaves United States territory at 1:30 p.m. on June 1st would complete the required 48-hour period at 1:30 p.m. on June 3rd. This time limitation does not apply if you are returning from Mexico or the U.S. Virgin Islands.
- You have not used this $300 exemption, or any part of it, within the preceding 30-day period. Also, your exemption is not cumulative. If you use a portion of your exemption on entering the United States, then you must wait for 30 days before you are entitled to another exemption other than a $25 exemption.
- Articles are not prohibited or restricted.

b. **$600 Exemption**

If you return directly or indirectly from the U.S. Virgin Islands, American Samoa or Guam (referred to as our "insular possessions"), you may receive a Customs exemption of $600 (based on the fair retail value of the articles in the country where acquired), provided not more than $300 of this exemption may be applied to merchandise obtained elsewhere than in these islands.

Residents, 21 years of age or older, may enter one U.S. gallon of alcoholic beverages (128 fluid ounces) free of duty and tax, *provided* not more than one quart of this amount is acquired elsewhere.

This personal exemption also applies to articles purchased in any U.S. possession and mailed home, as well as carried. Also, the next $600 worth of goods sent home will only be assessed a flat five percent rate of duty. This is comparatively new legislation, known as the "to-follow" privilege and U.S. Customs advises U.S. residents to follow these steps:

- At the time of purchase advise the storekeeper NOT TO MAIL your parcels until he receives a copy of your Customs Form CF-255 (Declaration of Unaccompanied Articles);
- When you clear Customs upon your return, list all articles acquired abroad (except your $40 gift provision);

- Fill out Customs Form (CF-255) on each unaccompanied article.
- Be certain parcel is marked by storekeeper "UNACCOMPANIED TOURIST PURCHASE."
- KEEP YOUR SALES SLIPS!

c. **$25 Exemption**—If you cannot claim the $300 or $600 exemption because of the 30-day or 48-hour minimum limitations, you may bring in free of duty and tax articles acquired abroad for your personal or household use if the total fair retail value does not exceed $25. This is an individual exemption and may not be grouped with other members of a family on one Customs declaration.

U.S. Customs Facilities Airports

Important: You should contact the AOPA Flight Operations Department for detailed Customs information contained in the U.S. Customs Flight Report.

No clearance is necessary for noncommercial outbound flights from the United States, but Customs inspection is required for flights entering from another country.

Aircraft entering the United States have access to Customs facilities at two basic types of airports. One is the international airport, commonly called airport of entry, and the other is an airport located near a Customs Office where, for the convenience of the pilot, landing rights will normally be granted by the Customs Office. For both types, advance notice of ETA must be transmitted to the U.S. Customs officer at or nearest the airport. At a number of these airports the "Communications-Operations Plan" is authorized. This provides a flight notification service for the pilot and allows him to advise Customs of his ETA by adding the abbreviation "ADCUS" (Advise Customs) to his flight plan. The necessary notification will then be transmitted for him.

Landings may be made at international airports at any time, day or night, without prior permission to land, but prior request for landing permission must be transmitted for landing rights airports. However, with certain exceptions, Customs will ordinarily treat notices of ETA also as application for the required landing permission.

Hours of operation for Customs facilities are normally 8 a.m. to 5 p.m., Monday through Friday including Sundays and holidays. Overtime charges will accrue after regular hours of duty on weekdays and before 8 a.m. and after 5 p.m. on Sundays and holidays. Pilots are urged to telephone Customs at the intended airport of entry for current information regarding hours of available Customs service. Telephone numbers of Customs are listed in the AOPA Customs Flight Report. The Customs Flight Report also provides information regarding special arrangements or requirements for each customs airport.

The Customs Flight Report can be obtained from the AOPA Flight Department by AOPA members at no cost. Charge for the publication for nonmembers is $7.00. Detailed customs information is also in AOPA's Airports U.S.A.

Rules for Mexico Border Crossings

Flights from Mexico are required to report to U.S. Customs or the FAA at least 15 minutes prior to entering U.S. airspace, the following:

- Point and time of penetration
- ETA and airport of intended first landing (for Customs inspection)
- N-number and name of aircraft commander
- Number of US citizens and/or aliens aboard
- Point of foreign departure

Fourteen airports along the border have been designated as locations for the required customs inspection stop for private aircraft. They are: Brownsville (Texas) International; Calexico (Calif.) International; Del Rio (Texas) International; Bisbee-Douglas (Ariz.) International; Eagle Pass (Texas) Airport; El Paso (Texas) International; Laredo (Texas) International; Miller International, McAllen, Texas; Nogales (Ariz.) International; Brown Field, San Diego, Calif.; San Diego (Calif.) International; Tucson (Ariz.) International; Yuma (Ariz.) International; and Presidio-Lely (Texas) International.

Certain exemptions to these rules may be granted by the U.S. Customs Service.

U.S. International Airports

ALASKA: Juneau Mun; Juneau SPB; ·Ketchikan Harbor SPB; Wrangell SPB.

ARIZONA: Douglas (Bisbee-Douglas Intl); Nogales Intl; Tucson Intl; Yuma Intl.

CALIFORNIA: Calexico Intl; San Diego (Lindbergh) Intl.

FLORIDA: Ft. Lauderdale-Hollywood Intl; Key West Intl; Miami Intl; Miami Chalk SPB; Tampa Intl; West Palm Beach Intl.

ILLINOIS: Chicago (Midway) Arpt.

MAINE: Caribou Mun; Houlton Intl.

MICHIGAN: Detroit City; Detroit Metro (Wayne Cty); Port Huron (St. Clair Cty) Arpt; Sault Ste Marie Mun.

MINNESOTA: Baudette Intl; Duluth Intl; Duluth (Sky Harbor) Arpt; International Falls (Falls Intl); Ranier Intl SPB.

MONTANA: Cut Bank Arpt; Great Falls Intl; Havre City-County Arpt.

NEW YORK: Albany Co.; Massena (Richards Fld); Ogdensburg Intl; Ogdensburg Harbor; Rochester-Monroe Co.; Rouses Point SPB; Watertown New York Intl.

NORTH DAKOTA: Grand Forks Intl; Minot Intl; Pembina Mun; Portal Mun; Williston (Sloulin Fld Intl).

OHIO: Akron Mun; Cleveland Hopkins Intl; Sandusky (Griffing-Sandusky Arpt.

TEXAS: Brownsville Intl; Del Rio Intl; Eagle Pass Mun; El Paso Intl; Laredo Intl; McAllen (Miller Intl); Presidio-Lely Intl.

VERMONT: Burlington Intl.

WASHINGTON: Bellingham Intl; Friday Harbor SPB; Oroville (Dorothy Scott Arpt); Oroville (Dorothy Scott SPB); Port Townsend (Jefferson Cty Intl); Seattle (King Co.); Seattle (Lake Union Air Service SPB); Spokane (Felts Fld Arpt).

State Avgas Tax Refunds

The following table includes the standard state tax on all motor vehicle gasoline; the amount of tax applied to aviation gasoline (normally paid by the aircraft operator); and the amount of refund, if any.

No attempt is made here to give details on obtaining refunds; inquiries on the proper procedure should be made to the appropriate state official.

State	Standard Tax (cents/gal)	Tax on Avgas (cents/gal)	Exemption or Refund (cents/gal)
Alabama	7	2.7	0
Alaska	8	4	0
Arizona	8	8	7
Arkansas	8.5	0	0
California	7	7	5
Colorado	7	0	0
Connecticut	11	7	0
Delaware	9	9	9
Florida	8	0	0
Georgia	7.5	1	0
Hawaii	11.5 to 13.5	1	0
Iadho	9.5	3.5	0
Illinois	7.5	7.5	7.5
Indiana	8	0	0
Iowa	7	7	7
Kansas	8	8	8
Kentucky	9	9	8.55
Louisiana	8	8	8
Maine	9	9	5
Maryland	9	0	0
Massachusetts	8.5	0	0
Michigan	9	3	0
Minnesota	9	9	varies from 4 to 8.5
Mississippi	9	9	8
Missouri	7	7	7

Montana	8	1	0
Nebraska	8.5	5	2.5
Nevada	6	6	varies from 5.88 to 7.88
New Hampshire	10	4	0
New Jersey	8	8	8
New Mexico	7	7	7
New York	8	8	8
North Carolina	9	0	0
North Dakota	8	8	4% of sales price is deducted from 8¢/gal refund
Ohio	7	0	0
Oklahoma	6.58	8	0
Oregon	7	3	0
Pennsylvania	9	1.5	0
Rhode Island	10	10	10
South Carolina	7	0	0
South Dakota	8	4	1, 2, or 3
Tennessee	7	0	0
Texas	5	5	5
Utah	9	4	0
Vermont	9	9	0
Virginia	9	4	0
Washington	9	2	0
West Virginia	8.5	0	0
Wisconsin	7	7	2
Wyoming	8	4	2

Federal Use Tax on Civil Aircraft

The tax is imposed annually on the owner (or, in certain cases, the lessee) of civil engine-driven aircraft registered in the United States and *used* in the navigable airspace of the United States, exclusive of Puerto Rico or any possession, during the fiscal year July 1–June 30. The tax is composed of a "base tax" of $25, which cannot be prorated for part-year use, and a "weight tax" of two cents per pound of gross weight for piston aircraft, or 3½ cents per pound for turbine aircraft, which can be prorated in monthly decrements if first taxable use of the aircraft occurs after July. The first 2,500 pounds of piston-aircraft weight are exempt from the weight tax.

Tax returns are filed with the regional IRS service center for your address, on IRS Form 4638, and are due the last day of the month following the month in which *first taxable use* occurs. Tax payment is made in full with the return, or in quarterly installments.

To calculate tax for a full year, use the appropriate formula below. To prorate for part-year use, multiply the weight-tax amount by $x/12$ where x equals the number of months remaining in the fiscal year; e.g., if first use occurs in October, multiply by $9/12$.

Piston Aircraft: $\$25.00 + .02(\text{Gross Weight} - 2,500) = \text{Use Tax}$
Turbine Aircraft: $\$25.00 + .035(\text{Gross Weight}) = \text{Use Tax}$

Examples:

Cessna 172: $\$25.00 + .02(2,300 - 2,500) = \$25.00 + 0 = \$25.00$
Piper *Cherokee Six D*: $\$25.00 + .02(3,400 - 2,500) = \$25.00 + 18.00 = \$43.00$
Beech *King Air C-90*: $\$25.00 + .035(9,650) = \$25.00 + 337.75 = \$362.75$

Performance Computations and Conversion Tables

AERONAUTICAL CHART SCALES (in statute and nautical miles)

Sectional—8 sm or 7 nm per inch
WAC and ONC—16 sm or 14 nm per inch

MILEAGE

1 nautical mile (6,076 feet) = 1.15 statute miles
1 statute mile (5,280 feet) = 0.87 nautical mile
1 kilometer (3,280.8 feet) = .62137 statute mile or .54 nautical mile

SPEED

1 foot per second = 60 feet per minute = 3,600 feet per hour
1 mile per hour = 88 feet per minute = 1.46 feet per second
1 knot = 101.288 feet per minute = 1.688 feet per second

TEMPERATURE

$°F = °C \times 9/5 + 32$ $°C = 5/9(°F - 32)$

MILLIBARS—INCHES OF MERCURY

Millibars (mb)		Inches of Mercury (in. Hg.)	Millibars (mb)		Inches of Mercury (in Hg.)
1026.1	—	30.30	1013.2	Standard atmos.	29.92
1022.7	—	30.20	1012.5	—	29.90
1019.3	—	30.10	1009.1	—	29.80
1015.9	—	30.00	1005.7	—	29.70
			1002.3		29.60

WEIGHTS	U.S. GALLONS

1 gallon of gasoline = 6.0 lbs.
1 gallon of oil = 7.5 lbs.
1 gallon of kerosene = 6.75 lbs.
1 gallon of methanol = 6.62 lbs.
1 gallon of water = 8.33 lbs.

1 U.S. gallon = .83268 imperial gallon
1 gallon = 231 cubic inches = 0.134 cubic feet = 3.785 liters.
1 cubic foot = 7.5 U.S. gallons

Groundspeed

(using section lines spaced one statute mile apart)

Time between section lines	True course 360°—180° 090°—270°	True course 045°—135° 225°—315°
20 secs	180 mph	255 mph
25 secs	144 mph	204 mph
30 secs	120 mph	170 mph
35 secs	103 mph	146 mph
40 secs	90 mph	127 mph
45 secs	80 mph	113 mph
50 secs	72 mph	102 mph
55 secs	65 mph	93 mph
60 secs	60 mph	85 mph

Statute or nautical miles per minute	Min. & sec. to go 10 miles	Speed (m.p.h. or knots)	Statute or nautical miles per minute	Min. & sec. to go 10 miles	Speed (m.p.h. or knots)
1	10:00	60	3	3:20	180
1¼	8:00	75	3¼	3:05	195
1½	6:40	90	3½	2:51	210
1¾	5:43	105	3¾	2:40	225
2	5:00	120	4	2:30	240
2¼	4:26	135	4¼	2:21	255
2½	4:00	150	4½	2:13	270
2¼	3:38	165	4¾	2:06	285
			5	2:00	300

For quick estimates of groundspeed, measure the distance traveled over a period of 36 seconds then multiply by 100. The result will be a very close approximation of the groundspeed. (3600 seconds = 1 hour.)

Slant range to the DME site does not appreciably alter these calculations at and below 18,000 feet altitude and in excess of 10 nautical miles from the navaid.

Crosswind Component Chart

The crosswind component chart may be used to determine the crosswind and headwind component for any runway. If a maximum crosswind or headwind is an operational consideration for either the aircraft or the pilot's abilities, then draw vertical and horizontal lines at these maximum wind velocities. Color shading may be used to differentiate between safe and unsafe areas. Any wind that plots outside the recommended safe area means use a different runway or another airport.

Enter chart with wind angle and velocity relative to runway to determine both headwind and crosswind components. Example: Active runway 09; tower-reported wind, 140° at 25K. Relative wind angle = 50°; X-wind = 19K; Headwind = 16K.

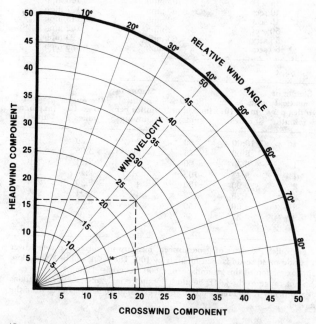

Maneuvering Speed

Maneuvering speed is the highest safe speed for abrupt control deflection or for operation in rough air. Upon encountering severe gusts, the pilot should reduce airspeed to maneuvering speed in order to lessen the strain upon the aircraft structure. For airplanes in which the maneuvering speed is not specified, it can be safely computed as 70 percent greater than normal stalling speed (stalling speed multiplied by 1.7).

Stall Speed Chart

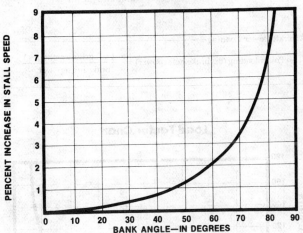

Aircraft Load Factors

(Source: FAA)

CATEGORIES OF AIRPLANES: Airplanes are designed to withstand the limit-load factors shown in the table that follows. The limit loads should not be exceeded in actual operation.

Category of Aircraft	Positive Limit Load
Normal (nonacrobatic)	3.8 times gross weight
Utility (normal operations and limited acrobatic maneuvers)	4.4 times gross weight
Acrobatic	6.0 times gross weight

Note: The negative limit-load factors shall not be less than -0.4 times the positive load factor for the N and U categories, and shall not be less than -0.5 times the positive load factor for the A category.

Formulas

Aircraft Wing Loading

$$\text{Wing loading (lb./sq. ft.)} = \frac{\text{aircraft gross weight (lbs.)}}{\text{wing area (sq. ft.)}}$$

Aircraft Power Loading

$$\text{Power loading (lb./brake horsepower)} = \frac{\text{aircraft gross weight (lbs.)}}{\text{brake horsepower}}$$

Load Factor Chart

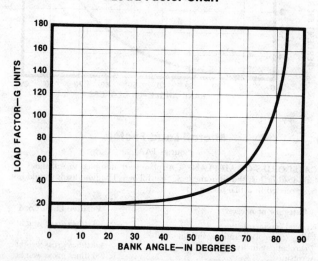

Density Altitude

With increased density altitude, engine horsepower decreases and the propeller loses efficiency, causing an increased takeoff roll and decreased rate of climb. High density altitude is most hazardous when combined with heavy loads, calm winds, short runways, unfavorable runway conditions and obstructions near the runway end. Remember: For each 1,000 feet above sea level, your true airspeed on landing will increase about 2% (although your indicated airspeeds will remain the same). The result is a longer landing roll due to the increased landing speed. As a general rule of thumb, for each thousand feet above sea level, your takeoff run increases by approximately 10%. With normally aspirated aircraft engines, *at 10,000 feet approximately 30% of the horsepower is lost; at 14,000 feet approximately 40% of the horsepower is lost.* It should be stressed, though, that this is a rule of thumb which may be inaccurate under certain circumstances. Pilots should consult their pilots' operating handbook, aircraft flight manual or aircraft owners manual to be sure.

The FAA has a pamphlet available entitled "Density Altitude" (FAA-P-8740-2) which contains information on the effects of density altitude on aircraft performance and an approximate method for computing takeoff distance and rate of climb at various altitudes and temperatures. To obtain a free copy, contact the nearest FAA General Aviation District Office (GADO) (See Section 5).

The Density Altitude Table on the next page, developed by the National Weather Service Forecast Office, Denver, CO, can be used to compute the additional runway required for takeoffs from high-altitude airfields.

To obtain a more exact pressure altitude for these computations you may read your altimeter when it is set at 29.92 in. Hg. However, field elevation may be used for pressure altitude because extreme pressure variations will seldom exceed 400 feet.

Example: Departure Airfield—Laramie, Wyo., elevation 7,276 ft.
Temperature—60° F.
Aircraft—Cessna 172 *Skyhawk.*
Using manufacturer's performance data, compute sea level takeoff distance: 865 ft.
From Density Altitude Table determine actual density altitude (9,300) for Laramie at the temperature of 60°. Note the multiplier, 2.9, in bold type. Multiply this number (2.9) times the sea level takeoff distance (865 ft.) to determine distance required for takeoff roll at Laramie (865 ft. times 2.9 equals 2,508.5 ft.).

Note: The bold-face numerals in the chart on the next page are the multipliers you use in arriving at your approximate takeoff run. Figures enclosed by parentheses represent the density altitude for the various Fahrenheit temperatures given at the left. *Long grass, sand, mud or deep snow can easily double your takeoff distance.*

DENSITY ALTITUDE CHART

PRESSURE ALTITUDE in feet (read your altimeter set at 29.92").

Temp. (F.)	4000	4500	5000	5500	6000	6500	7000	7500	8000	8500
105°	2.4 (7800)	2.6 (8300)	2.8 (9000)	3.2 (9600)	3.5 (10100)	— (10800)	— (11000)	— (11700)	— (12300)	— (13000)
100°	2.3 (7500)	2.4 (8000)	2.6 (8700)	3.0 (9300)	3.4 (9800)	3.5 (10500)	— (10800)	— (11400)	— (12000)	— (12700)
95°	2.2 (7200)	2.4 (7800)	2.6 (8300)	2.8 (9000)	3.2 (9500)	3.5 (10100)	3.7 (10500)	— (11200)	— (11700)	— (12500)
90°	2.1 (6900)	2.3 (7500)	2.5 (8100)	2.7 (8700)	3.0 (9200)	3.4 (9900)	3.5 (10200)	— (10800)	— (11400)	— (12000)
85°	2.0 (6600)	2.2 (7200)	2.4 (7800)	2.6 (8400)	2.9 (8900)	3.2 (9600)	3.4 (9900)	— (10500)	— (11100)	— (11800)
80°	2.0 (6300)	2.1 (6900)	2.3 (7500)	2.5 (8100)	2.8 (8600)	3.0 (9200)	3.2 (9700)	3.5 (10200)	— (10800)	— (11600)
75°	1.9 (6000)	2.0 (6600)	2.2 (7200)	2.4 (7800)	2.6 (8300)	2.8 (8900)	3.0 (9300)	3.3 (10000)	— (10500)	— (11200)
70°	1.9 (5700)	2.0 (6300)	2.1 (6900)	2.3 (7500)	2.5 (8000)	2.7 (8400)	2.8 (9000)	3.0 (9700)	3.6 (10200)	— (10900)
65°	1.8 (5400)	1.9 (6000)	2.0 (6600)	2.2 (7200)	2.4 (7800)	2.6 (8400)	2.8 (9000)	2.9 (9300)	3.5 (9800)	— (10600)
60°	1.7 (5100)	1.8 (5700)	2.0 (6200)	2.1 (6900)	2.3 (7400)	2.5 (8000)	2.7 (8400)	2.8 (9000)	3.4 (9800)	3.6 (10200)
55°	1.6 (4800)	1.8 (5300)	1.9 (6000)	2.0 (6500)	2.2 (7200)	2.4 (7800)	2.6 (8300)	2.7 (8700)	3.2 (9600)	3.5 (10000)
50°	1.6 (4400)	1.7 (5000)	1.8 (5700)	1.9 (6100)	2.1 (6900)	2.3 (7500)	2.5 (8100)	2.6 (8300)	3.0 (9200)	3.1 (9700)
45°	1.5 (4100)	1.6 (4700)	1.8 (5300)	1.9 (5900)	2.0 (6600)	2.2 (7100)	2.4 (7800)	2.5 (8100)	2.8 (8900)	2.9 (9200)
40°	1.5 (3800)	1.6 (4500)	1.7 (5000)	1.8 (5600)	2.0 (6100)	2.1 (6800)	2.3 (7500)	2.5 (8100)	2.6 (8600)	2.9 (9200)
35°	1.4 (3500)	1.5 (4000)	1.6 (4700)	1.7 (5200)	1.9 (6000)	2.0 (6500)	2.2 (7200)	2.4 (7800)	2.6 (8200)	2.8 (9000)

Metric Conversions

English to Metric

1 inch	25 millimeters or 2.54 centimeters
1 foot	0.3 meter
1 yard	0.9 meter
1 mile	1.6 kilometers or 1,609.3 meters
1 square inch	6.5 square centimeters
1 square foot	0.09 square meter
1 square yard	0.8 square meter
1 cubic inch	16 cubic centimeters
1 cubic foot	0.03 cubic meter
1 cubic yard	0.8 cubic meter
1 quart	0.95 liter
1 gallon	3.79 liters
1 ounce (avdp)	28 grams
1 pound (avdp)	0.45 kilogram
1 horsepower	0.75 kilowatt

Metric to English

1 millimeter	0.04 inch
1 centimeter	0.39 inch
1 meter	3.3 feet or 1.1 yard
1 kilometer	0.6 mile
1 square centimeter	0.16 square inch
1 square meter	11 square feet or 1.2 square yards
1 cubic centimeter	0.06 cubic inch
1 cubic meter	35 cubic feet or 1.3 cubic yards
1 liter	1.05 quarts (liquid)
1 cubic meter	35.31 cubic feet
1 gram	0.035 ounce (avdp)
1 kilogram	2.2 pounds (avdp)
1 kilowatt	1.3 horsepower

Kgs.	Kgs. or Lbs.	Lbs.	Kgs.	Kgs. or Lbs.	Lbs.
0.454	1	2.205	9.072	20	44.092
0.907	2	4.409	13.068	30	66.139
1.361	3	6.614	18.144	40	88.185
1.814	4	8.818	22.680	50	110.23
2.268	5	11.023	27.216	60	132.28
2.722	6	13.228	31.751	70	154.32
3.175	7	15.432	36.287	80	176.37
3.629	8	17.637	40.823	90	198.42
4.082	9	19.842	45.359	100	220.46
4.536	10	22.043			

Time Zones

Time is calculated from the Greenwich meridian. The Greenwich time zone extends 7½° east and west of the Greenwich meridian. Thus, twenty-four 15° arcs define the basic time zones around the earth. When the sun is directly above a meridian, the time at points on that meridian is noon. This is the basis on which time zones are established. As shown on the adjacent map, standard time zones are often modified to fit political boundaries of states and nations.

Greenwich Mean Time (GMT), often called "Z" or "Zulu" time, is frequently used in aviation to provide one standard time that helps eliminate confusion when aviation operations cross several time zones within a short time span. The 24-hour clock is also used as a convenient method for avoiding mistakes resulting from failure to specify "A.M." or "P.M."

Conversion to Greenwich Time from:

The 24-Hour Clock

Zone	Conversion	24-Hour		24-Hour	
Atlantic Standard	— Add 4 hrs.	0100 -	1 A.M.	1300 -	1 P.M.
Eastern Daylight	— " 4 "	0200 -	2 A.M.	1400 -	2 P.M.
Eastern Standard	— " 5 "	0300 -	3 A.M.	1500 -	3 P.M.
Central Daylight	— " 5 "	0400 -	4 A.M.	1600 -	4 P.M.
Central Standard	— " 6 "	0500 -	5 A.M.	1700 -	5 P.M.
Mountain		0600 -	6 A.M.	1800 -	6 P.M.
Daylight	— " 6 "	0700 -	7 A.M.	1900 -	7 P.M.
Mountain		0800 -	8 A.M.	2000 -	8 P.M.
Standard	— " 7 "	0900 -	9 A.M.	2100 -	9 P.M.
Pacific Daylight	— " 7 "	1000 - 10 A.M.		2200 - 10 P.M.	
Pacific Standard	— " 8 "	1100 - 11 A.M.		2300 - 11 P.M.	
Hawaii & Alaska		1200 - Noon		2400 - Midnight	
Standard	— " 10 "				
Westernmost					
Alaska &					
Aleutian Is.	— " 11 "				
(Bering Standard)					

Example: 1 P.M. EST (1300) = 1800Z

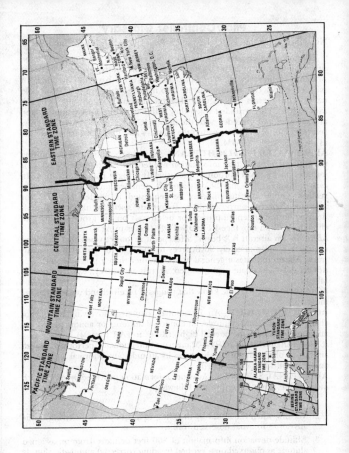

Standard Time Zones

Pilot/Controller Glossary

Note: See applicable Federal Aviation Regulations 91.5, 91.27 and 91.29.

The following glossary was compiled by the FAA to promote a common understanding of the terms used in the air traffic control system. Words are primarily defined in an operational sense. Terms basically intended for pilot/controller communications are also included and are printed in bold italics. Those terms published by the International Civil Aviation Organization (ICAO) are included when they differ from the FAA definition and are italicized and preceded with the initials ICAO. Included, too, are cross references to related items within the glossary and to other documents such as the FARs and the AIM.

ABBREVIATED IFR FLIGHT PLAN—An authorization by ATC requiring pilots to submit only that information needed for the purpose of ATC. It includes only a small portion of the usual IFR flight plan information. In certain instances, this may be only aircraft identification, location, and pilot request. Other information may be requested if needed by ATC for separation/control purposes. It is frequently used by airborne aircraft desiring an instrument approach, or by aircraft on the ground wishing to climb to VFR on top. (See VFR ON TOP) (Refer to AIM)

ABEAM—An aircraft is "abeam" a fix, point or object when that fix, point or object is approximately 90 degrees to the right or left of the aircraft track. Abeam indicates a general position rather than a precise point.

ABORT—To terminate a preplanned aircraft maneuver; e.g., an aborted takeoff.

ACKNOWLEDGE—Let me know that you have received and understand my message.

ACROBATIC FLIGHT—An intentional maneuver involving an abrupt change in an aircraft's attitude, an abnormal attitude, or abnormal acceleration, not necessary for normal flight. (Refer to FAR Part 91)

ICAO—ACROBATIC FLIGHT—Maneuvers intentionally performed by an aircraft involving an abrupt change in its attitude, an abnormal attitude, or an abnormal variation in speed.

ADDITIONAL SERVICES—Advisory information provided by ATC which includes but is not limited to the following:

1. Traffic advisories.

2. Vectors, when requested by the pilot, to assist aircraft receiving traffic advisories to avoid observed traffic.

3. Altitude deviation information of 300 feet or more from an assigned altitude as observed on a verified (reading correctly) automatic altitude readout (Mode C).

4. Advisories that traffic is no longer a factor.

5. Weather and chaff information.

6. Weather assistance.

7. Bird activity information.

8. Holding pattern surveillance.

Additional services are provided to the extent possible contingent only upon the controller's capability to fit it into the performance of higher priority duties and on the basis of limitations of the radar, volume of traffic, frequency congestion and controller workload. The controller has complete discretion for determining if he is able to provide or continue to provide a service in a particular case. The controller's reason not to provide or continue to provide a service in a particular case is not subject to question by the pilot and need not be made known to him. (See Duty Priorities, Traffic Advisories) (Refer to AIM)

ADMINISTRATOR—The Federal Aviation Administrator or any person to whom he has delegated his authority in the matter concerned.

ADVISE INTENTIONS—Tell me what you plan to do.

ADVISORY—Advice and information provided to assist pilots in the safe conduct of flight and aircraft movement. (See Advisory Service)

ADVISORY FREQUENCY—The appropriate frequency to be used for Airport Advisory Service. (See Airport Advisory Service and UNICOM) (Refer to Advisory Circular No. 90-42 and AIM)

ADVISORY SERVICE—Advice and information provided by a facility to assist pilots in the safe conduct of flight and aircraft movement. (See Airport Advisory Service, Traffic Advisories, Safety Advisories, Additional Services, Radar Advisory, En Route Flight Advisory Service) (Refer to AIM)

AERIAL REFUELING/INFLIGHT REFUELING—A procedure used by the military to transfer fuel from one aircraft to another during flight. (Refer to Graphic Notices and Supplementary Data)

AERODROME—A defined area on land or water (including any buildings, installations, and equipment) intended to be used either wholly or in part for the arrival, departure and movement of aircraft.

AERONAUTICAL BEACON—A visual navaid displaying flashes of white and/or colored light to indicate the location of an airport, a heliport, a landmark, a certain point of a Federal airway in mountainous terrain, or a hazard. (See Airport Rotating Beacon) (Refer to AIM)

AERONAUTICAL CHART—A map used in air navigation containing all or part of the following: topographic features, hazards and obstructions, navigation aids, navigation routes, designated airspace, and airports. Commonly used aeronautical charts are:

1. Sectional Charts—1:500,000—Designed for visual navigation of slow or medium speed aircraft. Topographic information on these charts features the portrayal of relief, and a judicious selection of visual check points for VFR flight. Aeronautical information includes visual and radio aids to navigation, airports, controlled airspace, restricted areas, obstructions and related data.

2. VFR Terminal Area Charts—1:250,000—Depict Terminal Control Area (TCA) airspace which provides for the control or segregation of all the aircraft within the TCA. The chart depicts topographic

information and aeronautical information which includes visual and radio aids to navigation, airports, controlled airspace, restricted areas, obstructions, and related data.

3. World Aeronautical Charts (WAC)—1:1,000,000—Provide a standard series of aeronautical charts covering land areas of the world, at a size and scale convenient for navigation by moderate speed aircraft. Topographic information includes cities and towns, principal roads, railroads, distinctive landmarks, drainage and relief. Aeronautical information includes visual and radio aids to navigation, airports, airways, restricted areas, obstructions and other pertinent data.

4. En Route Low Altitude Charts—Provide aeronautical information for en route instrument navigation (IFR) in the low altitude stratum. Information includes the portrayal of airways, limits of controlled airspace, position identification and frequencies of radio aids, selected airports, minimum en route and minimum obstruction clearance altitudes, airway distances, reporting points, restricted areas and related data. Area charts which are a part of this series furnish terminal data at a larger scale in congested areas.

5. En Route High Altitude Charts—Provide aeronautical information for en route instrument navigation (IFR) in the high altitude stratum. Information includes the portrayal of jet routes, identification and frequencies of radio aids, selected airports, distances, time zones, special use airspace and related information.

6. Area Navigation (RNAV) High Altitude Charts—Provide aeronautical information for en route IFR navigation for high altitude air routes established for aircraft equipped with RNAV systems. Information includes portrayal of RNAV routes, waypoints, track angles, changeover points, distances, selected navigational aids and airports, special use airspace, oceanic routes, and transitional information.

7. Instrument Approach Procedures (IAP) Charts—Portray the aeronautical data which is required to execute an instrument approach to an airport. These charts depict the Procedures, including all related data, and the airport diagram. Each procedure is designated for use with a specific type of electronic navigation system including NDB, TACAN, VOR, ILS, and RNAV. These charts are identified by the type of navigational aid(s) which provide final approach guidance.

8. Standard Instrument Departure (SID) Charts—Designed to expedite clearance delivery and to facilitate transition between take-off and en route operations. Each SID procedure is presented as a separate chart and may serve a single airport or more than one airport in a given geographical location.

9. Standard Terminal Arrival Route (STAR) Charts—Designed to expedite air traffic control arrival route procedures and to facilitate transition between en route and instrument approach operations. Each STAR procedure is presented as a separate chart and may serve

a single airport or more than one airport in a given geographical location.

10. Airport Taxi Charts—Designed to expedite the efficient and safe flow of ground traffic at an airport. These charts are identified by the official airport name, e.g., Washington National Airport.

ICAO—AERONAUTICAL CHART—A representation of a portion of the earth, its culture and relief, specifically designated to meet the requirements of air navigation.

AFFIRMATIVE—Yes.

AIR CARRIER DISTRICT OFFICE/ACDO—An FAA field office serving an assigned geographical area, staffed with Flight Standards personnel serving the aviation industry and the general public, on matters relating to the certification and operation of scheduled air carriers and other large aircraft operations.

AIRCRAFT—A device that is used or intended to be used for flight in the air and when used in air traffic control terminology may include the flight crew.

ICAO—AIRCRAFT—Any machine that can derive support in the atmosphere from the reactions of the air other than the reactions of the air against the earth's surface.

AIRCRAFT APPROACH CATEGORY—A grouping of aircraft based on a speed of 1.3 V_{so} (at maximum certificated landing weight), or on maximum certificated landing weight. V_{so} and the maximum certificated landing weight are those values as established for the aircraft by the certificating authority of the country of registry. If an aircraft falls into two categories, it is placed in the higher of the two. The categories are as follows:

1. Category A—Speed less than 91 knots; weight less than 30,001 pounds.
2. Category B—Speed 91 knots or more but less than 121 knots; weight 30,001 pounds or more but less than 60,001 pounds.
3. Category C—Speed 121 knots or more but less than 141 knots; weight 60,001 pounds or more but less than 150,001 pounds.
4. Category D—Speed 141 knots or more but less than 166 knots; weight 150,001 pounds or more.
5. Category E—Speed 166 knots or more; any weight.

(Refer to FAR Parts 1 and 97)

AIRCRAFT CLASSES—For the purposes of Wake Turbulence Separation Minima, ATC classifies aircraft as Heavy, Large and Small as follows:

1. Heavy—Aircraft capable of takeoff weights of 300,000 pounds or more whether or not they are operating at this weight during a particular phase of flight.
2. Large—Aircraft of more than 125,000 pounds, maximum certificated takeoff weight, up to 300,000 pounds.

3. Small—Aircraft of 12,500 pounds of less, maximum certificated takeoff weight. (Refer to AIM)

AIR DEFENSE EMERGENCY—A military emergency condition declared by a designated authority. This condition exists when an attack upon the continental U.S., Alaska, Canada, or U.S. installations in Greenland by hostile aircraft or missiles is considered probable, is imminent, or is taking place. (Refer to AIM)

AIR DEFENSE IDENTIFICATION ZONE/ADIZ—The area of airspace over land or water, extending upward from the surface, within which the ready identification, the location, and the control of aircraft are required in the interest of national security.

1. Domestic Air Defense Identification Zone—an ADIZ within the United States along an international boundary of the United States.

2. Coastal Air Defense Identification Zone—an ADIZ over the coastal waters of the United States.

3. Distant Early Warning Identification Zone (DEWIZ)—an ADIZ over the coastal waters of the State of Alaska.

ADIZ locations, and operating and flight plan requirements for civil aircraft operations are specified in FAR Part 99. (Refer to AIM)

AIRMAN'S INFORMATION MANUAL/AIM—A publication containing Basic Flight Information and ATC Procedures designed primarily as a pilot's instructional manual for use in the National Airspace System of the United States.

ICAO—AERONAUTICAL INFORMATION PUBLICATION—A publication issued by or with the authority of a state and containing aeronautical information of a lasting character essential to air navigation.

AIRMET/AIRMAN'S METEOROLOGICAL INFORMATION—Inflight weather advisories which cover moderate icing, moderate turbulence, sustained winds of 30 knots or more within 2,000 feet of the surface and the initial onset of phenomena producing extensive areas of visibilities below 3 miles or ceilings less than 1,000 feet. It concerns weather phenomena which are of operational interest to all aircraft and potentially hazardous to aircraft having limited capability because of lack of equipment, instrumentation or pilot qualifications. It concerns weather of less severity than SIGMETs or Convective SIGMETS. (See Convective SIGMETS or SIGMETS) (Refer to AIM)

AIR NAVIGATION FACILITY—Any facility used in, available for use in, or designed for use in, aid of air navigation, including landing areas, lights, any apparatus or equipment for disseminating weather information, for signaling, for radio-directional finding, or for radio or other electrical communication, and any other structure or mechanism having a similar purpose for guiding or controlling flight in the air or the landing and take-off of aircraft. (See Navigation Aid)

AIRPORT—An area of land or water that is used or intended to be used for the landing and takeoff of aircraft, and includes its buildings and facilities, if any.

AIRPORT ADVISORY AREA—The area within five statute miles of an airport not served by a control tower, i.e., there is no tower or the tower is not in operation, on which is located a Flight Service Station. (See Airport Advisory Service) (Refer to AIM)

AIRPORT ADVISORY SERVICE/AAS—A service provided by Flight Service Stations at airports not served by a control tower. This service consists of providing information to arriving and departing aircraft concerning wind direction and speed, favored runway, altimeter setting, pertinent known traffic, pertinent known field conditions, airport taxi routes and traffic patterns, and authorized instrument approach procedures. This information is advisory in nature and does not constitute an ATC clearance. (See Airport Advisory Area)

AIRPORT ELEVATION/FIELD ELEVATION—The highest point of an airport's usable runways measured in feet from mean sea level. (See Touchdown Zone Elevation)

ICAO—AERODROME ELEVATION—The elevation of the highest point of the landing area.

AIRPORT/FACILITY DIRECTORY—A publication designed primarily as a pilot's operational manual containing all airports, seaplane bases and heliports open to the public; including communications data, navigational facilities and certain special notices and procedures. This publication is issued in seven volumes according to geographical area.

AIRPORT INFORMATION DESK/AID—An airport unmanned facility designed for pilot self-service briefing, flight planning, and filing of flight plans. (Refer to AIM)

AIRPORT LIGHTING—Various lighting aids that may be installed on an airport. Types of airport lighting include:

1. Approach Light System/ALS—An airport lighting facility which provides visual guidance to landing aircraft by radiating light beams in a directional pattern by which the pilot aligns the aircraft with the extended centerline of the runway on his final approach for landing.

   Condenser-Discharge Sequential Flashing Lights/Sequenced Flashing Lights may be installed in conjunction with the ALS at some airports.

   Types of Approach Light Systems are:

   a. ALSF-I—Approach Light System with Sequenced Flashing Lights in ILS CAT-I configuration.

   b. ALSF-II—Approach Light System with Sequenced Flashing Lights in ILS CAT-II configuration.

   c. SSALF—Simplified Short Approach Light System with Sequenced Flashing Lights.

   d. SSALR—Simplified Short Approach Light System with Runway Alignment Indicator Lights,

   e. MALSF—Medium Intensity Approach Light System with Sequenced Flashing Lights,

f. MALSR—Medium Intensity Approach Light System with Runway Alignment Indicator Lights,

g. LDIN—Sequenced Flashing Lead-in Lights,

h. RAIL—Runway Alighment Indicator Lights (Sequenced Flashing Lights which are installed only in combination with other light systems).

2. Runway Lights/Runway Edge Lights—Lights having a prescribed angle of emission used to define the lateral limits of a runway. Runway lights are uniformly spaced at intervals of approximately 200 feet, and the intensity may be controlled or preset.

3. Touchdown Zone Lighting—Two rows of transverse light bars located symmetrically about the runway centerline normally at 100 foot intervals. The basic system extends 3,000 feet along the runway.

4. Runway Centerline Lighting—Flush centerline lights spaced at 50-foot intervals beginning 75 feet from the landing threshold and extending to within 75 feet of the opposite end of the runway.

5. Threshold Lights—Fixed green lights arranged symmetrically left and right of the runway centerline, identifying the runway threshold.

6. Runway End Identifier Lights/REIL—Two synchronized flashing lights, one on each side of the runway threshold, which provide rapid and positive identification of the approach end of a particular runway.

7. Visual Approach Slope Indicator/VASI—An airport lighting facility providing vertical visual approach slope guidance to aircraft during approach to landing by radiating a directional pattern of high intensity red and white focused light beams which indicate to the pilot that he is "on path" if he sees red/white, "above path" if white/white, and "below path" if red/red. Some airports serving large aircraft have three-bar VASIs which provide two visula glide paths to the same runway.

8. Boundary Lights—Lights defining the perimeter of an airport or landing area. (Refer to AIM)

AIRPORT ROTATING BEACON—A visual NAVAID operated at many airports. At civil airports alternating white and green flashes indicate the location of the airport. At military airports, the beacons flash alternately white and green, but are differentiated from civil beacons by dualpeaked (two quick) white flashes between the green flashes. (See Special VFR Operations, Instrument Flight Rules) (Refer to AIM Rotating Beacons) *ICAO—AERODROME BEACON*—Aeronautical beacon used to indicate the location of an aerodrome.

AIRPORT SURFACE DETECTION EQUIPMENT/ASDE—Radar equipment specifically designed to detect all principal features on the surface of an airport, including aircraft and vehicular traffic and to present the entire image on a radar indicator console in the control tower. Used to augment visual observation by tower personnel of aircraft and/or vehicular movements on runways and taxiways.

AIRPORT SURVEILLANCE RADAR/ASR—Approach control radar used to detect and display an aircraft's position in the terminal area. ASR provides range and azimuth information but does not provide elevation data. Coverage of the ASR can extend up to 60 miles.

AIRPORT TRAFFIC AREA—Unless otherwise specifically designated in FAR Part 93, that airspace within a horizontal radius of 5 statute miles from the geographical center of any airport at which a control tower is operating, extending from the surface up to, but not including, an altitude of 3,000 feet above the elevation of the airport. Unless otherwise authorized or required by ATC, no person may operate an aircraft within an airport traffic area except for the purpose of landing at, or taking off from, an airport within that area. ATC authorizations may be given as individual approval of specific operations or may be contained in written agreements between airport users and the tower concerned. (Refer to FAR Parts 1 and 91)

AIRPORT TRAFFIC CONTROL SERVICE—A service provided by a control tower for aircraft operating on the movement area and in the vicinity of an airport. (See Movement Area, Tower)

ICAO—AERODROME CONTROL SERVICE—Air traffic control service for aerodrome traffic.

AIR ROUTE SURVEILLANCE RADAR/ARSR—Air route traffic control center (ARTCC) radar, used primarily to detect and display an aircraft's position while en route between terminal areas. The ARSR enables controllers to provide radar air traffic control service when aircraft are within the ARSR coverage. In some instances, ARSR may enable an ARTCC to provide terminal radar services similar to, but usually more limited, than those provided by a radar approach control.

AIR ROUTE TRAFFIC CONTROL CENTER/ARTCC—A facility established to provide air traffic control service to aircraft operating on IFR flight plans within controlled airspace and principally during the en route phase of flight. When equipment capabilities and controller workload permit, certain advisory/assistance services may be provided to VFR aircraft. (See NAS Stage A, En Route Air Traffic Control Service) (Refer to AIM)

AIRSPEED—The speed of an aircraft relative to its surrounding air mass. The unqualified term "airspeed" means one of the following:

1. Indicated Airspeed—The speed shown on the aircraft airspeed indicator. This is the speed used in pilot/controller communications under the general term "airspeed." (Refer to FAR Part 1)

2. True Airspeed—The airspeed of an aircraft relative to undisturbed air. Used primarily in flight planning and the en route portion of flight. When used in pilot/controller communications, it is referred to as "true airspeed" and not shortened to "airspeed."

AIRSTART—The starting of an aircraft engine while the aircraft is airborne, preceded by engine shutdown during training flights or by actual engine failure.

AIR TRAFFIC—Aircraft operating in the air or on an airport surface, exclusive of loading ramps and parking areas.

ICAO—AIR TRAFFIC—All aircraft in flight or operating on the maneuvering area of an aerodrome.

AIR TRAFFIC CLEARANCE/ATC CLEARANCE—An authorization by air traffic control, for the purpose of preventing collision between known aircraft, for an aircraft to proceed under specific traffic conditions within controlled airspace. (See ATC Instructions)

ICAO—AIR TRAFFIC CONTROL CLEARANCE—Authorization for an aircraft to proceed under conditions specified by an air traffic control unit.

AIR TRAFFIC CONTROL/ATC—A service operated by appropriate authority to promote the safe, orderly and expeditious flow of air traffic.

ICAO—AIR TRAFFIC CONTROL SERVICE—A service provided for the purpose of:

1. Preventing collisions:
   a. Between aircraft, and
   b. On the maneuvering area between aircraft and obstructions, and
2. Expediting and maintaining an orderly flow of air traffic.

AIR TRAFFIC CONTROL SERVICE—(See Air Traffic Control)

AIR TRAFFIC CONTROL SPECIALIST/CONTROLLER—A person authorized to provide air traffic control service. (See Air Traffic Control Service, Flight Service Station)

ICAO—CONTROLLER—A person authorized to provide air traffic control services.

AIR TRAFFIC CONTROL SYSTEMS COMMAND CENTER/ATCSCC—An air traffic service facility consisting of four operational units.

1. Central Flow Control Function/CFCF—Responsible for coordination and approval of all major intercenter flow control restrictions on a system basis in order to obtain maximum utilization of the airspace. (See Quota Flow Control, Fuel Advisory Departure)
2. Central Altitude Reservation Function/CARF—Responsible for coordinating, planning and approving special user requirements under the Altitude Reservation (ALTRV) concept. (See Altitude Reservation)
3. Airport Reservation Office/ARO—Responsible for approving IFR flights at designated high density traffic airports (John F. Kennedy, La Guardia, O'Hare and Washington National) during specified hours. (Refer to FAR Part 93, Airport/Facility Directory)
4. ATC Contingency Command Post—A facility which enables the FAA to manage the ATC system when significant portions of the system's capabilities have been lost or are threatened.

AIRWAY BEACON—Used to mark airway segments in remote mountain areas. The light flashes Morse Code to identify the beacon site. (Refer to AIM)

AIRWAY/FEDERAL AIRWAY—A control area or portion thereof established in the form of a corridor, the centerline of which is defined by radio navigational aids. (Refer to FAR Part 71, AIM)

ICAO—AIRWAY—A control area or portion therof established in the form of corridor equipped with radio navigational aids.

ALERT AREA—(See Special Use Airspace)

ALERT NOTICE/ALNOT—A message sent by a Flight Service Station (FSS) or Air Route Traffic Control Center (ARTCC) that requests an extensive communication search for overdue, unreported or missing aircraft.

ALPHA-NUMERIC DISPLAY/DATA BLOCK—Letters and numerals used to show identification, altitude, beacon code and other information concerning a target on a radar display. (See Automated Radar Terminal Systems, NAS Stage A)

ALTERNATE AIRPORT—An airport at which an aircraft may land if a landing at the intended airport becomes inadvisable.

ICAO—ALTERNATE AERODROME—An aerodrome specified in the flight plan to which a flight may proceed when it becomes inadvisable to land at the aerodrome of intended landing.

ALTIMETER SETTING—The barometric pressure reading used to adjust a pressure altimeter for variations in existing atmospheric pressure or to the standard altimeter setting (29.92). (Refer to FAR Part 91, AIM)

ALTITUDE—The height of a level point or object measured in feet Above Ground Level (AGL) or from Mean Sea Level (MSC). (See Flight Level)

1. MSL Altitude—Altitude, expressed in feet measured from mean sea level.

2. AGL Altitude—Altitude expressed in feet measured above ground level.

3. Indicated Altitude—The altitude as shown by an altimeter. On a pressure or barometric altimeter it is altitude as shown uncorrected for instrument error and uncompensated for variation from standard atmospheric conditions.

ICAO—ALTITUDE—The vertical distance of a level, a point, or an object considered as a point, measured from a certain level.

ALTITUDE READOUT/AUTOMATIC ALTITUDE REPORT—An aircraft's altitude, transmitted via the Mode C transponder feature, that is visually displayed in 100-foot increments on a radar scope having readout capability. (See Automatic Radar Terminal Systems, NAS Stage A, Alpha Numeric Display) (Refer to AIM)

ALTITUDE RESERVATION/ALTRV—Airspace utilization under prescribed conditions normally employed for the mass movement of aircraft or other special user requirements which cannot otherwise be accomplished. ALTRVs are approved by the appropriate FAA facility. (See Air Traffic Control Systems Command Center)

ALTITUDE RESTRICTION—An altitude or altitudes stated in the order flown, which are to be maintained until reaching specific point or time.

Altitude restrictions may be issued by ATC due to traffic, terrain or other airspace considerations.

ALTITUDE RESTRICTIONS ARE CANCELLED—Adherence to previously imposed altitude restrictions is no longer required during a climb or descent.

APPROACH CLEARANCE—Authorization by ATC for a pilot to conduct an instrument approach. The type of instrument approach for which cleared and other pertinent information is provided in the approach clearance when required. (See Instrument Approach Procedure, Cleared for Approach) (Refer to AIM, FAR Part 91)

APPROACH CONTROL/APPROACH CONTROL FACILITY—A terminal air traffic control facility providing approach control service. (See Approach Control Service, Tower, Terminal Radar Approach Control, Radar Approach Control, Radar Air Traffic Control Facility.)

APPROACH CONTROL SERVICE—Air traffic control service provided by an approach control facility for arriving and departing VFR/IFR aircraft and, on occasion, en route aircraft. At some airports not served by an approach control facility, the ARTCC provides limited approach control service. (Refer to AIM)

ICAO—APPROACH CONTROL SERVICE—Air Traffic service for arriving or departing controlled flights.

APPROACH GATE—The point on the final approach course which is 1 mile from the final approach fix on the side away from the airport or 5 miles from landing threshold, whichever is farther from the landing threshold. This is an imaginary point used within ATC as a basis for final approach course interception for aircraft being vectored to the final approach course.

APPROACH LIGHT SYSTEM—(See Airport Lighting)

APPROACH SEQUENCE—The order in which aircraft are positioned while on approach or awaiting approach clearance. (See Landing Sequence)

ICAO—APPROACH SEQUENCE—The order in which two or more aircraft are cleared to approach to land at the aerodrome.

APPROACH SPEED—The recommended speed contained in aircraft manuals used by pilots when making an approach to landing. This speed will vary for different segments of an approach as well as for aircraft weight and configuration.

APRON/RAMP—A defined area, on a land airport, intended to accommodate aircraft for purposes of loading or unloading passengers or cargo, refueling, parking or maintenance. With regard to seaplanes, a ramp is used for access to the apron from the water.

ICAO—APRON—A defined area, on a land aerodrome, intended to accommodate aircraft for purposes of loading or unloading passengers or cargo, refueling, parking or maintenance.

ARC—The track over the ground of an aircraft flying at a constant distance from a navigational aid by reference to distance measuring equipment (DME).

AREA NAVIGATION/RNAV—A method of navigation that permits aircraft operations on any desired course within the coverage of station-referenced navigation signals or within the limits of self-contained system capability. (Refer to AIM, FAR Part 71)

1. Area Navigation Low Route—An area navigation route within the airspace extending upward from 1,200 feet above the surface of the earth to, but not including 18,000 feet MSL.

2. Area Navigation High Route—An area navigation route within the airspace extending upward from and including 18,000 feet MSL to flight level 450.

3. Random Area Navigation Routes/Random RNAV Routes—Direct routes, based on area navigation capability, between waypoints defined in terms of degree/distance fixes or offset from published or established routes/airways at specified distance and direction.

4. RNAV Waypoint/W/P—A predetermined geographical position used for route or instrument approach definition or progress reporting purposes that is defined relative to a VORTAC station position.

ICAO—AREA NAVIGATION/RNAV—A method of navigation which permits aircraft operation on any desired flight path within the coverage of station-referenced navigation aids or within the limits of the capability of self-contained aids or a combination of these.

ARMY AVIATION FLIGHT INFORMATION BULLETIN/USAFIB—A bulletin that provides air operation data covering Army, National Guard, and Army Reserve aviation activities.

ARMY RADAR APPROACH CONTROL/ARAC—An air traffic control facility located at a U.S. Army Airport utilizing surveillance and normally precision approach radar and air/ground communications equipment to provide approach control services to aircraft arriving, departing or transiting the airspace controlled by the facility. Service may be provided to both civil and military airports. Similar to TRACON (FAA), RAPCON (USAF) and RATCF (Navy). (See Approach Control, Approach Control Service, Departure Control)

ARRESTING SYSTEM—A safety device consisting of two major components, namely, engaging or catching devices, and energy absorption devices for the purpose of arresting both tail hook and/or non-tail hook equipped aircraft. It is used to prevent aircraft from overrunning runways when the aircraft cannot be stopped after landing or during aborted takeoff. Arresting systems have various names, e.g., arresting gear, hook, device, wire barrier, cable. (See Abort) (Refer to AIM)

ARRIVAL TIME—The time an aircraft touches down on arrival.

ARTCC—(See Air Route Traffic Control Center)

ASR APPROACH—(See Surveillance Approach)

ATC ADVISES—Used to prefix a message of noncontrol information when it is relayed to an aircraft by other than an air traffic controller. (See Advisory)

ATC ASSIGNED AIRSPACE/ATCAA—Airspace of defined vertical/lateral limits, assigned by ATC, for the purpose of providing air traffic segregation between the specified activities being conducted within the assigned airspace and other IFR air traffic. (See Military Operations Area, Alert Area)

ATC CLEARANCE—(See Air Traffic Clearance)

ATC CLEARS—Used to prefix an ATC clearance when it is relayed to an aircraft by other than an air traffic controller.

ATC INSTRUCTION—Directives issued by air traffic control for the purpose of requiring a pilot to take specific actions; e.g., "Turn left heading two five zero", "Go around," "Clear the runway." (Refer to FAR Part 91)

ATCRBS—(See Radar)

ATC REQUESTS—Used to prefix an ATC request when it is relayed to an aircraft by other than an air traffic controller.

AUTOMATED RADAR TERMINAL SYSTEMS/ARTS—The generic term for the ultimate in functional capability afforded by several automation systems. Each differs in functional capabilities and equipment. ARTS plus a suffix Roman Numeral denotes a specific system. A following letter indicates a major modification to that system. In general, an ARTS displays for the terminal controller aircraft identification, flight plan data, other flight associated information, e.g., altitude and speed, and aircraft position symbols in conjunction with his radar presentation. Normal radar co-exists with alphanumeric display. In addition to enhancing visualization of the air traffic situation, ARTS facilitate intra/inter-facility transfer and coordination of flight information. These capabilities are enabled by specially designed computers and subsystems tailored to the radar and communications equipments and operational requirements of each automated facility. Modular design permits adoption of improvements in computer software and electronic technologies as they become available while retaining the characteristics unique to each system:

1. ARTS IA—The functional capabilities and equipment of the New York Common IFR Room Terminal Automation System. It tracks primary as well as secondary targets derived from two radar sources. The aircraft targets are displayed on a radar type console by means of an alphanumeric generator. Aircraft identity is depicted in association with the appropriate aircraft target. When the aircraft is equipped with an encoded altimeter (Mode C), its altitude is also displayed. The system can exchange flight plan information with the ARTCC.

2. ART II—A programmable non-tracking, computer aided display subsystem capable of modular expansion. ARTS II systems provide a level of automated air traffic control capability at terminals having low to medium activity. Flight identification and altitude may be associated with the display of secondary radar targets. Also, flight plan information may be exchanged between the terminal and ARTCC.

3. ARTS III—The Beacon Tracking Level (BTL) of the modular programmable automated radar terminal system in use at medium to high activity terminals. ARTS III detects, tracks and predicts secondary radar derived aircraft targets. These are displayed by means of computer generated symbols and alphanumeric characters depicting flight identification, aircraft altitude, ground speed and flight plan data. Although it does not track primary targets, they are displayed coincident with the secondary radar as well as the symbols and

alphanumerics. The system has the capability of communicating with ARTCCs and other ARTS III facilities.

4. ARTS IIIA—The Radar Tracking and Beacon Tracking Level (RT& BTL) of the modular, programmable automated radar terminal system. ARTS IIIA detects, tracks and predicts primary as well as secondary radar derived aircraft targets. An enhancement of the ARTS III, this more sophisticated computer driven system will eventually replace the ARTS IA system and upgrade about half of the existing ARTS III systems. The enhanced system will provide improved tracking, continuous data recording and fail-soft capabilities.

AUTOMATIC ALTITUDE REPORTING—That function of a transponder which responds to Mode C interrogations by transmitting the aircraft's altitude in 100-foot increments.

AUTOMATIC CARRIER LANDING SYSTEM/ACLS—U.S. Navy final approach equipment consisting of precision tracking radar coupled to a computer data link to provide continuous information to the aircraft, monitoring capability to the pilot and a backup approach system.

AUTOMATIC DIRECTION FINDER/ADF—An aircraft radio navigation system which senses and indicates the direction to a L/MF nondirectional radio beacon (NDB) ground transmitter. Direction is indicated to the pilot as a magnetic bearing or as a relative bearing to the longitudinal axis of the aircraft depending on the type of indicator installed in the aircraft. In certain applications, such as military, ADF operations may be based on airborne and ground transmitters in the VHF/UHF frequency spectrum. (See Bearing, Nondirectional Beacon)

AUTOMATIC TERMINAL INFORMATION SERVICE/ATIS—The continuous broadcast of recorded noncontrol information in selected terminal areas. It purpose is to improve controller effectiveness and to relieve frequency congestion by automating the repetitive transmission of essential but routine information, e.g. "Los Angeles Information Alpha. 1300 Greenwich Weather, measured ceiling 2000 overcast, visibility three, haze, smoke, temperature seven zero, wind two five zero at five, altimeter two niner niner six, ILS runway two five left approach in use, runway two five right closed, advise you have Alpha." (Refer to AIM)

ICAO—AUTOMATIC TERMINAL INFORMATION SERVICE—The provision of current, routine information to arriving and departing aircraft by means of continuous and repetitive broadcasts through the day or a specified portion of the day.

AUTOROTATION—A rotorcraft flight condition in which the lifting rotor is driven entirely by action of the air when the rotorcraft is in motion.

1. Autorotative Landing/Touchdown Autorotation—Used by a pilot to indicate that he will be landing without applying power to the rotor.

2. Low Level Autorotation—Commences at an altitude well below the traffic pattern, usually below 100 feet AGL and is used primarily for tactical military training.

3. 180 degree Autorotation—Initiated from a downwind heading and is commenced well inside the normal traffic pattern. "Go around" may not be possible during the later part of this maneuver.

AVIATION WEATHER SERVICE—A service provided by the National Weather Service (NWS) and FAA which collects and disseminates pertinent weather information for pilots, aircraft operators and ATC. Available aviation weather reports and forecasts are displayed at each NWS office and FAA FSS. (See En Route Flight Advisory Service, Transcribed Weather Broadcasts, Scheduled Weather Broadcasts, Inflight Weather Advisories, Pilots Automatic Telephone Weather Answering Service) (Refer to AIM)

BASE LEG—(See Traffic Pattern)

BEACON—(See Radar, Nondirectional Beacon, Marker Beacon, Airport Rotating Beacon, Aeronautical Beacon, Airway Beacon)

BEARING—The horizontal direction to or from any point, usually measured clockwise from true north, magnetic north or some other reference point, through 360 degrees. (See Nondirectional Beacon)

BELOW MINIMUMS—Weather conditions below the minimums prescribed by regulation for the particular action involved, e.g., landing minimums, takeoff minimums.

BLAST FENCE—A barrier that is used to divert or dissipate jet or propeller blast.

BLIND SPEED—The rate of departure or closing of a target relative to the radar antenna at which cancellation of the primary radar target by moving target indicator (MTI) circuits in the radar equipment causes a reduction or complete loss of signal.

ICAO—BLIND VELOCITY—The radial velocity of a moving target such that the target is not seen on primary radars fitted with certain forms of fixed echo suppression.

BLIND SPOT/BLIND ZONE—An area from which radio transmissions and/or radar echoes cannot be received. The term is also used to describe portions of the airport not visible from the control tower.

BOUNDARY LIGHTS—(See Airport Lighting)

BREAKING ACTION (GOOD, MEDIUM OR FAIR, POOR, NIL)—A report of conditions on the airport movement area providing a pilot with a degree/quality of braking that he might expect. Braking action is reported in terms of good, medium (or fair), poor or nil. (See Runway Condition Reading).

BROADCAST—Transmission of information for which an acknowledgement is not expected.

ICAO—BROADCAST—A transmission of information relating to air navigation that is not addressed to a specific station or stations.

CALL-UP—Initial voice contact between a facility and an aircraft, using the identification of the unit being called and the unit initiating the call. (Refer to AIM)

CARDINAL ALTITUDES OR FLIGHT LEVELS—"Odd" or "Even" thousand-foot altitudes or flight levels; e.g., 5000, 6000, 7000, FL250, FL 260,

FL 270. (See Altitude, Flight Levels)

CEILING—The height above the earth's surface of the lowest layer of clouds or obscuring phenomena that is reported as "broken," "overcast," or "obscuration," and not classified as "thin" or "partial."

ICAO—CEILING—The height above the ground or water of the base of the lowest layer of cloud below 6000 meters (20,000 feet) covering more than half the sky.

CELESTIAL NAVIGATION—The determination of geographical position by reference to celestial bodies. Normally used in aviation as a secondary means of position determination.

CENTER—(See Air Route Traffic Control Center)

CENTER'S AREA—The specified airspace within which an air route traffic control center (ARTCC) provides air traffic control and advisory service. (See Air Route Traffic Conrtol Center) (Refer to AIM)

CHAFF—Thin, narrow metallic reflectors of various lengths and frequency responses, used to reflect radar energy. These reflectors when dropped from aircraft and allowed to drift downward result in large targets on the radar display.

CHASE/CHASE AIRCRAFT—An aircraft flown in proximity to another aircraft normally to observe its performance during training or testing.

CIRCLE TO LAND MANEUVER/CIRCLING MANEUVER—A maneuver initiated by the pilot to align the aircraft with a runway for landing when a straight-in landing from an instrument approach is not possible or is not desirable. This maneuver is made only after ATC authorization has been obtained and the pilot has established required visual reference to the airport (See Circle to Runway, Landing Minimums) (Refer to AIM)

CIRCLE TO RUNWAY (RUNWAY NUMBERED)—Used by ATC to inform the pilot that he must circle to land because the runway in use is other than the runway aligned with the instrument approach procedure. When the direction of the circling maneuver in relation to the airport/runway is required, the controller will state the direction (eight cardinal compass points) and specify a left or right downwind or base leg as appropriate; e.g., "Cleared VOR Runway 36 approach circle to Runway 22" or "Circle northwest of the airport for a right downwind to Runway 22." (See Circle to Land Maneuver, Landing Minimums) (Refer to AIM)

CIRCLING APPROACH—(See Circle-to-land Maneuver)

CIRCLING MINIMA—(See Landing Minimums)

CLEAR-AIR TURBULENCE/CAT—Tuburlence encountered in air where no clouds are present. This term is commonly applied to high-level tuburlence associated with wind shear. CAT is often encountered in the vicinity of the jet stream. (See Wind Shear, Jet Stream)

CLEARANCE—(See Air Traffic Clearance)

CLEARANCE LIMIT—The fix, point, or location to which an aircraft is cleared when issued an air traffic clearance.

ICAO—CLEARANCE LIMIT—The point of which an aircraft is granted an air traffic control clearance.

CLEARANCE VOID IF NOT OFF BY (TIME)—Used by ATC to advise an aircraft that the departure clearance is automatically cancelled if takeoff is not made prior to a specified time. The pilot must obtain a new clearance or cancel his IFR flight plan if not off by the specified time.

ICAO—CLEARANCE VOID TIME—A time specified by an air traffic control unit at which a clearance ceases to be valid unless the aircraft concerned has already taken action to comply therewith.

CLEARED AS FILED—Means the aircraft is cleared to proceed in accordance with the route of flight filed in the flight plan. This clearance does not include the altitude, SID, or SID Transition. (See Request Full Route Clearance) (Refer to AIM)

CLEARED FOR (TYPE OF) APPROACH—ATC authorization for an aircraft to execute a specific instrument approach procedure to an airport; e.g., "Cleared for ILS runway 36 approach." (See Instrument Approach Procedure, Approach Clearance) (Refer to AIM, FAR Part 91)

CLEARED FOR APPROACH—ATC authorization for an aircraft to execute any standard or special instrument approach procedure for that airport. Normally, an aircraft will be cleared for a specific instrument approach procedure. (See Instrument Approach Procedure, Cleared for (type of) Approach) (Refer to AIM, FAR Part 91)

CLEARED FOR TAKE-OFF—ATC authorization for an aircraft to depart. It is predicated on known traffic and known physical airport conditions.

CLEARED FOR THE OPTION—ATC authorization for an aircraft to make a touch-and-go, low approach, missed approach, stop and go, or full stop landing at the discretion of the pilot. It is normally used in training so that an instructor can evaluate a student's performance under changing situations. (See Option Approach) (Refer to AIM)

CLEARED THROUGH—ATC authorization for an aircraft to make intermediate stops at specified airports without refiling a flight plan while en route to the clearance limit.

CLEARED TO LAND—ATC authorization for an aircraft to land. It is predicated on known traffic and known physical airport conditions.

CLEAR OF TRAFFIC—Previously issued traffic is no longer a factor.

CLEARWAY—An area beyond the takeoff runway under control of airport authorities within which terrain or fixed obstacles may not extend above specified limits. These areas may be required for certain turbine powered operators and the size and upward slope of the clearway will differ depending on when the aircraft was certified. (Refer to FAR Part 1)

CLIMBOUT—That portion of flight operation between takeoff and the initial cruising altitude.

CLIMB TO VFR—ATC authorization for an aircraft to climb to VFR conditions within a control zone when the only weather limitation is restricted visibility. The aircraft must remain clear of clouds while climbing to VFR (See Special VFR) (Refer to AIM)

CLOSED RUNWAY—A runway that is unusable for aircraft operations. Only the airport management/military operations office can close a runway.

CLOSED TRAFFIC—Successive operations involving takeoffs and landings or low approaches where the aircraft does not exit the traffic pattern.

CLUTTER—In radar operations, clutter refers to the reception and visual display of radar returns caused by precipitation, chaff, terrain, numerous aircraft targets, or other phenomena. Such returns may limit or preclude ATC from providing services based on radar. (See Ground Clutter, Chaff, Precipitation, Target)

ICAO—RADAR CLUTTER—The visual indication on a radar display of unwanted signals.

COASTAL FIX—A navigation aid or intersection where an aircraft transitions between the domestic route structure and the oceanic route structure.

CODES/TRANSPONDER CODES—The number assigned to a particular multiple pulse reply signal transmitted by a transponder. (See Discrete Code)

COMBINED CENTER-RAPCON/CERAP—An air traffic control facility which combines the functions of an ARTCC and a RAPCON. (See Air Route Traffic Control Center/ARTCC, Radar Approach Control/RAPCON)

COMBINED STATION/TOWER/CS/T—An air traffic control facility which combines the functions of a flight service station and an airport traffic control tower. (See Tower, Flight Service Station) (Refer to AIM)

COMMON ROUTE/COMMON PORTION—That segment of a North American route between the inland navigation facility and the coastal fix.

COMPASS LOCATOR— A low power, low or medium frequency (L/MF) radio beacon install in conjunction with the outer or middle marker of an instrument landing system (ILS). It can be used for navigation at distances of approximately 15 miles or as authorized in the approach procedure.

1. Outer Compass Locator/LOM—A compass locator installed in conjunction with the outer marker of an instrument landing system. (See Outer Marker)

2. Middle Compass Locator/LMM—A compass locator installed in conjunction with the middle marker of an instrument landing system. (See Middle Marker)

ICAO—LOCATOR—An LF/MF NDB used as an aid to final approach.

COMPASS ROSE—A circle graduated in degrees, printed on some charts or marked on the ground at an airport. It is used as a reference to either true or magnetic direction.

COMPOSITE FLIGHT PLAN—A flight plan which specifies VFR operation for one portion of flight and IFR for another portion. It is used primarily in military operations. (Refer to AIM)

COMPOSITE ROUTE SYSTEM—An organized oceanic route structure, incorporating reduced lateral spacing between routes, in which composite separation is authorized.

COMPOSITE SEPARATION—A method of separating aircraft in a composite route system where, by management of route and altitude assignments, a combination of half the lateral minimum specified for the area concerned and half the vertical minimum is applied.

COMPULSORY REPORTING POINTS—Reporting points which must be reported to ATC. They are designated on aeronautical charts by solid triangles or filed in a flight plan as fixes selected to define direct routes.

These points are geographical locations which are defined by navigation aids/fixes. Pilots should discontinue position reporting over compulsory reporting points when informed by ATC that their aircraft is in "radar contact."

CONFLICT ALERT—A function of certain air traffic control automated systems designed to alert radar controllers to existing or pending situations recognized by the program parameters that require his immediate attention/action.

CONSOLAN—A low frequency, long-distance NAVAID used principally for transoceanic navigations.

CONTACT—

1. Establish communication with (followed by the name of the facility and, if appropriate, the frequency to be used).

2. A flight condition wherein the pilot ascertains the attitude of his aircraft and navigates by visual reference to the surface. (See Contact Approach, Radar Contact)

CONTACT APPROACH—An approach wherein an aircraft on an IFR flight plan, operating clear of clouds with at least 1 mile flight visibility and having received an air traffic control authorization, may deviate from the instrument approach procedure and proceed to the airport of destination by visual reference to the surface. This approach will only be authorized when requested by the pilot and the reported ground visibility at the destination airport is at least 1 statute mile. (See Visual Approach) (Refer to AIM)

CONTERMINOUS U.S.—The forty-eight adjoining states and the District of Columbia.

CONTINENTAL CONTROL AREA—(See Controlled Airspace)

CONTINENTAL UNITED STATES—The 49 states located on the continent of North America and the District of Columbia.

CONTROL AREA—(See Controlled Airspace)

CONTROLLED AIRSPACE—Airspace, designated as a continental control area, control area, control zone, terminal control area, or transition area, within which some or all aircraft may be subject to air traffic control. (Refer to AIM, FAR Part 71)

ICAO—CONTROLLED AIRSPACE—Airspace of defined dimensions within which air traffic control service is provided to controlled flights.

Types of U.S. Controlled Airspace:

1. Continental Control Area—The airspace of the 48 contiguous states, the District of Columbia and Alaska, excluding the Alaska peninsula west of Long. 160° 00' 00"W, at and above 14,500 feet MSL, but does not include:

   a. The airspace less than 1,500 feet above the surface of the earth or,

   b. Prohibited and restricted areas, other than the restricted areas listed in FAR Part 71.

2. Control Area—Airspace designated as Colored Federal Airways, VOR

Federal Airways, Terminal Control Areas, Additional Control Areas, and Control Area Extensions, but not including the Continental Control Area. Unless otherwise designated, control areas also include the airspace between a segment of a main VOR airway and its associated alternate segments. The vertical extent of the various categories of airspace contained in control areas are defined in FAR Part 71.

*ICAO—Control Area—*A controlled airspace extending upward from a specified limit above the earth.

3. Control Zone—Controlled airspace which extends upward from the surface and terminates at the base of the continental control area. Control zones that do not underlie the continental control area have no upper limit. A control zone may include one or more airports and is normally a circular area within a radius of 5 statute miles and any extensions necessary to include instrument approach and departure paths.
   *ICAO—Control Zone—*A controlled airspace extending upwards from the surface of the earth to a specified upper limit.

4. Terminal Control Area/TCA—Controlled airspace extending upward from the surface or higher to specified altitudes, within which all aircraft are subject to operating rules and pilot and equipment requirements specified in FAR Part 91. TCA's are depicted on Sectional World Aeronautical, En Route Low Altitude, DOD FLIP, and TCA charts. (Refer to FAR Part 91, AIM)
   *ICAO—Terminal Control Area—*A control area normally established at the confluence of ATS routes in the vicinity of one or more major aerodromes.

5. Transition Area—Controlled airspace extending upward from 700 feet or more above the surface of the earth when designated in conjunction with an airport for which an approved instrument approach procedure has been prescribed, or from 1,200 feet or more above the surface of the earth when designated in conjunction with airway route structures or segments. Unless otherwise limited, transition areas terminate at the base of the overlying controlled airspace. Transition areas are designed to contain IFR operations in controlled airspace during portions of the terminal operation and while transiting between the terminal and en route environment.

CONTROLLER—(See Air Traffic Control Specialist)
CONTROL SECTOR—An airspace area of defined horizontal and vertical dimensions for which a controller, or group of controllers, has air traffic control responsibility, normally within an air route traffic control center or an approach control facility. Sectors are established based on predominant traffic flows, altitude strata, and controller workload. Pilot-controller communications during operations within a sector are normally maintained on discrete frequencies assigned to the sector. (See Discrete Frequency)
CONTROL SLASH—A radar beacon slash representing the actual position of the associated aircraft. Normally, the control slash is the one closest to the

interrogating radar beacon site. When ARTCC radar is operating in narrowband (digitized) mode, the control slash is converted to a target symbol.

CONTROL ZONE—(See Controlled Airspace)

CONVECTIVE SIGMET/CONVECTIVE SIGNIFICANT METEOROLOGICAL INFORMATION—A weather advisory concerning convective weather significant to the safety of all aircraft. Convective SIGMETs are issued for tornadoes, lines of thunderstorms, embedded thunderstorms of any intensity level, isolated thunderstorms for intensity level 5 and above, areas of thunderstorms containing intensity level 4 and above, and hail ¾ inch or greater. (See SIGMET and AIRMET) (Refer to AIM)

COORDINATES—The intersection of lines of reference, usually expressed in degrees/minutes/seconds of latitude and longitude, used to determine position or location.

COORDINATION FIX—The fix in relation to which facilities will handoff, transfer control of an aircraft, or coordinate flight progress data. For terminal facilities it may also serve as a clearance limit for arriving aircraft.

CORRECTION—An error has been made in the transmission and the correct version follows.

COURSE

1. The intended direction of flight in the horizontal plane measured in degrees from north.

2. The ILS localizer signal pattern usually specified as front course or back course. (See Bearing, Radial, Instrument Landing Systems)

CRITICAL ENGINE—The engine which, upon failure, would most adversely affect the performance or handling qualities of an aircraft.

CROSS (FIX) AT (ALTITUDE)—Used by ATC when a specific altitude restriction at a specified fix is required.

CROSS (FIX) AT OR ABOVE (ALTITUDE)—Used by ATC when an altitude restriction at a specified fix is required. It does not prohibit the aircraft from crossing the fix at a higher altitude than specified; however, the higher altitude may not be one that will violate a succeeding altitude restriction or altitude assignment. (See Altitude Assignment, Altitude Restriction) (Refer to AIM)

CROSS (FIX) AT OR BELOW (ALTITUDE)—Used by ATC when a maximum crossing altitude at a specific fix is required. It does not prohibit the aircraft from crossing the fix at a lower altitude; however, it must be at or above the minimum IFR altitude. (See Minimum IFR Altitude, Altitude Restriction) (Refer to FAR Part 91)

CROSSWIND—

1. When used concerning the traffic pattern, the word means "crosswind leg." (See Traffic Pattern)

2. When used concerning wind conditions, the word means a wind not parallel to the runway or the path of an aircraft. (See Crosswind Component)

CROSSWIND COMPONENT—The wind component measured in knots at 90 degrees to the longitudinal axis of the runway.

CRUISE—Used in an ATC clearance to authorize a pilot to conduct flight at any altitude from the minimum IFR altitude up to and including the altitude specified in the clearance. The pilot may level off at any intermediary altitude within this block of airspace. Climb/descent within the block is to be made at the discretion of the pilot. However, once the pilot starts descent and reports leaving an altitude in the block he may not return to that altitude without additional ATC clearance. Further, it is approval for the pilot to proceed to and make an approach at destination airport and can be used in conjunction with:

1. An airport clearance limit at locations with a standard/special instrument approach procedure. The FARs require that if an instrument letdown to an airport is necessary the pilot shall make the letdown in accordance with a standard/special instrument approach procedure for that airport, or

2. An airport clearance limit at locations that are within/below/outside controlled airspace and without a standard/special instrument approach procedure. Such a clearance is NOT AUTHORIZATION for the pilot to descend under IFR conditions below the applicable minimum IFR altitude nor does it imply that ATC is exercising control over aircraft in uncontrolled airspace; however, it provides a means for the aircraft to proceed to destination airport, descend and land in accordance with applicable FARs governing VFR flight operations. Also, this provides search and rescue protection until such time as the IFR flight plan is closed. (See Instrument Approach Procedure)

CRUISING ALTITUDE/LEVEL—An altitude or flight level maintained during en route level flight. This is a constant altitude and should not be confused with a cruise clearance. (See Altitude)

ICAO—CRUISING LEVEL—A level maintained during a significant portion of a flight.

DECISION HEIGHT/DH—With respect to the operation of aircraft means, the height at which a decision must be made, during an ILS or PAR instrument approach, to either continue the approach or to execute a missed approach.

ICAO—DECISION HEIGHT—A specified height at which a missed approach must be initiated if the required visual reference to continue the approach to land has not been established.

DECODER—The device used to decipher signals received from ATCRBS and SIF transponders to effect their display as select codes. (See Codes, Radar)

DEFENSE VISUAL FLIGHT RULES/DVFR—Rules applicable to flights within an ADIZ conducted under the visual flight rules in FAR Part 91. (See Air Defense Identification Zone) (Refer to FAR Part 99)

DELAY INDEFINITE (REASON IF KNOWN) EXPECT APPROACH/ FURTHER CLEARANCE (TIME)—Used by ATC to inform a pilot when an accurate estimate of the delay time and the reason for the delay cannot immediately be determined; e.g., a disabled aircraft on the runway, terminal or center area saturation, weather below landing minimums. (See Expect Approach Clearance, Expect Further Clearance)

DEPARTURE CONTROL—A function of an approach control facility providing air traffic control service for departing IFR and, under certain conditions, VFR aircraft. (See Approach Control) (Refer to AIM)

DEPARTURE TIME—The time an aircraft becomes airborne.

DEVIATION—

1. A departure from a current clearance; such as an off course maneuver to avoid weather or turbulence.

2. Where specifically authorized in the FAR's and requested by the pilot ATC may permit pilots to deviate from certain regulations. (Refer to AIM)

DF APPROACH PROCEDURE—Used under emergency conditions where another instrument approach procedure cannot be executed. DF guidance for an instrument approach is given by ATC facilities with DF Capability. (See DF Guidance, Direction Finder) (Refer to AIM)

DF FIX—The geographical location of an aircraft obtained by one or more direction finders. (See Direction Finder)

DF GUIDANCE/DF STEER—Headings provided to aircraft by facilities equipped with direction finding equipment. These headings, if followed, will lead the aircraft to a predetermined point such as the DF station or an airport. DF guidance is given to aircraft in distress or to other aircraft which request the service. Practice DF guidance is provided when workload permits. (See Direction Finder, DF Fix) (Refer to AIM)

DIRECT—Straight line flight between two navigational aids, fixes, points or any combination thereof. When used by pilots in describing off-airway routes, points defining direct route segments become compulsory reporting points unless the aircraft is under radar contact.

DIRECTION FINDER/DF/UDF/VDF/UVDF—A radio receiver equipped with a directional sensing antenna used to take bearings on a radio transmitter. Specialized radio direction finders are used in aircraft as air navigation aids, others are ground based primarily to obtain a "fix" on a pilot requesting orientation assistance, or to locate downed aircraft. A location "fix" is established by the intersection of two or more bearing lines plotted on a navigational chart using either two separately located Direction Finders to obtain a fix on an aircraft or by a pilot plotting the bearing indications of his DF on two separately located ground based transmitters both of which can be identified on his chart. UDFs receive signals in the ultra high frequency radio broadcast band. VDFs in the very high frequency band, UVDFs in both bands. ATC provides DF service at those air traffic control towers and Flight Service Stations listed in AIM Part 2, and DOD FLIP IFR En Route Supplement. (See DF Guidance, DF Fix)

DISCRETE CODE/DISCRETE BEACON CODE—As used in the Air Traffic Control Radar Beacon System (ATCRBS), any one of the 4096 selectable Mode 3/A aircraft transponder codes except those ending in zero zero; e.g., discrete codes: 0010, 1201, 2317, 7777; non-discrete codes: 0100, 1200, 7700. Non-discrete codes are normally reserved for radar facilities that are not equipped with discrete decoding capability and for other purposes such as emergencies (7700), VFR aircraft (1200), etc. (See Radar) (Refer to AIM)

DISCRETE FREQUENCY—A separate radio frequency for use in direct pilot-controller communications in air traffic control which reduces frequency congestion by controlling the number of aircraft operating on a particular frequency at one time. Discrete frequencies are normally designated for each control sector in en route/terminal ATC facilities. Discrete frequencies are listed in the Airport/Facilities Directory, AIM Part 3, and DOD FLIP IFR En Route Supplement. (See Control Sector)

DISPLACED THRESHOLD—A threshold that is located at a point on the runway other than the designated beginning of the runway. (See Threshold) (Refer to AIM)

DISTANCE MEASURING EQUIPMENT/DME—Equipment (airborne and ground) used to measure, in nautical miles, the slant range distance of an aircraft from the DME navigation aid. (See TACAN, VORTAC)

DME FIX—A geographical position determined by reference to a navigational aid which provides distance and azimuth information. It is defined by a specific distance in nautical miles and a radial or course (i.e., localizer) in degrees magnetic from that aid. (See Distance Measuring Equipment, Fix)

DME SEPARATION—Spacing of aircraft in terms of distances (nautical miles) determined by reference to distance measuring equipment (DME) (See Distance Measuring Equipment).

DOD FLIP—Department of Defense Flight Information Publications used for flight planning, en route, and terminal operations. FLIP is produced by the Defense Mapping Agency for world-wide use. United States Government Flight Information Publications (en route charts and instrument approach procedure charts) are incorporated in DOD FLIP for use in the National Airspace System (NAS).

DOWNWIND LEG—(See Traffic Pattern)

DRAG CHUTE—A parachute device installed on certain aircraft which is deployed on landing roll to assist in deceleration of the aircraft.

EMERGENCY LOCATOR TRANSMITTER/ELT—A radio transmitter attached to the aircraft structure which operates from its own power source on 121.5 MHz and 243.0 MHz. It aids in locating downed aircraft by radiating a downward sweeping audio tone, 2–4 times per second. It is designed to function without human action after an accident. (Refer to FAR Part 91, AIM)

EMERGENCY SAFE ALTITUDE—(See Minimum Safe Altitude)

EN ROUTE AIR TRAFFIC CONTROL SERVICES—Air traffic control service provided aircraft on an IFR flight plan, generally by centers, when these aircraft are operating between departure and destination terminal areas. When equipment capabilities and controller workload permit, certain advisory/assistance services may be provided to VFR aircraft. (See NAS

Stage A, Air Route Traffic Control Center) (Refer to AIM)

EN ROUTE AUTOMATED RADAR TRACKING SYSTEM/EARTS—An automated radar and radar beacon tracking system. Its functional capabilities and design are essentially the same as the terminal ARTS IIIA system except for the EARTS capability of employing both short-range (ASR) and long-range (ARSR) radars, use of full digital radar displays, and fail-safe design. (See Automated Radar Terminal Systems/ARTS)

EN ROUTE CHARTS—(See Aeronautical Charts)

EN ROUTE DESCENT—Descent from the en route cruising altitude which takes place along the route of flight.

EN ROUTE FLIGHT ADVISORY SERVICE/FLIGHT WATCH— A service specifically designed to provide, upon pilot request, timely weather information pertinent to his type of flight, intended route of flight and altitude. The FSSs providing this service are listed in the Airport/Facility Directory. (See Flight Watch) (Refer to AIM)

EXECUTE MISSED APPROACH—Instructions issued to a pilot making an instrument approach which means continue inbound to the missed approach point and execute the missed approach procedure as described on the Instrument Approach Procedure Chart, or as previously assigned by ATC. The pilot may climb immediately to the altitude specified in the missed approach procedure upon making a missed approach. No turns should be initiated prior to reaching the missed approach point. When conducting an ASR or PAR approach, execute the assigned missed approach procedure immediately upon receiving instructions to "execute missed approach." (Refer to AIM)

EXPECT APPROACH CLEARANCE (TIME)/EAC—The time at which it is expected that an arriving aircraft will be cleared to commence an approach for landing. It is issued when the aircraft clearance limit is a designated Initial, Intermediate, or Final Approach Fix for the approach in use and the aircraft is to be held. If delay is anticipated, the pilot should be advised of his EAC at least 5 minutes before the aircraft is estimated to reach the clearance limit.

EXPECT (ALTITUDE) AT (TIME) or (FIX)—Used under certain conditions in a departure clearance to provide a pilot with an altitude to be used in the event of two-way communications failure. (Refer to AIM)

EXPECT DEPARTURE CLEARANCE (TIME)/EDCT—Used in Fuel Advisory Departure (FAD) program. The time the operator can expect a gate release. Excluding long distance flight, an EDCT will always be assigned even though it may be the same as the Estimated Time of Departure (ETD). The EDCT is calculated by adding the ground delay factor. (See Fuel Advisory Departure)

EXPECT FURTHER CLEARANCE (TIME)/EFC—The time at which it is expected that additional clearance will be issued to an aircraft. It is issued when the aircraft clearance limit is a fix not designated as part of the approach procedure to be executed and the aircraft will be held. If delay is anticipated the pilot should be advised of his EFC at least 5 minutes before the aircraft is estimated to reach the clearance limit.

EXPECT FURTHER CLEARANCE VIA (AIRWAYS, ROUTES OR FIXES)—
Used to inform a pilot of the routing he can expect if any part of the route
beyond a short range clearance limit differs from that filed.

EXPEDITE—Used by ATC when prompt compliance is required to avoid
the development of an imminent situation.

FAST FILE—A system whereby a pilot files a flight plan via telephone that
is tape recorded and then transcribed for transmission to the appropriate
air traffic facility. Locations having a fast file capability are contained in the
Airport/Facility Directory. (Refer to AIM)

FEATHERED PROPELLER—A propeller whose blades have been rotated
so that the leading and trailing edges are nearly parallel with the aircraft
flight path to stop or minimize drag and engine rotation. Normally used to
indicate shutdown of a reciprocating or turboprop engine due to malfunction.

FEEDER ROUTE—A route depicted on instrument approach procedure
charts to designate routes for aircraft to proceed from the en route structure
to the initial approach fix (IAF). (See Instrument Approach Procedure)

FERRY FLIGHT— A flight for the purpose of:

1. returning an aircraft to base;

2. delivering an aircraft from one location to another; or

3. moving an aircraft to and from a maintenance base.

Ferry flights, under certain conditions may be conducted under terms of a
special flight permit.

FILED—Normally used in conjunction with flight plans, meaning a flight
plan has been submitted to ATC.

FINAL—Commonly used to mean that an aircraft is on the final approach
course or is aligned with a landing area. (See Final Approach Course, Final
Approach—IFR, Traffic Pattern, Segments of an Instrument Approach
Procedure)

FINAL APPROACH COURSE—A straight line extension of a localizer, a final
approach radial/bearing, or a runway centerline, all without regard to
distance. (See Final Approach—IFR, Traffic Pattern)

FINAL APPROACH FIX/FAF—The designated fix from or over which the
final approach (IFR) to an airport is executed. The FAF identifies the
beginning of the final approach segment of the instrument approach. (See
Final Approach Point, Segments of an Instrument Approach Procedure,
Glide Slope Intercept Altitude)

FINAL APPROACH—IFR—The flight path of an aircraft which is inbound
to an airport on a final instrument approach course, beginning at the final
approach fix or point and extending to the airport or the point where a
circle to land maneuver or a missed approach is executed. (See Segments of
an Instrument Approach Procedure, Final Approach Fix, Final Approach
Course, Final Approach Point)

ICAO—FINAL APPROACH—That part of an instrument approach procedure from the time the aircraft has:

1. completed the last procedure turn or base turn, where one is specified,
or

2. crossed a specified fix, or

3. intercepted the last track specified for the procedures; until it has crossed a point in the vicinity of an aerodrome from which:

    a. a landing can be made; or

    b. a missed approach procedure is initiated.

FINAL APPROACH POINT—The point, within prescribed limits of an instrument approach procedure, where the aircraft is established on the final approach course and final approach descent may be commenced. A final approach point is applicable only in non-precision approaches where a final approach fix has not been established. In such instances, the point identifies the beginning of the final approach segment of the instrument approach. (See Final Approach Fix, Segments of an Instrument Approach Procedure, Glide Slope Intercept Altitude)

FINAL APPROACH SEGMENT—(See Segments of an Instrument Approach Procedure)

FINAL APPROACH—VFR—(See Traffic Pattern)

FINAL CONTROLLER—The controller providing information and final approach guidance during PAR and ASR approaches utilizing radar equipment. (See Radar Approach)

FIX—A geographical position determined by visual reference to the surface, by reference to one or more radio NAVAIDs, by celestial plotting, or by another navigational device.

FIXED-WING SPECIAL IFR—Aircraft operating in accordance with a waiver and a Letter of Agreement within control zones specified in FAR 93.113. These operations are conducted by IFR qualified pilots in IFR equipped aircraft and by pilots of agricultural and industrial aircraft.

FLAG/FLAG ALARM—A warning device incorporated in certain airborne navigation and flight instruments indicating that:

1. instruments are inoperative or otherwise not operating satisfactorily, or

2. signal strength or quality of the received signal falls below acceptable values.

FLAMEOUT—Unintended loss of combustion in turbine engines resulting in the loss of engine power.

FLIGHT INFORMATION REGION/FIR—An airspace of defined dimensions within which Flight Information Service and Alerting Service are provided.

1. Flight Information Service—A service provided for the purpose of giving advice and information useful for the safe and efficient conduct of flights.

2. Alerting Service—A service provided to notify appropriate organizations regarding aircraft in need of search and rescue aid, and assist such organizations as required.

FLIGHT INSPECTION/FLIGHT CHECK—Inflight investigation and evaluation of a navigational aid to determine whether it meets established tolerances. (See Navigational Aid)

FLIGHT LEVEL—A level of constant atmospheric pressure related to a reference datum of 29.92 inches of mercury. Each is stated in three digits that represent hundreds of feet. For example, flight level 250 represents a barometric altimeter indication of 25,000 feet; flight level 255, an indication of 25,500 feet.

ICAO—FLIGHT LEVELS—Surfaces of constant atmospheric pressure which are related to a specific pressure datum, 1013.2 mb (29.92 inches) and are separated by specific pressure intervals.

FLIGHT PATH—A line, course, or track along which an aircraft is flying or intended to be flown. (See Track, Course)

FLIGHT PLAN—Specified information relating to the intended flight of an aircraft, that is filed orally or in writing with an FSS or an ATC facility. (See Fast File, Filed) (Refer to AIM)

FLIGHT RECORDER—A general term applied to any instrument or device that records information about the performance of an aircraft in flight, or about conditions encountered in flight. Flight recorders may make records of airspeed, outside air temperature, vertical acceleration, engine RPM, manifold pressure, and other pertinent variables for a given flight.

ICAO—FLIGHT RECORDER—Any type of recorder installed in the aircraft for the purpose of complementing accident/incident investigation.

FLIGHT SERVICE STATION/FSS—Air traffic facilities which provide pilot briefing, en route communications and VFR search and rescue services, assist lost aircraft and aircraft in emergency situations, relay ATC clearances, originate Notices to Airmen, broadcast aviation weather and NAS information, receive and process IFR flight plans, and monitor NAVAIDS. In addition, at selected locations FSSs provide Enroute Flight Advisory Service (Flight Watch), take weather observations, issue airport advisories, and advise Customs and Immigration of transborder flights. (Refer to AIM)

FLIGHT STANDARDS DISTRICT OFFICE/FSDO—An FAA field office serving an assigned geographical area, staffed with Flight Standards personnel, who serve the aviation industry and the general public on matters relating to the certification and operation of air carrier and general aviation aircraft. Activites include general surveillance of operational safety, certification of airmen and aircraft, accident prevention, investigation, enforcement, etc.

FLIGHT TEST—A flight for the purpose of:

1. Investigating the operation/flight characteristics of an aircraft or aircraft component.
2. Evaluating an applicant for a pilot certificate or rating.

FLIGHT VISIBILITY—(See Visibility)

FLIGHT WATCH—A shortened term for use in air-ground contacts on frequency 122.0 MHz to identify the flight service station providing En

Route Flight Advisory Service; e.g., "Oakland Flight Watch." (See En Route Flight Advisory Service)

FLIP—(See DOD FLIP)

FLOW CONTROL—Measures designed to adjust the flow of traffic into a given airspace, along a given route, or bound for a given aerodrome (airport) so as to ensure the most effective utilization of the airspace. (See Quota Flow Control) (Refer to Airport/Facility Directory)

FLY HEADING (DEGREES)—Informs the pilot of the heading he should fly. The pilot may have to turn to , or continue on, a specific compass direction in order to comply with the instructions. The pilot is expected to turn in the shorter direction to the heading, unless otherwise instructed by ATC.

FORMATION FLIGHT—More than one aircraft which, by prior arrangement between the pilots, operate as a single aircraft with regard to navigation and position reporting. Separation between aircraft within the formation is the responsibility of the flight leader and the pilots of the other aircraft in the flight. This includes transition periods when aircraft within the formation are maneuvering to attain separation from each other to effect individual control and during join-up and breakaway.

1. A standard formation is one in which a proximity of more than 1 mile laterally or longitudinally and within 100 feet vertically from the flight leader is maintained by each wingman.

2. Nonstandard formations are those operating under any of the following conditions:

   a. When the flight leader has requested and ATC has approved other than standard formation dimensions.

   b. When operating within an authorized altitude reservation (ALTRV) or under the provisions of a Letter of Agreement.

   c. When the operations are conducted in airspace specifically designed for a special activity. (See Altitude Reservation) (Refer to FAR Part 91)

FSS—(See Flight Service Station)

FUEL ADVISORY DEPARTURE/FAD—Procedures to minimize engine running time for aircraft destined for an airport experiencing prolonged arrival delays. (Refer to AIM)

FUEL DUMPING—Airborne release of usuable fuel. This does not include the dropping of fuel tanks. (See Jettisoning of External Stores)

FUEL SIPHONING/FUEL VENTING—Unintentional release of fuel caused by overflow, puncture, loose cap, etc.

GATE HOLD PROCEDURES—Procedures at selected airports to hold aircraft at the gate or other ground location whenever departure delays exceed or are anticipated to exceed 5 minutes. The sequence for departure will be maintained in accordance with initial call up unless modified by Flow Control restrictions. Pilots should monitor the ground control/clearance delivery frequency for engine startup advisories or new proposed start time if the delay changes. (See Flow Control)

GENERAL AVIATION—That portion of civil aviation which encompasses all facets of aviation except air carriers holding a certificate of public convenience and necessity from the Civil Aeronautics Board, and large aircraft commercial operators.

ICAO—GENERAL AVIATION—All civil aviation operations other than scheduled air services and nonscheduled air transport operations for remuneration or hire.

GENERAL AVIATION DISTRICT OFFICE/GADO—An FAA field office serving a designated geographical area, staffed with Flight Standards personnel, who have responsibility for serving the aviation industry and the general public on all matters relating to the certification and operation of general aviation aircraft.

GLIDE PATH, (ON/ABOVE/BELOW)—Used by ATC to inform an aircraft making a PAR approach of its vertical position (elevation) relative to the descent profile. The terms "slightly" and "well" are used to describe the degree of deviation; e.g., "slightly above glidepath." Trend information is also issued with respect to the elevation of the aircraft and may be modified by the terms "rapidly" and "slowly;" e.g., "well above glidepath, coming down rapidly." (See PAR Approach)

GLIDE SLOPE/GS—Provides vertical guidance for aircraft during approach and landing. The glide slope consists of the following:

1. Electronic components emitting signals which provide vertical guidance by reference to airborne instruments during instrument approaches such as ILS; or

2. Visual ground aids such as VASI which provides vertical guidance for VFR approach or for the visual portion of an instrument approach and landing.

ICAO—GLIDE PATH—A descent profile determined for vertical guidance during a final approach.

GLIDE SLOPE INTERCEPT ALTITUDE—The minimum altitude of the intermediate approach segment prescribed for a precision approach which assures required obstacle clearance. It is depicted on instrument approach procedure charts. (See Segments of an Instrument Approach Procedure, Instrument Landing System)

GO AHEAD—Proceed with your message. Not to be used for any other purpose.

GO AROUND—Instructions for a pilot to abandon his approach to landing. Additional instructions may follow. Unless otherwise advised by ATC, a VFR aircraft or an aircraft conducting visual approach should overfly the runway while climbing to traffic pattern altitude and enter the traffic pattern via the crosswind leg. A pilot on an IFR flight plan making an instrument approach should execute the published missed approach procedure or proceed as instructed by ATC; e.g., "Go Around" (additional instructions, if required). (See Low Approach, Missed Approach)

GRAPHIC NOTICES AND SUPPLEMENTAL DATA—A publication designed primarily as a pilot's operational manual containing a tabulation of parachute jump areas, special notice-area graphics, terminal radar service area graphics, civil flight test areas, military refueling tracks and areas, and other data not requiring frequent change.

GROUND CLUTTER—A pattern produced on the radar scope by ground returns which may degrade other radar returns in the affected area. The effect of ground clutter is minimized by the use of moving target indicator (MTI) circuits in the radar equipment resulting in a radar presentation which displays only targets which are in motion. (See Clutter)

GROUND CONTROLLED APPROACH/GCA—A radar approach system operated from the ground by air traffic control personnel transmitting instructions to the pilot by radio. The approach may be conducted with surveillance radar (ASR) only or with both surveillance and precision approach radar (PAR). Usage of the term "GCA" by pilots is discouraged except when referring to a GCA facility. Pilots should specifically request a "PAR" approach when a precision radar approach is desired or request an "ASR" or "surveillance" approach when a nonprecision radar approach is desired. (See Radar Approach)

GROUNDSPEED—The speed of an aircraft relative to the surface of the earth.

GROUND VISIBILITY—(See Visibility)

HANDOFF—Transfer of radar identification of an aircraft from one controller to another, either within the same facility or interfacility. Actual transfer of control responsibility may occur at the time of the handoff, or at a specified time, point or altitude.

HAVE NUMBERS—Used by pilots to inform ATC that they have received runway, wind and altimeter information only.

HEAVY (AIRCRAFT)—(See Aircraft Classes)

HEIGHT ABOVE AIRPORT/HAA—The height of the Minimum Descent Altitude above the published airport elevation. This is published in conjunction with circling minimums. (See Minimum Descent Altitude)

HEIGHT ABOVE LANDING/HAL—The height above a designated helicopter landing area used for helicopter instrument approach procedures. (Refer to FAR Part 97)

HEIGHT ABOVE TOUCHDOWN/HAT—The height of the Decision Height or Minimum Descent Altitude above the highest runway elevation in the touchdown zone (first 3,000 feet of the runway). HAT is published on instrument approach charts in conjunction with all straight-in minimums. (See Decision Height, Minimum Descent Altitude)

HELICOPTER/COPTER—Rotorcraft that, for its horizontal motion, depends principally on its engine-driven rotors.

ICAO—HELICOPTER—A heavier-than-air aircraft supported in flight by the reactions of the air on one or more power-driven rotors on substantially vertical axes.

HELIPAD—That part of the landing and takeoff area designed for helicopters.

HELIPORT—An area of land, water, or structure used or intended to be used for the landing and takeoff of helicopters.

HERTZ/Hz—The standard radio equivalent of frequency in cycles per second of an electromagnetic wave. Kilohertz (kHz) is a frequency of one thousand cycles per second. Megahertz (MHz) is a frequency of one million cycles per second.

HIGH FREQUENCY COMMUNICATIONS/HF COMMUNICATIONS—High radio frequencies (HF) between 3 and 30 MHz used for air-to-ground voice communication in overseas operations.

HIGH FREQUENCY/HF—The frequency band between 3 and 30 MHz. (See High Frequency Communications)

HIGH SPEED TAXIWAY/EXIT/TURNOFF—A long radius taxiway designed and provided with lighting or marking to define the path of aircraft, traveling at high speed (up to 60 knots), from the runway center to a point on the center of a taxiway. Also referred to as long radius exit or turn-off taxiway. The high speed taxiway is designed to expedite aircraft turning off the runway after landing, thus reducing runway occupancy time.

HOLD/HOLDING PROCEDURE—A predetermined maneuver which keeps aircraft within a specified airspace while awaiting further clearance from air traffic control. Also used during ground operations to keep aircraft within a specified area or at a specified point while awaiting further clearance from air traffic control. (See Holding Fix) (Refer to AIM)

HOLDING FIX—A specified fix identifiable to a pilot by NAVAIDS or visual reference to the ground used as a reference point in establishing and maintaining the position of an aircraft while holding. (See Fix, Hold, Visual Holding) (Refer to AIM)

ICAO—HOLDING POINT—A specified location, identified by visual or other means, in the vicinity of which the position of an aircraft in flight is maintained in accordance with air traffic control clearances.

HOMING—Flight toward a NAVAID, without correcting for wind, by adjusting the aircraft heading to maintain a relative bearing of zero degrees. (See Bearing)

ICAO—HOMING—The procedure of using the direction-finding equipment of one radio station with the emission of another radio station, where at least one of the stations is mobile, and whereby the mobile station proceeds continuously towards the other station.

HOW DO YOU HEAR ME?—A question relating to the quality of the transmission or to determine how well the transmission is being received.

IDENT—A request for a pilot to activate the aircraft transponder identification feature. This will help the controller to confirm an aircraft identity or to identify an aircraft. (Refer to AIM)

IDENT FEATURE—The special feature in the Air Traffic Control Radar Beacon System (ATCRBS) equipment and the "I/P" feature in certain Selective Identification Feature (SIF) equipment. It is used to immediately distinguish one displayed beacon target from other beacon targets. (See IDENT)

IF FEASIBLE, REDUCE SPEED TO (SPEED)—(See Speed Adjustment)

IF NO TRANSMISSION RECEIVED FOR (TIME)—Used by ATC in radar approaches to prefix procedures which should be followed by the pilot in event of lost communications. (See Lost Communications)

IFR AIRCRAFT/IFR FLIGHT—An aircraft conducting flight in accordance with instrument flight rules.

IFR CONDITIONS—Weather conditions below the minimum for flight under visual flight rules. (See Instrument Meteorological Conditions)

IFR DEPARTURE PROCEDURE—(See IFR Takeoff Minimums and Departure Procedures) (Refer to AIM)

IFR MILITARY TRAINING ROUTES (IR)—Routes used by the Department of Defense and associated Reserve and Air Guard units for the purpose of conducting low-altitude navigation and tactical training in both IFR and VFR weather conditions below 10,000 feet MSL at airspeeds of 250 kts IAS.

IFR OVER THE TOP—The operation of an aircraft over the top of an IFR flight plan when cleared by air traffic control to maintain "VFR conditions" or "VFR conditions on top." (See VFR on Top)

IFR TAKEOFF MINIMUMS AND DEPARTURE PROCEDURES—FAR, Part 91, prescribes standard takeoff rules for certain civil users. At some airports, obstructions or other factors require the establishment of nonstandard takeoff minimums, departure procedures, or both, to assist pilots in avoiding obstacles during climb to the minimum en route altitude. Those airports are listed in NOS/DOD Instrument Approach Charts (IAPs) under a section entitled "IFR Takeoff Minimums and Departure Procedures." The NOS/DOD IAP chart legend illustrates the symbol used to alert the pilot to nonstandard takeoff minimums and departure procedures. When departing IFR from such airports, or from any airports where there are no departure procedures, SIDs, or ATC facilities available, pilots should advise ATC of any departure limitations. Controllers may query a pilot to determine acceptable departure directions, turns, or headings after takeoff. Pilots should be familiar with the departure procedures and must assure that their aircraft can meet or exceed any specified climb gradients.

ILS CATEGORIES—

1. ILS Category I—An ILS approach procedure which provides for approach to a height above touchdown of not less than 200 feet and with runway visual range of not less than 1800 feet.

2. ILS Category II—An ILS approach procedure which provides for approach to a height above touchdown of not less than 100 feet and with runway visual range of not less than 1200 feet.

3. ILS Category III
   a. IIIA—An ILS approach procedure which provides for approach without a decision height minimum and with runway visual range of not less than 700 feet.
   b. IIIB—An ILS approach procedure which provides for approach without a decision height minimum and with runway visual range of not less than 150 feet.
   c. IIIC—An ILS approach procedure which provides for approach without a decision height minimum and without runway visual range minimum.

IMMEDIATELY—Used by ATC when such action is required to avoid an imminent situation.

INCREASE SPEED TO (SPEED)—(See Speed Adjustment)

INFORMATION REQUEST/INREQ—A request originated by an FSS for information concerning an overdue VFR aircraft.

INITIAL APPROACH FIX/IAF—The fix(es) depicted on instrument approach procedure charts that identifies the beginning of the initial approach segment(s). (See Fix, Segments of an Instrument Approach Procedure)

INITIAL APPROACH SEGMENT—(See Segments of an Instrument Approach Procedure)

INNER MARKER/IM/INNER MARKER BEACON—A marker beacon used with an ILS (CAT II) precision approach located between the middle marker and the end of the ILS runway, transmitting a radiation pattern keyed at six dots per second and indicating to the pilot, both aurally and visually, that he is at the designated decision height (DH), normally 100 feet above the touchdown zone elevation, on the ILS CAT II approach. It also marks progress during a CAT III approach. (See Instrument Landing System) (Refer to AIM)

INSTRUMENT APPROACH PROCEDURE/IAP/INSTRUMENT APPROACH—A series of predetermined maneuvers for the orderly transfer of an aircraft under instrument flight conditions from the beginning of the initial approach to a landing, or to a point from which a landing may be made visually. It is prescribed and approved for a specific airport by competent authority. (See Segments of an Instrument Approach Procedure) (Refer to FAR Part 91, AIM)

1. U.S. civil standard instrument approach procedures are approved by the FAA as prescribed under FAR, Part 97, and are available for public use.

2. U.S. military standard instrument approach procedures are approved and published by the Department of Defense.

3. Special instrument approach procedures are approved by the FAA for individual operators, but are not published in FAR, Part 97, for public use.

ICAO—INSTRUMENT APPROACH PROCEDURE—A series of predetermined maneuvers for the orderly transfer of an aircraft under instrument flight conditions from the beginning of the initial approach to a landing, or to a point from which a landing may be made visually.

INSTRUMENT FLIGHT RULES/IFR—Rules governing the procedures for conducting instrument flight. Also a term used by pilots and controllers to indicate type of flight plan. (See Visual Flight Rules, Instrument Meteorological Conditions, Visual Meteorological Conditions) (Refer to AIM)

ICAO—INSTRUMENT FLIGHT RULES—A set of rules governing the conduct of flight under instrument meteorological conditions.

INSTRUMENT LANDING SYSTEM/ILS—A precision instrument approach system which normally consists of the following electronic components and visual aids:

1. Localizer (See Localizer)
2. Glide Slope (See Glide Slope)
3. Outer Marker (See Outer Marker)
4. Middle Marker (See Middle Marker)
5. Approach lights (See Airport Lighting)

(Refer to FAR Part 91, AIM)

INSTRUMENT METEOROLOGICAL CONDITIONS/IMC—Meteorological conditions expressed in terms of visibility, distance from cloud, and ceiling less than the minima specified for visual meteorological conditions. (See Visual Meteorological Conditions, Instrument Flight Rules, Visual Flight Rules)

INSTRUMENT RUNWAY—A runway equipped with electronic and visual navigation aids for which a precision or nonprecision approach procedure having straight-in landing minimums has been approved.

ICAO—INSTRUMENT RUNWAY—A runway intended for the operation of aircraft using nonvisual aids and comprising:

1. Instrument Approach Runway—An instrument runway served by a nonvisual aid providing at least directional guidance adequate for a straight-in approach.

2. Precision Approach Runway, Category I—An instrument runway served by ILS or GCA approach aids and visual aids intended for operations down to 60 meters (200 feet) decision height and down to an RVR of the order of 800 meters (2600 feet.)

3. Precision Approach Runway, Category II—An instrument runway served by ILS and visual aids intended for operations down to 30 meters (100 feet) decision height and down to an RVR of the order of 400 meters (1200 feet.)

4. Precision Approach Runway, Category III—An instrument served by ILS (no decision height being applicable) and:

   a. By visual aids intended for operations down to an RVR of the order of 200 meters 700 feet;

   b. By visual aids intended for operations down to an RVR of the order of 50 meters (150 feet);

   c. Intended for operations without reliance on external visual reference.

INTERMEDIATE APPROACH SEGMENT—(See Segments of an Instrument Approach Procedure)

INTERMEDIATE FIX/IF—The fix that identifies the beginning of the intermediate approach segment of an instrument approach procedure. The fix is not normally identified on the instrument approach chart as an intermediate fix (IF). (See Segments of an Instrument Approach Procedure)

INTERNATIONAL AIRPORT—Relating to international flights, it means:

1. An airport of entry which has been designated by the Secretary of Treasury or Commissioner of Customs as an international airport for customs service,

2. A landing rights airport at which specific permission to land must be obtained from customs authorities in advance of contemplated use,

3. Airports designated under the Convention on International Civil Aviation as an airport for use by international commercial air transport and/or international general aviation. (Refer to Airport/Facility Directory and IFIM)

ICAO—INTERNATIONAL AIRPORT—Any airport designated by the Contracting State in whose territory it is situated as an airport of entry and departure for international air traffic, where the formalities incident to customs, immigration, public health, animal and plant quarantine and similar procedures are carried out.

INTERNATIONAL CIVIL AVIATION ORGANIZATION/ICAO—A specialized agency of the United Nations whose objective is to develop the principles and techniques of international air navigation and to foster planning and development of international civil air transport.

INTERNATIONAL FLIGHT INFORMATION MANUAL/IFIM—A publication designed primarily as a pilot's preflight planning guide for flights into foreign airspace and for flights returning to the U.S. from foreign locations.

INTERROGATOR—The ground-based surveillance radar beacon transmitter-receiver which normally scans in synchronism with a primary radar, transmitting discrete radio signals which repetitiously requests all transponders, on the mode being used, to reply. The replies received are mixed with the primary radar returns and displayed on the same plan position indicator (radar scope). Also applied to the airborne element of the TACAN/DME system. (See Transponder) (Refer to AIM)

INTERSECTING RUNWAYS—Two or more runways which cross or meet within their lengths. (See Intersection)

INTERSECTION—

1. A point defined by any combination of courses, radials or bearings of two or more navigational aids.

2. Used to describe the point where two runways cross, a taxiway and a runway cross, or, two taxiways cross.

INTERSECTION DEPARTURE/INTERSECTION TAKEOFF—A takeoff or proposed takeoff on a runway from an intersection. (See Intersection)

I SAY AGAIN—The message will be repeated.

JAMMING—Electronic or mechanical interference which may disrupt the display of aircraft on radar or the transmission/reception of radio communications/navigation.

JET BLAST—Jet engine exhaust (thrust stream turbulence). (See Wake Turbulence)

JET ROUTE—A route designed to serve aircraft operations from 18,000 feet MSL up to and including flight level 450. The routes are referred to as "J" routes with numbering to identify the designated route; e.g., J 105. (See Route) (Refer to FAR Part 71)

JET STREAM—A migrating stream of high-speed winds present at high altitudes.

JETTISONING OF EXTERNAL STORES—Airborne release of external stores; e.g., tiptanks, ordnances. (See Fuel Dumping) (Refer to FAR Part 91)

JOINT USE RESTRICTED AREA—(See Restricted Area)

KNOWN TRAFFIC—With respect to ATC clearances, means aircraft whose altitude, position and intentions are known to ATC.

LANDING AREA—Any locality either of land or water, including airports and intermediate landing fields, which is used, or intended to be used, for the landing and takeoff of aircraft, whether or not facilities are provided for the shelter, servicing, or repair of aircraft, or for receiving or discharging passengers or cargo.

ICAO—LANDING AREA—That part of the movement area intended for the landing and takeoff of aircraft.

LANDING DIRECTION INDICATOR—A device which visually indicates the direction in which landings and takeoffs should be made. (See Tetrahedron) (Refer to AIM)

LANDING MINIMUMS/IFR LANDING MINIMUMS—The minimum visibility prescribed for landing a civil aircraft while using an instrument approach procedure. The minimum applies with other limitations set forth in FAR Part 91, with respect to the Minimum Descent Altitude (MDA) or Decision Height (DH) prescribed in the instrument approach procedures as follows:

1. Straight-in landing minimums—A statement of MDA and visibility, or DH and visibility, required for straight-in landing on a specified runway; or

2. Circling minimums—A statement of MDA and visibility required for the circle-to-land maneuver.

Descent below the established MDA or DH is not authorized during an approach unless the aircraft is in a position from which a normal approach to the runway of intended landing can be made, and adequate visual reference to required visual cues is maintained. (See Straight-in Landing, Circle-to-Land Maneuver, Decision Height, Minimum Descent Altitude, Visibility, Instrument Approach Procedure) (Refer to FAR Part 91)

LANDING ROLL—The distance from the point of touchdown to the point where the aircraft can be brought to a stop, or exit the runway.

LANDING SEQUENCE—The order in which aircraft are positioned for landing. (See Approach Sequence)

LAST ASSIGNED ALTITUDE—The last altitude/flight level assigned by ATC and acknowledged by the pilot. (See Maintain) (Refer to FAR Part 91)

LATERAL SEPARATION—The lateral spacing of aircraft at the same altitude by requiring operation on different routes or in different geographical locations. (See Separation)

LIGHTED AIRPORT—An airport where runway and obstruction lighting is available. (See Airport Lighting) (Refer to AIM)

LIGHT GUN—A handheld directional light signaling device which emits a brilliant narrow beam of white, green, or red light as selected by the tower controller. The color and type of light transmitted can be used to approve or disapprove anticipated pilot actions where radio communication is not available. The light gun is used for controlling traffic operating in the vicinity of the airport and on the airport movement area. (Refer to AIM)

LIMITED REMOTE COMMUNICATIONS OUTLET/LRCO—An unmanned satellite air/ground communications facility which may be associated with a VOR. These outlets effectively extend the service range of the FSS and provide greater communications reliability. LRCOs are depicted on En Route Charts. (See Remote Communications Outlet)

LOCALIZER—The component of an ILS which provides course guidance to the runway. (See Instrument Landing System) (Refer to AIM)

ICAO—LOCALIZER COURSE (ILS)—The locus of points, in any given horizontal point, at which the DDM (difference in depth of modulation) is zero.

LOCALIZER TYPE DIRECTIONAL AID/LDA—A NAVAID, used for nonprecision instrument approaches with utility and accuracy comparable to a localizer but which is not a part of a complete ILS and is not aligned with the runway. (Refer to AIM)

LOCALIZER USABLE DISTANCE—The maximum distance from the localizer transmitter at a specified altitude, as verified by flight inspection, at which reliable course information is continuously received. (Refer to AIM)

LOCAL TRAFFIC—Aircraft operating in the traffic pattern or within sight of the tower, or aircraft known to be departing or arriving from flight in local practice areas, or, aircraft executing practice instrument approaches at the airport. (See Traffic Pattern)

LONGITUDINAL SEPARATION—The longitudinal spacing of aircraft at the same altitude by a minimum distance expressed in units of time or miles. (See Separation) (Refer to AIM)

LORAN/LONG RANGE NAVIGATION—An electronic navigational system by which hyperbolic lines of position are determined by measuring the difference in the time of reception of synchronized pulse signals from two fixed transmitters. Loran A operates in the 1750–1950 kHz frequency band. Loran C and D operate in the 100–110 kHz frequency band. (Refer to AIM)

LOST COMMUNICATIONS/TWO-WAY RADIO COMMUNICATIONS FAILURE—Loss of the ability to communicate by radio. Aircraft are sometimes referred to as NORDO (No Radio). Standard pilot procedures are specified in FAR Part 91. Radar controllers issue procedures for pilots to follow in the event of lost communications during a radar approach, when weather reports indicate that an aircraft will likely encounter IFR weather conditions during the approach. (Refer to FAR Part 91, AIM)

LOW ALTITUDE AIRWAY STRUCTURE/FEDERAL AIRWAYS—The network of airways serving aircraft operations up to but not including 18,000 feet MSL. (See Airway) (Refer to AIM)

LOW ALTITUDE ALERT, CHECK YOUR ALTITUDE IMMEDIATELY—(See Safety Advisory)

LOW APPROACH—An approach over an airport or runway following an instrument approach or a VFR approach including the go-around maneuver where the pilot intentionally does not make contact with the runway (Refer to AIM)

LOW FREQUENCY/LF—The frequency band between 30 and 300 kHz. (Refer to AIM)

MACH NUMBER—The ratio of true airspeed to the speed of sound, e.g., MACH .82, MACH 1.6. (See Airspeed)

MAINTAIN—

1. Concerning altitude/flight level, the term means to remain at the altitude/flight level specified. The phrase "climb and" or "descend and" normally precedes "maintain" and the altitude assignment; e.g., "descend and maintain 5000."

2. Concerning other ATC instructions, the term is used in its literal sense; e.g., maintain VFR.

MAKE SHORT APPROACH—Used by ATC to inform a pilot to alter his traffic pattern so as to make a short final approach. (See Traffic Pattern)

MANDATORY ALTITUDE—An altitude depicted on an Instrument Approach Procedure Chart requiring the aircraft to maintain altitude at the depicted value.

MARKER BEACON—An electronic navigation facility transmitting a 75 MHz vertical fan or boneshaped radiation pattern. Marker beacons are identified by their modulation frequency and keying code and when received by compatible airborne equipment, indicate to the pilot, both aurally and visually, that he is passing over the facility. (See Outer Marker, Middle Marker, Inner Marker) (Refer to AIM)

MAXIMUM AUTHORIZED ALTITUDE/MAA—A published altitude representing the maximum usable altitude or flight level for an airspace structure or route segment. It is the highest altitude on a Federal airway, Jet route, area navigation low or high route, or other direct route for which an MEA is designated in FAR Part 95, at which adequate reception of navigation and signals is assured.

MAYDAY—The international radio–telephony distress signal. When repeated three times, it indicates imminent and grave danger and that immediate assistance is requested. (See PAN) (Refer to AIM)

METERING—A method of time regulating arrival traffic flow into a terminal area so as not to exceed a predetermined terminal acceptance rate.

METERING FIX—A fix along an established arrival route from over which aircraft will be metered prior to entering terminal airspace. Normally, this fix should be established at a distance from the airport which will facilitate a profile descent 10,000 feet above airport elevation (AAE) or above.

MICROWAVE LANDING SYSTEM/MLS—An instrument landing system operating in the microwave spectrum which provides lateral and vertical guidance to aircraft having compatible avionics equipment. (See Instrument Landing System) (Refer to AIM)

MIDDLE COMPASS LOCATOR—(See Compass Locator)

MIDDLE MARKER/MM—A marker beacon that defines a point along the glide slope of an ILS normally located at or near the point of decision height (ILS Category I). It is keyed to transmit alternate dots and dashes, two per second, on a 1300 HZ tone which is received aurally and visually by compatible airborne equipment. (See Marker Beacon, Instrument Landing System) (Refer to AIM)

MID RVR—(See Visibility)

MILITARY AUTHORITY ASSUMES RESPONSIBILITY FOR SEPARATION OF AIRCRAFT/MARSA—A condition whereby the military services involved assume reponsibility for seperation between participating military aircraft in the ATC system. It is used only for required IFR operations which are specified in Letters of Agreement or other appropriate FAA military documents.

MILITARY OPERATIONS AREA/MOA—(See Special Use Airspace)

MILITARY TRAINING ROUTES/MTR—Airspace of defined vertical and lateral dimensions established for the conduct of military flight training at airspeeds in excess of 250 knots IAS. (See IFR (IR) and VFR (VR) Military Training Routes)

MINIMUM CROSSING ALTITUDE/MCA—The lowest altitude at certain fixes at which an aircraft must cross when preceding in the direction of a higher minimum en route IFR altitude (MEA). (See Minimum En Route IFR Altitude)

MINIMUM DESCENT ALTITUDE/MDA—The lowest altitude, expressed in feet above mean sea level, to which descent is authorized on final approach or during circle-to-land maneuvering in execution of a standard instrument approach procedure where no electronic glide scope is provided. (See Nonprecision Approach Procedure)

MINIMUM EN ROUTE IFR ALTITUDE/MEA—The lowest published altitude between radio fixes which assures acceptable navigational signal coverage and meets obstacle clearance requirements between those fixes. The MEA prescribed for a Federal airway or segment thereof, area navigation low or high route, or other direct route, applies to the entire width of the airway, segment or route between the radio fixes defining the airway, segment or route. (Refer to FAR Parts 91 and 95, AIM)

MINIMUM FUEL—Indicates that an aircraft's fuel supply has reached a state where, upon reaching the destination, it can accept little or no delay. This is not an emergency situation but merely indicates an emergency situation is possible should any undue delay occur.

MINIMUM HOLDING ALTITUDE/MHA—The lowest altitude prescribed for a holding pattern which assures navigational signal coverage, communications, and meets obstacle clearance requirements.

MINIMUM IFR ALTITUDES—Minimum altitudes for IFR operations as prescribed in FAR Part 91. These altitudes are published on aeronautical charts and prescribed in FAR Part 95, for airways and routes, and FAR Part 97, for standard instrument approach procedures. If no applicable minimum altitude is prescribed in FAR Parts 95 or 97, the following minimum IFR altitude applies:

1. In designated mountainous areas, 2000 feet above the highest obstacle within a horizontal distance of 5 statute miles from the course to be flown; or

2. Other than mountainous areas, 1000 feet above the highest obstacle within a horizontal distance of 5 statute miles from the course to be flown; or

3. As otherwise authorized by the Administrator or assigned by ATC. (See Minimum En Route IFR Altitude, Minimum Obstruction Clearance Altitude, Minimum Crossing Altitude, Minimum Safe Altitude, Minimum Vectoring Altitude) (Refer to FAR Part 91)

MINIMUM OBSTRUCTION CLEARANCE ALTITUDE/MOCA—The lowest published altitude in effect between radio fixes on VOR airways, off-airway routes, or route segments which meets obstacle clearance requirements for the entire route segment and which assures acceptable navigational signal coverage only within 22 nautical miles of a VOR. (Refer to FAR Part 91 and 95).

MINIMUM RECEPTION ALTITUDE/MRA—The lowest altitude at which an intersection can be determined. (Refer to FAR Part 95)

MINIMUM SAFE ALTITUDE/MSA—

1. The minimum altitude specified in FAR Part 91, for various aircraft operations.

2. Altitudes depicted on approach charts which provide at least 1,000 feet of obstacle clearance for emergency use within a specified distance from the navigation facility upon which a procedure is predicated. These altitudes will be identified as MINIMUM SECTOR ALTITUDES or EMERGENCY SAFE ALTITUDES and are established as follows:

MINIMUM SECTOR ALTITUDES—Altitudes depicted on approach charts which provide at least 1,000 feet of obstacle clearance within a 25-mile radius of the navigation facility upon which the procedure is predicated. Sectors depicted on approach charts must be at least 90 degrees in scope. These altitudes are for emergency use only and do not necessarily assure acceptable navigational signal coverage.

EMERGENCY SAFE ALTITUDES—Altitudes depicted on approach charts which provide at least 1,000 feet of obstacle clearance within a 100-mile radius of the navigation facility upon which the procedure is predicated, and are normally used only in military procedures. These altitudes are identified on published procedures as "Emergency Safe Altitudes."

ICAO—MINIMUM SECTOR ALTITUDE—The lowest altitude which may be used under emergency conditions which will provide a minimum clearance of 300 meters (1000 feet) above all obstacles located in an area contained within a sector of a circle of 25 nautical miles radius centered on a radio aid to navigation.

MINIMUM SAFE ALTITUDE WARNING (MSAW)—A function of the ARTS III computer that aids the controller by alerting him when a tracked Mode C equipped aircraft is below or is predicted by the computer to go below a predetermined minimum safe altitude. (Refer to AIM)

MINIMUMS/MINIMA—Weather condition requirements established for a particular operation or type of operation; e.g., IFR takeoff or landing, alternate airport for IFR flight plans, VFR flight. (See Landing Minimums, IFR Takeoff Minimums, VFR Conditions, IFR Conditions) (Refer to FAR Part 91, AIM)

MINIMUM VECTORING ALTITUDE/MVA—The lowest MSL altitude at which an IFR aircraft will be vectored by a radar controller, except as otherwise authorized for radar approaches, departures and missed approaches. The altitude meets IFR obstacle clearance criteria. It may be lower than the published MEA along an airway or J-route segment. It may be utilized for radar vectoring only upon the controllers' determination that an adequate radar return is being received from the aircraft being controlled. Charts depicting minimum vectoring altitudes are normally available only to the controllers and not to pilots. (Refer to AIM)

MISSED APPROACH—

1. A maneuver conducted by a pilot when an instrument approach cannot be completed to a landing. The route of flight and altitude are shown on instrument approach procedure charts. A pilot executing a missed approach prior to the Missed Approach Point (MAP) must continue along the final approach to the MAP. The pilot may climb immediately to the altitude specified in the missed approach procedure.

2. A term used by the pilot to inform ATC that he is executing the missed approach.

3. At locations where ATC radar service is provided the pilot should conform to radar vectors, when provided by ATC, in lieu of the published missed approached procedure. (See Missed Approach Point) (Refer to AIM)

ICAO—MISSED APPROACH PROCEDURE—The procedure to be followed if, after an instrument approach, a landing is not effected and occurring normally:

1. When the aircraft has descended to the decision height and has not established visual contact, or

2. When directed by air traffic control to pull up or to go around again.

MISSED APPROACH POINT/MAP—A point prescribed in each instrument approach procedure at which a missed approach procedure shall be executed if the required visual reference does not exist. (See Missed Approach, Segments of an Instrument Approach Procedure)

MISSED APPROACH SEGMENT—(See Segments of an Instrument Approach Procedure)

MODE—The letter or number assigned to a specific pulse spacing of radio signals transmitted or received by ground interrogator or airborne transponder components of the Air Traffic Control Radar Beacon System (ATCRBS). Mode A (military Mode 3) and Mode C (altitude reporting) are used in air traffic control. (See Transponder, Interrogator, Radar) (Refer to AIM)

ICAO—MODE (SSR MODE)—The letter or number assigned to a specific pulse spacing of the interrogation signals transmitted by an interrogator. There are 4 modes, A, B, C and D corresponding to four different interrogation pulse spacings.

MOVEMENT AREA—The runways, taxiways, and other areas of an airport which are utilized for taxiing, takeoff, and landing of aircraft, exclusive of loading ramp and parking areas. At those airports with a tower, specific approval for entry onto the movement area must be obtained from ATC.

ICAO—MOVEMENT AREA—That part of an aerodrome intended for the surface movement of aircraft, including maneuvering area and aprons.

MOVING TARGET INDICATOR/MTI—An electronic device which will permit radar scope presentation only from targets which are in motion. A partial remedy for ground clutter.

MSAW—(See Minimum Safe Altitude Warning)

NAS STAGE A—The en route ATC system's radar, computers and computer programs, controller plan view displays (PVDs/Radar Scopes), input/output devices, and the related communications equipment which are integrated to form the heart of the automated IFR air traffic control system. This equipment performs Flight Data Processing (FDP) and Radar Data Processing (RDP). It interfaces with automated terminal systems and is used in the control of en route IFR aircraft. (Refer to AIM)

NATIONAL AIRSPACE SYSTEM/NAS—The common network of U.S. airspace; air navigation facilities, equipment and services, airports or landing areas; aeronautical charts, information and services; rules, regulations and procedures, technical information, and manpower and material. Included are system components shared jointly with the military.

NATIONAL BEACON CODE ALLOCATION PLAN AIRSPACE/NBCAP AIRSPACE—Airspace over United States territory located within the North American continent between Canada and Mexico, including adjacent territorial waters outward to abut boundaries of oceanic control areas (CTA)/Flight Information Regions (FIR). (See Flight Information Region)

NATIONAL FLIGHT DATA CENTER/NFDC—A facility in Washington, DC, established by FAA to operate a central aeronautical information service for the collection, validation, and dissemination of aeronautical data in support of the activities of government, industry, and the aviation community. The information is published in the National Flight Data Digest. (See National Flight Data Digest)

NATIONAL FLIGHT DATA DIGEST/NFDD—A daily (except weekends and federal holidays) publication of flight information appropriate to aeronautical charts, aeronautical publications, Notices to Airmen or other media serving the purpose of providing operational flight data essential to safe and efficient aircraft operations.

NATIONAL SEARCH AND RESCUE PLAN—An interagency agreement which provides for the effective utilization of all available facilities in all types of search and rescue missions.

NAVAID CLASSES—VOR, VORTAC, and TACAN aids are classed according to their operational use. The three classes of NAVAIDS are:

    T—Terminal

    L—Low altitude

    H—High altitude

The normal service range for T, L, and H class aids is found in AIM. Certain operational requirements make it necessary to use some of these aids at greater service ranges than specified. Extended range is made possible through flight inspection determinations. Some aids also have lesser service range due to location, terrain, frequency protection, etc. Restrictions to service range are listed in Airport/Facility Directory.

NAVIGABLE AIRSPACE—Airspace at and above the minimum flight altitudes prescribed in the FARs including airspace needed for safe take-off and landing. (Refer to FAR Part 91)

NAVIGATIONAL AID/NAVAID—Any visual or electronic device airborne or on the surface which provides point to point guidance information or position data to aircraft in flight. (See Air Navigation Facility)

NDB—(See Nondirectional beacon)

NEGATIVE—"No" or "Permission not granted" or "That is not correct."

NEGATIVE CONTACT—Used by pilots to inform ATC that:

1. Previously issued traffic is not in sight. It may be followed by the pilot's request for the controller to provide assistance in avoiding the traffic.

2. They were unable to contact ATC on a particular frequency.

NIGHT—The time between the end of evening civil twilight and the beginning of morning civil twilight, as published in the American Air Almanac, converted to local time.

ICAO—NIGHT—The hours between the end of evening civil twilight and the beginning of morning civil twilight or such other period between sunset and sunrise as may be specified by the appropriate authority.

NO GYRO APPROACH/VECTOR—A radar approach/vector provided in case of a malfunctioning gyrocompass or directional gyro. Instead of providing the pilot with headings to be flown, the controller observes the radar track and issues control instructions "turn right/left" or "stop turn" as appropriate. (Refer to AIM)

NON-COMPOSITE SEPARATION—Separation in accordance with minima other than the composite separation minimum specified for the area concerned.

NONDIRECTIONAL BEACON/RADIO BEACON/NDB—An L/MF or UHF radio beacon transmitting nondirectional signals whereby the pilot of an aircraft equipped with direction finding equipment can determine his bearing to or from the radio beacon and "home" on or track to or from the station. When the radio beacon is installed in conjunction with the Instrument Landing System marker, it is normally called a Compass Locator. (See Compass Locator, Automatic Direction Finder)

NONPRECISION APPROACH PROCEDURE/NONPRECISION APPROACH—A standard instrument approach procedure in which no electronic glide slope is provided; e.g., VOR, TACAN, NDB, LOC, ASR, LDA, or SDF approaches.

NONRADAR—Precedes other terms and generally means without the use of radar, such as:

1. Nonradar Route—A flight path or route over which the pilot is performing his own navigation. The pilot may be receiving radar separation, radar monitoring or other ATC services while on a nonradar route. (See Radar Route)

2. Nonradar Approach—Used to describe instrument approaches for which course guidance on final approach is not provided by ground based precision or surveillance radar. Radar vectors to the final approach course may or may not be provided by ATC. Examples of nonradar approaches are VOR, ADF, TACAN, and ILS, approaches. (See Final Approach—IFR, Final Approach Course, Radar Approach, Instrument Approach Procedure)

3. Nonradar Separation—The spacing of aircraft in accordance with established minima without the use of radar; e.g., vertical, lateral, or longitudinal separation. (See Radar Separation)

ICAO—Non-Radar Separation The separation used when aircraft position information is derived from sources other than radar.

4. Nonradar Arrival—An arriving aircraft that is not being vectored to the final approach course for an instrument approach or towards the airport for a visual approach. The aircraft may or may not be in a radar environment and may or may not be receiving radar separation, radar monitoring or other services provided by ATC. (See Radar Arrival, Radar Environment)

NONRADAR APPROACH CONTROL—An ATC facility providing approach control service without the use of radar. (See Approach Control, Approach Control Service)

NORDO—(See Lost Communications)

NORTH AMERICAN ROUTE—A numerically coded route preplanned over existing airway and route systems to and from specific coastal fixes serving the North Atlantic. North American Routes consist of the following:

1. Common Route/Portion—That segment of a North American route between the inland navigation facility and the coastal fix.

2. Non-Common Route/Portion—That segment of a North American

route between the inland navigation facility and a designated North American terminal.

3. Inland Navigation Facility—A navigation aid on a North American route at which the common route and/or the non-common route begins or ends.

4. Coastal Fix—A navigation aid or intersection where an aircraft transitions between the domestic route structure and the oceanic route structure.

NOTICES TO AIRMEN/PUBLICATION—A publication designed primarily as a pilot's operational manual containing current NOTAM information (see Notice to Airmen—NOTAM) considered essential to the safety of flight as well as supplemental data to other aeronautical publications.

NOTICE TO AIRMEN/NOTAM—A notice containing information (not known sufficiently in advance to publicize by other means) concerning the establishment, condition or change in any component (facility, service, or procedure of, or hazard in the National Airspace System) the timely knowledge of which is essential to personnel concerned with flight operations.

1. NOTAM(D)—A NOTAM given (in addition to local dissemination) distant dissemination via teletypewriter beyond the area of responsibility of the Flight Service Station. These NOTAMS will be stored and repeated hourly until cancelled.

2. NOTAM(L)—A NOTAM given local dissemination by voice, (Teletypewriter where applicable), and a wide variety of means such as: Teleautograph, teleprinter, facsimile reproduction, hot line, telecopier, telegraph, and telephone to satisfy local user requirements.

3. FDC NOTAM—A notice to airmen, regulatory in nature, transmitted by NFDC and given all-circuit dissemination.

ICAO—NOTAM—A notice, containing information concerning the establishment, condition or change in any aeronautical facility, service, procedure or hazard, the timely knowledge of which is essential to personnel concerned with flight operations.

NUMEROUS TARGETS VICINITY (LOCATION)—A traffic advisory issued by ATC to advise pilots that targets on the radar scope are too numerous to issue individually. (See Traffic Advisories)

OBSTACLE—An existing object, object of natural growth, or terrain at a fixed geographical location, or which may be expected at a fixed location within a prescribed area, with reference to which vertical clearance is or must be provided during flight operation.

OBSTRUCTION—An object which penetrates an imaginary surface described in FAR Part 77. (Refer to FAR Part 77)

OBSTRUCTION LIGHT—A light, or one of a group of lights, usually red or white, frequently mounted on a surface structure or natural terrain to warn pilots of the presence of an obstruction.

OFF-ROUTE VECTOR—A vector by ATC which takes an aircraft off a previously assigned route. Altitudes assigned by ATC during such vectors provide required obstacle clearance.

OFFSET PARALLEL RUNWAYS—Staggered runways having centerlines which are parallel.

ON COURSE—

1. Used to indicate that an aircraft is established on the route centerline.

2. Used by ATC to advise a pilot making a radar approach that his aircraft is lined up on the final approach course. (See On-Course Indication)

ON-COURSE INDICATION—An indication on an instrument which provides the pilot a visual means of determining that the aircraft is located on the centerline of a given navigational track; or an indication on a radar scope that an aircraft is on a given track.

OPTION APPROACH—An approach requested and conducted by a pilot which will result in either a touch-and-go, missed approach, low approach, stop-and-go or full stop landing. (See Cleared for option) (Refer to **AIM**)

ORGANIZED TRACK SYSTEM—A moveable system of oceanic tracks that traverses the North Atlantic between Europe and North America the physical position of which is determined twice daily taking the best advantage of the winds aloft.

OUT—The conversation is ended and no response is expected.

OUTER COMPASS LOCATOR—(See Compass Locator)

OUTER FIX—A general term used within ATC to describe fixes in the terminal area, other than the final approach fix. Aircraft are normally cleared to these fixes by an Air Route Traffic Control Center or an Approach Control Facility. Aircraft are normally cleared from these fixes to the final aproach fix or final approach course.

OUTER MARKER/OM—A marker beacon at or near the glide slope intercept altitude of an ILS approach. It is keyed to transmit two dashes per second on a 400 Hz tone which is received aurally and visually by compatible airborne equipment. The OM is normally located four to seven miles from the runway threshold on the extended centerline of the runway. (See Marker Beacon, Instrument Landing System) (Refer to AIM)

OVER—My transmission is ended; I expect a response.

OVERHEAD APPROACH/360 OVERHEAD—A series of predetermined maneuvers prescribed for VFR arrival of military aircraft (often in formation) for entry into the VFR traffic pattern and to proceed to a landing. The pattern usually specifies the following:

1. The ratio contact required of the pilot.

2. The speed to be maintained.

3. An initial approach 3 to 5 miles in length.

4. An elliptical pattern consisting of two 180 degree turns.

5. A break point at which the first 180 degree turn is started.

6. The direction of turns.

7. Altitude (at least 500 feet above the conventional pattern).

8. A "Roll-out" on final approach not less than ¼ mile from the land threshold and not less than 300 feet above the ground.

PAN—The international radio-telephony urgency signal. When repeated three times indicates uncertainty or alert, followed by nature of urgency. (See MAYDAY) (Refer to AIM)

PARALLEL ILS APPROACHES—ILS approaches to parallel runways by IFR aircraft which, when established inbound toward the airport on the adjacent localizer courses, are radar-separated by at least 2 miles. (See Simultaneous ILS Approaches)

PARALLEL OFFSET ROUTE—A parallel track to the left or right of the designated or established airway/route. Normally associated with Area Navigation (RNAV) operations. (See Area Navigation)

PARALLEL RUNWAYS—Two or more runways at the same airport whose centerlines are parallel. In addition to runway number, parallel runways are designated as L (left) and R (right) or, if three parallel runways exist, L (left) C (center), and R (right).

PAR APPROACH—A precision instrument approach wherein the air traffic controller issues guidance instructions, for pilot compliance, based on the aircraft's position in relation to the final approach course (azimuth), the glide scope (elevation), and the distance (range) from the touchdown point on the runway as displayed on the controller's radar scope. (See Precision Approach Radar, Glide Path) (Refer to AIM)

PERMANENT ECHO—Radar signals reflected from fixed objects on the earth's surface; e.g., buildings, towers, terrain. Permanent echoes are distinguished from "ground clutter" by being definable locations rather than large areas. Under certain conditions they may be used to check radar alignment.

PHOTO RECONNAISSANCE (PR)—Military activity that requires locating individual photo targets and navigating to the targets at a preplanned angle and altitude. The activity normally requires a lateral route width of 16NM and altitude range of 1,500 feet to 10,000 feet AGL.

PILOT BRIEFING/PRE-FLIGHT PILOT BRIEFING—A service provided by the FSS to assist pilots in flight planning. Briefing items may include weather information, NOTAMS, military activities, flow control information and other items as requested. (Refer to AIM)

PILOT IN COMMAND—The pilot responsible for the operation and safety of an aircraft during flight time. (Refer to FAR Part 91)

PILOTS AUTOMATIC TELEPHONE WEATHER ANSWERING SERVICE/PATWAS—A continuous telephone recording containing current and forecast weather information for pilots. (See Flight Service Station) (Refer to AIM)

PILOT'S DISCRETION—When used in conjunction with altitude assignments, means that ATC has offered the pilot the option of starting climb or descent whenever he wishes and conducting the climb or descent at any rate he wishes. He may temporarily level off at any intermediary altitude. However, once he has vacated an altitude he may not return to that altitude.

PILOT WEATHER REPORT/PIREP—A report of meteorological phenomena encountered by aircraft in flight. (Refer to AIM)

POSITION REPORT/PROGRESS REPORT—A report over a known

location as transmitted by an aircraft to ATC. (Refer to AIM)

POSITION SYMBOL—A computer generated indication shown on a radar display to indicate the mode of tracking.

POSITIVE CONTROL—The separation of all air traffic, within designated airspace, by air traffic control. (See Positive Control Area)

POSITIVE CONTROL AREA/PCA—Airspace designated in FAR Part 71 wherein aircraft are required to be operated under Instrument Flight Rules (IFR). Vertical extent of PCA is from 18,000 feet to and including flight level 600 throughout most of the conterminous United States. In Alaska, it includes the airspace over the State of Alaska from 18,000 feet to and including FL 600, but not including the airspace less than 1,500 feet above the surface of the earth and the Alaskan Peninsula west of longitude 160° 00' W. Rules for operating in positive control area are found in FARs 91.97 and 91.24.

PRECIPITATION—Any or all forms of water particles (rain, sleet, hail, or snow), that fall from the atmosphere and reach the surface.

PRECISION APPROACH PROCEDURE/PRECISION APPROACH—A standard instrument approach procedure in which an electronic glide slope is provided; e.g., ILS and PAR. (See Instrument Landing System, Precision Approach Radar)

PRECISION APPROACH RADAR/PAR—Radar equipment in some ATC facilities serving military airports, which is used to detect and display the azimuth, range, and elevation of an aircraft on the final approach course to a runway. It is used by air traffic controllers to provide the pilot with a precision approach, or to monitor certain nonradar approaches. (See PAR Approach)

ICAO—PRECISION APPROACH RADAR/PAR—Primary radar equipment used to determine the position of an aircraft during final approach, in terms of lateral and vertical deviations relative to a nominal approach path, and in range relative to touchdown.

PREFERENTIAL ROUTES—Preferential routes (PDRs, PARs, and PDARs) are adapted in ARTCC computers to accomplish inter/intra-facility controller coordination and to assure that flight data are posted at the proper control positions. Locations having a need for these specific inbound and outbound routes normally publish such routes in local facility bulletins and their use by pilots minimizes flight plan route amendments. When the workload or traffic situation permits, controllers normally provide radar vectors or assign requested routes to minimize circuitous routing. Preferential routes are usually confined to one ARTCC's area and are referred to by the following names or acronyms:

1. Preferential Departure Route/PDR—A specific departure route from an airport or terminal area to an en route point where is no further need for flow control. It may be included in a Standard Instrument Departure (SID) or a Preferred IFR Route.

2. Preferential Arrival Route/PAR—A specific arrival route from an appropriate en route point to an airport or terminal area. It may be included in a Standard Terminal Arrival Route (STAR) or a Preferred

IFR Route. The abbreviation "PAR" is used primarily within the ARTCC and should not be confused with the abbreviation for Precision Approach Radar.

3. Preferential Departure and Arrival Route/PDAR—A route between two terminals which are within or immediately adjacent to one ARTCC's area. PDARs are not synonomous with Preferred IFR Routes but may be listed as such as they do accomplish essentially the same purpose. (See Preferred IFR Routes, NAS Stage A)

PREFERRED IFR ROUTES—Routes established between busier airports to increase system efficiency and capacity. They normally extend through one or more ARTCC areas and are designed to achieve balanced traffic flows among high density terminals. IFR clearances are issued on the basis of these routes except when severe weather avoidance procedures or other factors dictate otherwise. Preferred IFR Routes are listed in the Airport/Facility Directory. If a flight is planned to or from an area having such routes but the departure or arrival point is not listed in the Airport/Facility Directory, pilots may use that part of a preferred IFR Route which is appropriate for the departure or arrival point that is listed. Preferred IFR Routes are correlated with SIDs and STARs and may be defined by airways, jet routes, direct routes between NAVAIDS. Waypoints NAVAID radials/DME, or any combinations thereof. (See Standard Instrument Departure, Standard Terminal Arrival Route, Preferential Routes, Center Area) (Refer to Airport/Facility Directory and Notices to Airmen)

PREVAILING VISIBILITY—(See Visibility)

PROCEDURE TURN INBOUND—That point of a procedure turn maneuver where course reversal has been completed and an aircraft is established inbound on the intermediate approach segment or final approach course. A report of "procedure turn inbound" is normally used by ATC as a position report for separation purposes. (See Final Approach Course, Procedure Turn, Segments of an Instrument Approach Procedure)

PROCEDURE TURN/PT—The maneuver prescribed when it is necessary to reverse direction to establish an aircraft on the intermediate approach segment or final approach course. The outbound course, direction of turn, distance within which the turn must be completed, and minimum altitude are specified in the procedure. However, the point at which the turn may be commenced, and the type and rate of turn, are left to the discretion of the pilot.

ICAO—PROCEDURE TURN—A maneuver in which a turn is made away from a designated track followed by a turn in the opposite direction, both turns being executed so as to permit the aircraft to intercept and proceed along the reciprocal of the designated track.

PROFILE DESCENT—An uninterrupted descent (except where level flight is required for speed adjustment; e.g., 250 knots at 10,000 feet MSL) from cruising altitude/level to interception of a glide slope or to a minimum altitude specified for the initial or intermediate approach segment of a nonprecision instrument approach. The profile descent normally terminates at the approach gate or where the glide slope or other appropriate minimum altitude is intercepted.

PROHIBITED AREA—(See Special Use Airspace)

ICAO—PROHIBITED AREA—An airspace of defined dimensions, above the land areas or territorial waters of a state, within which the flight of aircraft is prohibited.

PROPOSED BOUNDARY CROSSING TIME/PBCT—Each center has a PBCT parameter for each internal airport. Proposed internal flight plans are transmitted to the adjacent center if the flight time along the proposed route from the departure airport to the center boundary is less than or equal to the value of PBCT or if airport adaption specifies transmission regardless of PBCT.

PUBLISHED ROUTE—A route for which an IFR altitude has been established, and published; e.g., Federal Airways, Jet Routes, Area Navigation Routes, Specified Direct Routes. (See Published)

QUADRANT—A quarter part of a circle, centered on a NAVAID, oriented clockwise from magnetic north as follows: NE quadrant 000–089, SE quadrant 090–179, SW quadrant 180–269, NW quadrant 270–359.

QUICK LOOK—A feature of NAS Stage A and ARTS which provides the controller the capability to display full data blocks of tracked aircraft from other control positions.

QUOTA FLOW CONTROL/QFLOW—A flow control procedure by which the Central Flow Control Facility (CFCF) restricts traffic to the ARTC Center area having an impacted airport thereby avoiding sector/area saturation. (See Air Traffic Control Systems Command Center) (Refer to Airport/Facility Director)

RADAR ADVISORY—The provision of advice and information based on radar observations. (See Advisory Service)

RADAR AIR TRAFFIC CONTROL FACILITY/RATCF—An air traffic control facility, located at a U.S. Navy or Marine Corps Air Station, utilizing surveillance and, normally, precision approach radar and air/ground communications equipment to provide approach control services to aircraft arriving, departing or transiting the airspace controlled by the facility. The facility may be operated by the FAA, the USN, or USMC and service may be provided to both civil and military airports. Similar to TRACON (FAA), RAPCON (USAF), RATCF (Navy), and ARAC (Army) (See Approach Control, Approach Control Service, Departure Control)

RADAR APPROACH—An instrument approach procedure which utilizes Precision Approach Radar (PAR) or Airport Surveillance Radar (ASR). (See PAR Approach, Surveillance Approach, Airport Surveillance Radar, Precision Approach Radar, Instrument Approach Procedure) (Refer to AIM)

ICAO—RADAR APPROACH—An approach, executed by an aircraft, under the direction of a radar controller.

RADAR APPROACH CONTROL/RAPCON—An air traffic control facility, located at a U.S. Air Force Base, utilizing surveillance and, normally, precision approach radar and air/ground communications equipment to provide approach control services to aircraft arriving, departing or transiting the airspace controlled by the facility. The facility may be operated by the FAA or the USAF and service may be provided to both civil and military airports. Similar to TRACON (FAA), RATCF (Navy) and ARAC (Army). (See Approach Control, Approach Control Service, Departure Control)

RADAR ARRIVAL—An arriving aircraft which is being vectored to the final approach course for an instrument approach, or for a visual approach to the airport. (See Radar Approach, Visual Approach)

RADAR BEACON—(See Radar)

RADAR CONTACT—

1. Used by ATC to inform an aircraft that it is identified on the radar display and radar flight following will be provided until radar identification is terminated. Radar service may also be provided within the limits of necessity and capability. When a pilot is informed of "radar contact" he automatically discontinues reporting over compulsory reporting points.

2. The term an air traffic controller uses to inform the transferring controller that the target being transferred is identified on his radar display.

ICAO—RADAR CONTACT—The situation which exists when the radar blip of a particular aircraft is seen and identified on a radar display.

RADAR CONTACT LOST—Used by ATC to inform a pilot that radar identification of his aircraft has been lost. The loss may be attributed to several things including the aircraft merging with weather or ground clutter, the aircraft flying below radar line of sight, the aircraft entering an area of poor radar return or a failure of the aircraft transponder or ground radar equipment. (See Clutter, Radar Contact)

RADAR ENVIRONMENT—An area in which radar service may be provided. (See Radar Contact, Radar Service, Additional Services, Traffic Advisories)

RADAR FLIGHT FOLLOWING—The observation of the progress of radar identified aircraft, whose primary navigation is being provided by the pilot, wherein the controller retains and correlates the aircraft identity with the appropriate target or target symbol displayed on the radar scope. (See Radar Contact, Radar Service) (Refer to AIM)

RADAR IDENTIFICATION—The process of ascertaining that an observed radar target is the radar return from a particular aircraft. (See Radar Contact, Radar Service)

ICAO—RADAR IDENTIFICATION—The process of correlating a particular radar blip with a specific aircraft.

RADAR IDENTIFIED AIRCRAFT—An aircraft, the position of which has been correlated with an observed target or symbol on the radar display. (See Radar Contact, Radar Contact Lost)

RADAR MONITORING—(See Radar Service)

RADAR NAVIGATIONAL GUIDANCE—(See Radar Service)

RADAR POINT OUT/POINT OUT—Used between controllers to indicate radar handoff action where the initiating controller plans to retain communications with an aircraft penetrating the other controller's airspace and additional coordination is required.

RADAR/RADIO DETECTION AND RANGING—A device which by measuring the time interval between transmission and reception of radio pulses and correlating the angular orientation of the radiated antenna beam or beams in azimuth and/or elevation, provides information range, azimuth and/or elevation of objects in the path of the transmitted pulses.

1. Primary Radar—A radar system in which a minute portion of a radio pulse transmitted from a site is reflected by an object and then received back at that site, for processing and display at an air traffic control facility.

2. Secondary Radar/Radar Beacon/ATCRBS—A radar system in which the object to be detected is fitted with cooperative equipment in the form of a radio receiver/transmitter (transponder). Radar pulses transmitted from the searching transmitter/receiver (interrogator) site are received in the cooperative equipment and used to trigger a distinctive transmission from the transponder. This reply transmission rather than a reflected signal, is then received back at the transmitter/receiver site for processing and display at an air traffic control facility. (See Transponder, Interrogator) (Refer to AIM)

ICAO—RADAR—A radio detection device which provides information on range, azimuth and/or elevation of objects.

1. *Primary Radar*—A radar system which uses reflected radio signals.

2. *Secondary Radar*—A radar system wherein a radio signal transmitted from a radar station initiates the transmission of a radio signal from another station.

RADAR ROUTE—A flight path or route over which an aircraft is vectored. Navigational guidance and altitude assignments are provided by ATC. (See Flight Path, Route, Radar Vector)

RADAR SEPARATION—(See Radar Service)

RADAR SERVICE—A term which encompasses one or more of the following services based on the use of radar which can be provided by a controller to a pilot of a radar identified aircraft.

1. Radar Separation—Radar spacing of aircraft in accordance with established minima.

2. Radar Navigational Guidance—Vectoring aircraft to provide course guidance.

3. Radar Monitoring—The radar flight following of aircraft, whose primary navigation is being performed by the pilot, to observe and note deviations from its authorized flight path, airway, or route. When being applied specifically to radar monitoring of instrument approaches, i.e., with precision approach radar (PAR) or radar monitoring or simultaneous ILS approaches, it includes advice and instructions whenever an aircraft nears or exceeds the prescribed PAR safety limit

or simultaneous ILS no transgression zone. (See Additional Services, Traffic Advisories, Duty Priority)

ICAO—RADAR SERVICE—Term used to indicate a service provided directly by means of radar.

ICAO—RADAR SEPARATION—The separation used when aircraft position information is derived from radar sources.

ICAO—RADAR MONITORING—The use of radar for the purpose of providing aircraft with information and advice relative to significant deviations from nominal flight path.

RADAR SERVICE TERMINATED—Used by ATC to inform a pilot that he will no longer be provided any of the services that could be received while under radar contact. Radar service is automatically terminated and the pilot is not advised in the following cases:

1. An aircraft cancels its IFR flight plan, except within a TCA, TRSA, or where Stage II service is provided.

2. At the completion of a radar approach.

3. When an arriving aircraft receiving Stage I, II, or III service is advised to contact the tower.

4. When an aircraft conducting a visual approach is advised to contact the tower.

5. When an aircraft vectored to a final approach course for an instrument approach has landed or the tower has the aircraft in sight, whichever occurs first.

RADAR SURVEILLANCE—The radar observation of a given geographical area for the purpose of performing some radar function

RADAR TRAFFIC ADVISORIES—(See Traffic Advisories)

RADAR TRAFFIC INFORMATION SERVICE—(See Traffic Advisories)

RADAR WEATHER ECHO INTENSITY LEVELS—Existing radar systems cannot detect turbulence. However, there is a direct correlation between the degree of turbulence and other weather features associated with thunderstorms, and the radar weather echo intensity. The National Weather Service has categorized six (6) levels of radar weather echo intensity. The following list gives the weather features likely to be associated with these levels during thunderstorm weather situations:

1. Level 1 (WEAK) and Level 2 (MODERATE). Light to moderate turbulence is possible with lightning.

2. Level 3 (STRONG). Severe turbulence possible, lightning.

3. Level 4 (VERY STRONG). Severe turbulence likely, lightning.

4. Level 5 (INTENSE). Severe turbulence, lightning, organized wind gusts. Hail likely.

5. Level 6 (EXTREME). Severe turbulence, large hail, lightning, extensive wind gusts and turbulence.

RADIAL—A magnetic bearing extending from a VOR/VORTAC/TACAN navigation facility.

RADIO—

1. A device used for communication.
2. Used to refer to a Flight Service Station, e.g., "Seattle Radio" is used to call Seattle FSS.

RADIO ALTIMETER/RADAR ALTIMETER—Aircraft equipment which makes use of the reflection of radio waves from the ground to determine the height of the aircraft above the surface.

RADIO BEACON—(See Nondirectional Beacon)

RADIO MAGNETIC INDICATOR/RMI—An aircraft navigational instrument coupled with a gyro compass or similar compass that indicates the direction to a selected NAVAID and indicates bearing with respect to the heading of the aircraft.

RAMP—(See Apron)

READ BACK—Repeat my message back to me.

RECEIVING CONTROLLER/FACILITY—A controller/facility receiving control of an aircraft from another controller/facility.

REDUCE SPEED TO (SPEED)—(See Speed Adjustment)

RELEASE TIME—A departure time restriction issued to a pilot by ATC when necessary to separate a departing aircraft from other traffic.

ICAO—RELEASE TIME—Time prior to which an aircraft should be given further clearance or prior to which it should not proceed in case of radio failure.

REMOTE COMMUNICATIONS AIR/GROUND FACILITY/RCAG—An unmanned VHF/UHF transmitter/receiver facility which is used to expand ARTCC air/ground communications coverage and to facilitate direct contact between pilots and controllers. RCAG facilities are sometimes not equipped with emergency frequencies 121.5 MHz and 243.0 MHz. (Refer to AIM)

REMOTE COMMUNICATIONS OUTLET/RCO—An unmanned air/ground communications station remotely controlled, providing UHF and VHF transmit and receive capability to extend the service range of the FSS.

REPORT—Used to instruct pilots to advise ATC of specified information, e.g., "Report passing Hamilton VOR."

REPORTING POINT—A geographical location in relation to which the position of an aircraft is reported. (See Compulsory Reporting Point) (Refer to AIM)

ICAO—REPORTING POINT—A specified geographical location in relation to which the position of an aircraft can be reported.

REQUEST FULL ROUTE CLEARANCE/FRC—Used by pilots to request that the entire route of flight be read verbatim in an ATC clearance. Such request should be made to preclude receiving an ATC clearance based on the originally filed flight plan when a filed IFR flight plan has been revised by the pilot, company, or operations prior to departure.

RESCUE COORDINATION CENTER/RCC—A search and rescue (SAR) facility equipped and manned to coordinate and control SAR operations in an area designated by the SAR plan. The U.S. Coast Guard and the U.S. Air Force have responsibility for the operation of RCCs.

*ICAO—RESCUE CO-ORDINATION CENTER—*A unit responsible for promoting efficient organization of search and rescue service and for coordinating the conduct of search and rescue region.

RESTRICTED AREA—(See Special Use Airspace)

*ICAO—RESTRICTED AREA—*Airspace of defined dimensions, above the land areas or territorial waters of a State, within which the flight of aircraft is restricted in accordance with certain specified conditions.

*RESUME OWN NAVIGATION—*Used by ATC to advise a pilot to resume his own navigational responsibility. It is issued after completion of a radar vector or when radar contact is lost while the aircraft is being radar vectored. (See Radar Contact Lost, Radar Service Terminated)

RNAV—(See Area Navigation)

RNAV APPROACH—An instrument approach procedure which relies on aircraft area navigation equipment for navigational guidance. (See Instrument Approach Procedure, Area Navigation)

ROAD RECONNAISSANCE (RC)—Military activity requiring navigation along roads, railroads and rivers. Reconnaissance route/route segments are seldom along a straight line and normally require a lateral route width of 10NM to 30NM and altitude range of 500 feet to 10,000 feet AGL.

*ROGER—*I have received all of your last transmission. It should not be used to answer a question requiring a yes or no answer. (See Affirmative, Negative)

ROLLOUT RVR—(See Visibility)

ROUTE—A defined path, consisting of one or more courses in a horizontal plane, which aircraft traverse over the surface of the earth. (See Jet Route, Airway, Published Route, Unpublished Route)

ROUTE SEGMENT—As used in Air Traffic Control, a part of a route that can be defined by two navigational fixes, two NAVAIDs, or a fix and a NAVAID. (See Route, Fix)

*ICAO—ROUTE SEGMENT—*A portion of a route to be flown, as defined by two consecutive significant points specified in a flight plan.

RUNWAY—A defined rectangular area, on a land airport prepared for the landing and takeoff run of aircraft along its length. Runways are normally numbered in relation to their magnetic direction rounded off to the nearest 10 degrees, e.g., Runway 25, Runway 01. (See Parallel Runways)

*ICAO—RUNWAY—*A defined rectangular area, on a land aerodrome prepared for the landing and takeoff run of aircraft along its length.

RUNWAY CENTERLINE LIGHTING—(See Airport Lighting)

RUNWAY CONDITION READING/RCR—Numerical decelerometer readings relayed by air traffic controllers at USAF and certain civil bases for use by the pilot in determining runway braking action. These readings are routinely relayed only to USAF and Air National Guard Aircraft. (See Braking Action)

RUNWAY END IDENTIFIER LIGHTS—(See Airport Lighting)

RUNWAY GRADIENT—The average slope, measured in percent, between two ends or points on a runway. Runway gradient is depicted on Government aerodrome sketches when total runway gradient exceeds 0.3%.

RUNWAY IN USE/ACTIVE RUNWAY/DUTY RUNWAY—Any runway or runways currently being used for takeoff or landing. When multiple runways are used, they are all considered active runways.

RUNWAY LIGHTS—(See Airport Lighting)

RUNWAY MARKINGS—

1. Basic marking—Markings on runways used for operations under visual flight rules consisting of centerline marking and runway direction numbers and, if required, letters.

2. Instrument marking—Markings on runways served by nonvisual navigation aids and intended for landings under instrument weather conditions, consisting of basic marking plus threshold marking.

3. All-weather (precision instrument) marking—Markings on runways served by nonvisual precision approach aids and on runways having special operational requirements, consisting of instrument markings plus landing zone marking and side strips. (Refer to AIM)

RUNWAY PROFILE DESCENT—An instrument flight rules (IFR) air traffic control arrival procedure to a runway published for pilot use in graphic and/or textual form and may be associated with a STAR. RUNWAY PROFILE DESCENTs provide routing, and may depict crossing altitudes, speed restrictions, and headings to be flown from the en route structure to the point where the pilot will receive clearance for and execute an instrument approach procedure. A RUNWAY PROFILE DESCENT may apply to more than one runway if so stated on the chart. (Refer to AIM)

RUNWAY USE PROGRAM—Action initiated by the airport proprietor, with assistance from the users and FAA, to reduce the effect of noise on residents surrounding an airport through the use of specific runways when wind, weather, and other safety related factors permit.

RUNWAY VISIBILITY VALUE—(See Visibility)

RUNWAY VISUAL RANGE—(See Visibility)

SAFETY ADVISORY—A safety advisory issued by ATC to aircraft under their control if ATC is aware the aircraft is at an altitude which, in the controller's judgment, places the aircraft in unsafe proximity to terrain, obstructions or other aircraft. The controller may discontinue the issuance of further advisories if the pilot advises he is taking action to correct the situation or has the other aircraft in sight.

1. Terrain/Obstruction Advisory—A safety advisory issued by ATC to aircraft under their control if ATC is aware the aircraft is at an altitude which, in the controller's judgment, places the aircraft in unsafe proximity to terrain/obstructions; e.g., "Low Altitude Alert, check your altitude immediately."

2. Aircraft Conflict Advisory—A safety advisory issued by ATC to aircraft under their control if ATC is aware of an aircraft that is not under their control at an altitude which, in the controller's judgment, places both aircraft in unsafe proximity to each other. With the alert, ATC will offer the pilot an alternate course of action when feasible, e.g.,

"Traffic Alert, advise you turn right heading zero niner zero or climb to eight thousand immediately."

The issuance of a safety advisory is contingent upon the capability of the controller to have an awareness of an unsafe condition. The course of action provided will be predicated on other traffic under ATC control. Once the advisory is issued, it is solely the pilot's prerogative to determine what course of action, if any, he will take.

SAY AGAIN—Used to request a repeat of the last transmission. Usually specifies transmission or portion thereof not understood or not received, e.g., "Say again all after ABRAM VOR."

SAY ALTITUDE—Used by ATC to ascertain an aircraft's specific altitude/flight level. When the aircraft is climbing or descending, the pilot should state the indicated altitude rounded to the nearest 100 feet.

SAY HEADING—Used by ATC to request an aircraft heading. The pilot should state the actual heading of the aircraft.

SEARCH AND RESCUE FACILITY—A facility responsible for maintaining and operating a search and rescue (SAR) service to render aid to persons and property in distress. It is any SAR unit, station, NET or other operational activity which can be usefully employed during an SAR Mission, e.g., a Civil Air Patrol Wing or a Coast Guard Station. (See Search and Rescue)

SEARCH AND RESCUE/SAR—A service which seeks missing aircraft and assists those found to be in need of assistance. It is a cooperative effort using the facilities and services of available Federal, state and local agencies. The U.S. Coast Guard is responsible for coordination of search and rescue for the Maritime Region and the U.S. Air Force is responsible for search and rescue for the Inland Region. Information pertinent to search and rescue should be passed through any air traffic facility or be transmitted directly to the Rescue Coordination Center by telephone. (See Flight Service Station, Rescue Coordination Center) (Refer to AIM)

SEE AND AVOID—A visual procedure wherein pilots of aircraft flying in visual meteorological conditions (VMC), regardless of type of flight plan, are charged with the responsibility to observe the presence of other aircraft and to maneuver their aircraft as required to avoid the other aircraft. Right-of-way rules are contained in FAR, Part 91. (See Instrument Flight Rules, Visual Flight Rules, Visual Meteorological Conditions, Instrument Meteorological Conditions)

SEGMENTED CIRCLE—A system of visual indicators designed to provide traffic pattern information at airports without operating control towers. (Refer to AIM)

SEGMENTS OF AN INSTRUMENT APPROACH PROCEDURE—An instrument approach procedure may have as many as four separate segments depending on how the approach procedure is structured.

1. Initial Approach—The segment between the initial approach fix and the intermediate fix or the point where the aircraft is established on the intermediate course or final approach course.

2. Intermediate Approach—The segment between the intermediate fix

or point and the final approach fix.

3. Final Approach—The segment between the final approach fix or point and the runway, airport or missed approach point.

4. Missed Approach—The segment between the missed approach point, or point of arrival at decision height, and the missed approach fix at the prescribed altitude. (Refer to FAR Part 97)

ICAO

1. *Initial Approach*—That part of an instrument approach procedure consisting of the first approach to the first navigational facility associated with the procedure, or to a predetermined fix.

2. *Intermediate Approach*—That part of an instrument approach procedure from the first arrival at the first navigational facility or predetermined fix, to the beginning of the final approach.

3. *Final Approach*—That part of an instrument approach procedure from the time the aircraft has:

   a. Completed the last procedure turn or base turn where one is specified, or

   b. crossed a specified fix, or

   c. intercepted the last track specified for the procedures; until it has crossed a point in the vicinity of an aerodrome from which:
   (1) a landing can be made; or
   (2) a missed approach procedure is initiated.

4. *Missed Approach Procedure*—The procedure to be followed if, after an instrument approach, a landing is not effected and occuring normally:

   a. When the aircraft has descended to the decision height and has not established visual contact, or

   b. when directed by air traffic control to pull up or to go around again.

SEPARATION—In air traffic control, the spacing of aircraft to achieve their safe and orderly movement in flight and while landing and taking off. (See Separation Minima)

ICAO—SEPARATION—Spacing between aircraft, levels or tracks.

SEPARATION MINIMA—The minimum longitudinal, lateral, or vertical distances by which aircraft are spaced through the application of air traffic control procedures. (See Separation)

SEVERE WEATHER AVOIDANCE PLAN/SWAP—A plan to reroute traffic to avoid severe weather in the New York ARTCC area to provide the least disruption to the ATC system when large portions of airspace are unusable due to severe weather. (Refer to Airport/Facility Directory)

SHORT RANGE CLEARANCE—A clearance issued to a departing IFR flight which authorizes IFR flight to a specific fix short of the destination while air traffic control facilities are coordinating and obtaining the complete clearance.

SHORT TAKEOFF AND LANDING AIRCRAFT/STOL AIRCRAFT—An

aircraft which, at some weight within its approved operating weight, is capable of operating from a STOL runway in compliance with the applicable STOL characteristics, airworthiness, operations, noise, and pollution standards. (See Vertical Takeoff and Landing Aircraft)

SIDESTEP MANEUVER—A visual maneuver accomplished by a pilot at the completion of an instrument approach to permit a straight-in landing on a parallel runway not more than 1200 feet to either side of the runway to which the instrument approach was conducted. (Refer to AIM)

SIGMET/SIGNIFICANT METEOROLOGICAL INFORMATION—A weather advisory issued concerning weather significant to the safety of all aircraft. SIGMET advisories cover tornadoes, lines of thunderstorms, embedded thunderstorms, large hail, severe and extreme turbulence, severe icing, and widespread dust or sandstorms that reduce visibility to less than 3 miles. (See Convective SIGMET and AIRMET) (Refer to AIM)

ICAO—SIGMET INFORMATION—Information prepared by a meteorological watch office regarding the occurrence or expected occurrence of one or more of the following phenomena:

1. At subsonic cruising levels:
   Active thunderstorm area
   Tropical revolving storm
   Severe line squall
   Heavy hair
   Severe turbulence
   Severe icing
   Marked mountain waves
   Widespread sandstorm/duststorm.

2. At transonic levels and supersonic cruising levels:
   Moderate or severe turbulence
   Cumulonimbus clouds
   Hail

SIMPLIFIED DIRECTIONAL FACILITY/SDF—A NAVAID used for non-precision instrument approaches. The final approach course is similar to that of an ILS localizer except that the SDF course may be offset from the runway, generally not more than 3 degrees, and the course may be wider than the localizer, resulting in a lower degree of accuracy. (Refer to AIM)

SIMULATED FLAMEOUT/SFO—A practice approach by a jet aircraft (normally military) at idle thrust to a runway. The approach may start at a relatively high altitude over a runway (high key) and may continue on a relatively high and wide downwind leg with a high rate of descent and a continuous turn to final. It terminates in a landing or low approach. The purpose of this approach is to simulate a flameout. (See Flameout)

SIMULTANEOUS ILS APPROACHES—An approach system permitting simultaneous ILS approaches to airports having parallel runways separated by at least 4,300 feet between centerlines. Integral parts of a total system are ILS, radar, communications, ATC procedures, and appropriate airborne equipment. (See Parallel Runways) (Refer to AIM)

SINGLE DIRECTION ROUTES—Preferred IFR routes which are sometimes depicted on high altitude en route charts and which are normally flown in one direction only. (See Preferred IFR Route) (Refer to Airport/Facility Directory)

SINGLE FREQUENCY APPROACH/SFA—A service provided under a Letter of Agreement to military single-piloted turbojet aircraft which permits use of a single UHF frequency during approach for landing. Pilots will not normally be required to change frequency from the beginning of the approach to touchdown except that pilots conducting an en route descent are required to change frequency when control is transferred from the air route traffic control center to the terminal facility. The abbreviation "SFA" in the DOD FLIP IFR Supplement under "Communications" indicates this service is available at an aerodrome.

SINGLE FREQUENCY OUTLETS/SFO and SIMULTANEOUS SINGLE FREQUENCY OUTLETS/SSFO—Frequency Outlets commissioned at locations in Alaska not served by air traffic control facilities and remotely controlled by adjacent FSSs. They are subject to undetected and prolonged outages.

SINGLE-PILOTED AIRCRAFT—A military aircraft possessing one set of flight controls, tandem cockpits or two sets of flight controls but operated by one pilot is considered single-piloted by ATC when determining the appropriate air traffic service to be applied. (See Single Frequency Approach)

SLASH—A radar beacon reply displayed as an elongated target.

SPEAK SLOWER—Used in verbal communications as a request to reduce speech rate.

SPECIAL EMERGENCY—A condition of air piracy, or other hostile act by a person(s) aboard an aircraft which threatens the safety of the aircraft or its passengers.

SPECIAL IFR—(See Fixed-Wing Special IFR)

SPECIAL INSTRUMENT APPROACH PROCEDURE—(See Instrument Approach Procedure)

SPECIAL USE AIRSPACE—Airspace of defined dimensions identified by an area on the surface of the earth wherein activities must be confined because of their nature and/or wherein limitations may be imposed upon aircraft operations that are not a part of those activities.

Types of special use airspace:

1. Alert Area—Airspace which may contain a high volume of pilot training activities or an unusual type of aerial activity—neither of which is hazardous to aircraft. Alert Areas are depicted on aeronautical charts for the information of nonparticipating pilots. All activities within an Alert Area are conducted in accordance with Federal Aviation Regulations and pilots of participating aircraft as well as pilots transiting the area are equally responsible for collision avoidance.

2. Controlled Firing Areas—Airspace wherein activities are conducted under conditions so controlled as to eliminate hazards to nonpartici-

pating aircraft and to ensure the safety of persons and property on the ground.

3. Military Operations Area (MOA)—An MOA is an airspace assignment of defined vertical and lateral dimensions established outside positive control areas to separate/segregate certain military activities from IFR traffic and to identify for VFR traffic where these activities are conducted. (Refer to AIM)

4. Prohibited Area—Designated airspace within which the flight of aircraft is prohibited. (Refer to En Route Charts, AIM)

5. Restricted Area—Airspace designated under FAR, Part 73, within which the flight of aircraft, while not wholly prohibited, is subject to restriction. Most restricted areas are designated joint use and IFR/VFR operations in the area may be authorized by the controlling ATC facility when it is not being utilized by the using agency. Restricted areas are depicted on en route charts. Where joint use is authorized, the name of the ATC controlling facility is also shown. (Refer to FAR Part 73; AIM)

6. Warning Area—Airspace which may contain hazards to nonparticipating aircraft in international airspace.

SPECIAL VFR CONDITIONS—Weather conditions in a control zone which are less than basic VFR and in which some aircraft are permitted flight under Visual Flight Rules. (See Special VFR Operations) (Refer to FAR Part 91)

SPECIAL VFR OPERATIONS—Aircraft operating in accordance with clearances within control zones in weather conditions less than the basic VFR weather minima. Such operations must be requested by the pilot and approved by ATC. (See Special VFR Conditions)

ICAO—SPECIAL VFR FLIGHT—A controlled VFR flight authorized by air traffic control to operate within a control zone under meteorological conditions below the visual meteorological conditions.

SPEED—(See Airspeed, Groundspeed)

SPEED ADJUSTMENT—An ATC procedure used to request pilots to adjust aircraft speed to a specific value for the purpose of providing desired spacing. Speed adjustments are always expressed as indicated airspeed and pilots are expected to maintain a speed of plus or minus to 10 knots of the specified speed.

Examples of Speed Adjustments are:

1. "Increase speed to (speed)" or "Increase speed (number of) knots"— Used by ATC to request a pilot to increase the indicated airspeed of the aircraft.

2. "Reduce speed to (speed)" or "Reduce speed (number of) knots"— Used by ATC to request a pilot to reduce the indicated airspeed of the aircraft.

3. "If feasible, reduce speed to (speed)" or "If feasible, reduce speed (number of) knots"—Used by ATC to request a pilot to reduce the

indicated airspeed of the aircraft below specified speeds. (Refer to AIM; FAR Part 91)

SPEED BRAKES/DIVE BRAKES—Moveable aerodynamic devices on aircraft that reduce airspeed during descent and landing.

SQUAWK (Mode, Code, Function)—Activate specific modes/codes/functions on the aircraft transponder, e.g., "Squawk Three/Alpha, Two one zero five, Low." (See Transponder)

STAGE I/II/III SERVICE—(See Terminal Radar Program)

STANDARD INSTRUMENT APPROACH PROCEDURE—(See Instrument Approach Procedure)

STANDARD INSTRUMENT DEPARTURE/SID—A preplanned instrument flight rule (IFR) air traffic control departure procedure printed for pilot use in graphic and/or textual form. SIDs provide transition from the terminal to the appropriate en route structure. (See IFR Takeoff Minema and Departure Procedures) (Refer to AIM)

STANDARD RATE TURN—A turn of three degrees per second.

STANDARD TERMINAL ARRIVAL ROUTE/STAR—A preplanned instrument flight rule (IFR) air traffic control arrival route published for pilot use in graphic and/or textual form. STARs provide transition from the en route structure to a fix or point from which an approach can be made. (See Preferential Routes) (Refer to AIM)

STAND BY—Means the controller or pilot must pause for a few seconds, usually to attend to other duties of a higher priority. Also means to "wait" as in "stand by for clearance." If a delay is lengthy, the caller should reestablish contact.

STATIONARY RESERVATIONS—Altitude reservations which encompass activities in a fixed area. Stationary reservations may include activities such as special test of weapons systems or equipment, certain U.S. Navy carrier, fleet, and anti-submarine operations, rocket, missile and drone operations, and certain aerial refueling or similar operations.

STEPDOWN FIX—A fix permitting additional descent within a segment of an instrument approach procedure by identifying a point at which a controlling obstacle has been safely overflown.

STOP ALTITUDE SQUAWK—Used by ATC to inform an aircraft to turn-off the automatic altitude reporting feature of its transponder. It is issued when the verbally reported altitude varies 300 feet or more from the automatic altitude report. (See Altitude Readout, Transponder)

STOP AND GO—A procedure wherein an aircraft will land, make a complete stop on the runway, and then commence a takeoff from that point. (See Low Approach, Option Approach)

STOP-OVER FLIGHT PLAN—A flight plan which includes to or more separate en route flight segments with a stopover at one or more intermediate airports.

STOP SQUAWK (Mode or Code).—Used by ATC to tell the pilot to turn specified functions of the aircraft transponder off. (See Stop Altitude Squawk, Transponder)

STOP STREAM/BURST/BUZZER—Used by ATC to request a pilot to suspend electronic countermeasure activity. (See Jamming)

STOPWAY—An area beyond the takeoff runway designated by the airport authorities as able to support an airplane during an aborted takeoff. (Refer to FAR Part 1)

STRAIGHT-IN APPROACH—IFR—An instrument approach wherein final approach is begun without first having executed a procedure turn. Not necessarily completed with a straight-in landing or made to straight-in landing minimums. (See Straight-in Landing, Landing Minimums, Straight-in Approach-VFR)

STRAIGHT-IN APPROACH—VFR—Entry into the traffic pattern by interception of the extended runway centerline (final approach course) without executing any other portion of the traffic pattern. (See Traffic Pattern)

STRAIGHT-IN LANDING—A landing made on a runway aligned within 30° of the final approach course following completion of an instrument approach. (See Straight-in Approach-IFR)

STRAIGHT-IN LANDING MINIMUM/STRAIGHT-IN MINIMUMS—(See Landing Minimums)

SUBSTITUTE ROUTE—A route assigned to pilots when any part of an airway or route is unusable because of NAVAID status. These routes consist of:

1. Substitute routes which are shown on U.S. Government Charts.

2. Routes defined by ATC as specific NAVAID radials of courses.

3. Routes defined by ATC as direct to or between NAVAIDs.

SUNSET AND SUNRISE—The mean solar times of sunset and sunrise as published in the Nautical Almanac, converted to local standard time for the locality concerned. Within Alaska, the end of evening civil twilight and the beginning of morning civil twilight, as defined for each locality.

SURVEILLANCE APPROACH—An instrument approach wherein the air traffic controller issues instructions, for pilot compliance, based on aircraft position in relation to the final approach course (azimuth), and the distance (range) from the end of the runway as displayed on the controller's radar scope. The controller will provide recommended altitudes on final approach if requested by the pilot. (See PAR Approach) (Refer to AIM)

SYSTEM STRATEGIC NAVIGATION (SN)—Military activity accomplished by navigating along a preplanned route using internal aircraft systems to maintain a desired track. This activity normally requires a lateral route width of 10NM and altitude range of 1,000 feet to 6,000 feet AGL with some route segments that permit terrain following.

TACAN ONLY AIRCRAFT—An aircraft, normally military, possessing TACAN with DME but no VOR navigational system capability. Clearances must specify TACAN or VORTAC fixes and approaches.

TACAN/TACTICAL AIR NAVIGATION—An ultra-high frequency electronic rho-theta air navigation aid which provides suitably equipped aircraft a continuous indication of bearing and distance to the TACAN station. (See VORTAC) (Refer to AIM)

TARGET—The indication shown on a radar display resulting from a primary radar return or a radar beacon reply. (See Target Symbol, Radar)
*ICAO—TARGET—*In radar:

1. Generally, any discrete object which reflects or retransmits energy back to the radar equipment;
2. Specifically, an object of radar search or surveillance.

TARGET SYMBOL—A computer generated indication shown on a radar display resulting from a primary radar return on a radar beacon reply.
*TAXI INTO POSITION AND HOLD—*Used by ATC to inform a pilot to taxi onto the departure runway in takeoff position and hold. It is not authorization for takeoff. It is used when takeoff clearance cannot immediately be issued because of traffic or other reasons. (See Hold, Cleared for Take-off)
TAXI PATTERNS—Patterns established to illustrate the desired flow of ground traffic for the different runways or airport areas available for use.
TERMINAL AREA—A general term used to describe airspace in which approach control service or airport traffic control service is provided.
TERMINAL AREA FACILITY—A facility providing air traffic control service for arriving and departing IFR, VFR, Special VFR, Special IFR aircraft and on occasion, en route aircrat. (See Approach Control, Tower)
TERMINAL CONTROL AREA—(See Controlled Airspace)
TERMINAL RADAR APPROACH CONTROL/TRACON—An FAA air traffic control facility using radar and air/ground communications to provide approach control services to aircraft arriving, departing or transiting the airspace controlled by the facility. Service may be provided to both civil and military airports. A TRACON is similar to a RAPCON (USAF), RATCF (Navy) and ARAC (Army). (See Approach Control Service, Departure Control)
TERMINAL RADAR PROGRAM—A national program instituted to extend the terminal radar services provided IFR aircraft to VFR aircraft. Pilot participation in the program is urged but is not mandatory. The progressive states of the program are referred to as Stage I, Stage II and Stage III. The stage service provided at a particular location is contained in Airport/Facility Directory.

1. Stage I/Radar Advisory Service for VFR Aircraft —Provides traffic information and limited vectoring to VFR aircraft on a workload permitting basis.
2. Stage II/Radar Advisory and Sequencing for VFR Aircraft—Provides, in addition Stage I service, vectoring and sequencing on a full-time basis to arriving VFR aircraft. The purpose is to adjust the flow of arriving IFR and VFR aircraft into the traffic pattern in a safe and orderly manner and to provide traffic advisory to departing VFR aircraft.
3. Stage III/Radar Sequencing and Separation Service for VFR Aircraft—Provides, in addition to Stage II services, separation between all

participating aircraft. The purpose is to provide separation between all participating VFR aircraft and all IFR aircraft operating within the airspace defined as Terminal Radar Service Area (TRSA), or Terminal Control Area (TCA). (See Terminal Radar Service Area, Controlled Airspace) (Refer to AIM, Airport/Facility Directory and Graphic Notices and Supplemental Data)

TERMINAL RADAR SERVICE AREA/TRSA—Airspace surrounding designated airports wherein ATC provides radar vectoring, sequencing and separation on a full-time basis for all IFR and participating VFR aircraft. Service provided in a TRSA is called Stage III Service. AIM contains an explanation of TRSA. Graphics depicting TRSA layouts and communications frequencies are shown in Graphic Notices and Supplemental Data. Pilot participation is urged but is not mandatory. (See Terminal Radar Program) (Refer to AIM, Airport/Facility Directory and Graphic Notices and Supplemental Data)

TERRAIN FOLLOWING (TF)—The flight of a military aircraft maintaining a constant AGL altitude above the terrain or the highest obstruction. The altitude of the aircraft will constantly change with the varying terrain and/or obstruction.

TETRAHEDRON—A device normally located on uncontrolled airports and used as a landing direction indicator. The small end of a tetrahedron points in the direction of landing. At controlled airports, the tetrahedron, if installed, should be disregarded because tower instructions supersede the indicator. (See Segmented Circle) (Refer to AIM)

THAT IS CORRECT—The understanding you have is right.

THRESHOLD—The beginning of that portion of the runway usable for landing. (See Airport Lighting, Displayed Threshold)

THRESHOLD CROSSING HEIGHT/TCH—The height of the glide slope above the runway threshold. (See Threshold, Glide Slope)

THRESHOLD LIGHTS—(See Airport Lighting)

TIME GROUP—Four digits representing the hour and minutes from the 24-hour clock. Time group without time zone indicators are understood to be GMT (Greenwich Mean Time); e.g., "0205." A time zone designator is used to indicate local time, e.g., "0205M." The end and beginning of the day are shown by "2400" and "0000," respectively.

TORCHING—The burning of fuel at the end of an exhaust pipe or stack of a reciprocating aircraft engine, the result of an excessive richness in the fuel air mixture.

TOUCH AND GO/TOUCH AND GO LANDING—An operation by an aircraft that lands and departs on a runway without stopping or exiting the runway.

TOUCHDOWN—

1. The point at which an aircraft first makes contact with the landing surface.

2. Concerning a precision radar approach (PAR), it is the point where the glide path intercepts the landing surface.

ICAO—TOUCHDOWN—The point where the nominal glide path intercepts the runway.

TOUCHDOWN RVR—(See Visibility)

TOUCHDOWN ZONE—The first 3,000 feet of the runway beginning at the threshold. The area is used for determination of Touch-down Zone Elevation in the development of straight-in landing minimums for instrument approaches.

TOUCHDOWN ZONE ELEVATION/TDZE—The highest elevation in the first 3,000 feet of the landing surface. TDZE is indicated on the instrument approach procedure chart when straight-in landing minimums are authorized. (See Touchdown Zone)

TOUCHDOWN ZONE LIGHTING—(See Airport Lighting)

TOWER/AIRPORT TRAFFIC CONTROL TOWER—A terminal facility that uses air/ground communications, visual signaling, and other devices, to provide ATC services to airborne aircraft operating in the vicinity of an airport or on the movement area. Authorizes aircraft to land or takeoff at the airport controlled by the tower or to transit the airport traffic area regardless of flight plan or weather conditions (IFR or VFR). A tower may also provide approach control services (radar or nonradar). (See Airport Traffic Area, Airport Traffic Control Service, Approach Control/Approach Control Facility, Approach Control Service, Movement Area, Tower En Route Control Service/Tower to Tower) (Refer to AIM)

ICAO—AERODROME CONTROL TOWER—A unit established to provide air traffic control service to aerodrome traffic.

TOWER EN ROUTE CONTROL SERVICE/TOWER TO TOWER—The control of IFR en route traffic within delegated airspace between two or more adjacent approach control facilities. This service is designed to expedite traffic and reduce control and pilot communication requirements.

TPX 42—A numeric beacon decoder equipment/system. It is designed to be added to terminal radar systems for beacon decoding. It provides rapid target identification, reinforcement of the primary radar target and altitude information from Mode C. (See Automatic Radar Terminal Systems, Transponder)

TRACK—The actual flight path of an aircraft over the surface of the earth. (See Course, Route, Flight Path)

ICAO—TRACK—The projection on the earth's surface of the path of an aircraft, the direction of which path at any point is usually expressed in degrees from north (true, magnetic or grid).

TRAFFIC ALERT, ADVISE YOU TURN RIGHT/LEFT HEADING (DEGREES) AND/OR CLIMB/DESCEND TO (ALTITUDE) IMMEDIATELY—(See Safety Advisory)

TRAFFIC ADVISORIES—Advisories issued to alert a pilot to other known or observed IFR/VFR air traffic which may be in such proximity to his aircraft's position or intended route of flight to warrant his attention. Such advisories may be based on:

1. Visual observation from a control tower,

2. Observation of radar identified and nonidentified aircraft targets on an ARTCC/Approach Control radar scope, or,

3. Verbal reports from pilots or other facilities.

Controllers use the word "traffic" followed by additional information, if known, to provide such advisories, e.g., "Traffic, 2 o'clock, one zero miles, southbound, fast moving, altitude readout seven thousand five hundred."

Traffic advisory service will be provided to the extent possible depending on higher priority duties of the controller or other limitations, e.g., radar limitations, volume of traffic, frequency congestion or controller workload. Radar/nonradar traffic advisories do not relieve the pilot of his responsibility for continual vigilance to see and avoid other aircraft. IFR and VFR aircraft are cautioned th at there are many times when he controller is not able to give traffic advisories concerning all traffic in the aircraft's proximity; in other words, when a pilot requests or is receiving traffic advisories, he should not assume that all traffic will be issued.

TRAFFIC INFORMATION—(See Traffic Advisories)

TRAFFIC IN SIGHT—Used by pilots to inform a controller that previously issued traffic is in sight. (See Negative Contact, Traffic Advisories)

TRAFFIC NO LONGER A FACTOR—Indicates that the traffic described in a previously issued traffic advisory is no longer a factor.

TRAFFIC PATTERN—The traffic flow that is prescribed for aircraft landing at, taxiing on, or taking off from an airport. The components of a typical traffic pattern are upwind leg, crosswind leg, downwind leg, base leg and final approach.

1. Upwind Leg—A flight path parallel to the landing runway in the direction of landing.

2. Crosswind Leg—A flight path at right angles to the landing runway off its takeoff end.

3. Downwind Leg—A flight path parallel to the landing runway in the direction opposite to landing. The downwind leg normally extends between the crosswind leg and the base leg.

4. Base Leg—A flight path at right angles to the landing runway off its approach end. The base leg normally extends from the downwind leg to the intersection of the extended runway centerline.

5. Final Approach—A flight path in the direction of landing along the extended runway centerline. The final approach normally extends from the base leg to the runway. An aircraft making a straight-in approach VFR is also considered to be on final approach.

(See Taxi Patterns. Straight-In Approach-VFR) (Refer to AIM, FAR Part 91)

ICAO—AERODROME TRAFFIC CIRCUIT—The specified path to be flow by aircraft operating in the vicinity of an aerodrome.

TRANSCRIBED WEATHER BROADCAST/TWEB—A continuous recording of meteorological and aeronautical information that is broadcast on L/MF and VOR facilities for pilots. (Refer to AIM)

TRANSFER OF CONTROL—That action whereby the responsibility for the separation of an aircraft is transferred from one controller to another. *ICAO—TRANSFER OF CONTROL*—Transfer of responsibility for providing air traffic control service.

TRANSFERRING CONTROLLER/FACILITY—A controller/facility transferring control of an aircraft to another controller/facility. *ICAO—TRANSFERRING UNIT/CONTROLLER*—Air Traffic Control Unit/Air Traffic Controller in the process of transferring the responsibility for providing air traffic control service to an aircraft to the next air traffic control unit/air traffic controller along the route of flight.

TRANSITION—

1. The general term that describes the change from one phase of flight or flight condition to another, e.g., transition from en route flight to the approach or transition from instrument flight to visual flight.

2. A published route (SID Transition) used to connect the basic SID to one of several en route airways/jet routes, or, a published procedure (STAR Transition) used to connect one of several en route airways/jet routes to the basic STAR. (Refer to SID/STAR Charts)

TRANSITION AREA—(See Controlled Airspace)

TRANSMISSOMETER—An apparatus used to determine visibility by measuring the transmission of light through the atmosphere. It is the measurement source for determining runway visual range (RVR) and runway visibility value (RVV). (See Visibility)

TRANSMITTING IN THE BLIND/BLIND TRANSMISSION—A transmission from one station to other stations in circumstances where two-way communication cannot be established, but where it is believed that the called stations may be able to receive the transmission.

TRANSPONDER—The airborne radar beacon receiver/transmitter portion of the Air Traffic Control Radar Beacon System (ATCRBS) which automatically receives radio signals from interrogators on the ground, and selectively replies with a specific reply pulse or pulse group only to those interrogations being received on the mode to which it is set to respond. (See Interrogator) (Refer to AIM)

ICAO—TRANSPONDER—A receiver/transmitter which will generate a reply signal upon proper interrogation; the interrogation and reply being on different frequencies.

TURBOJET AIRCRAFT—An aircraft having a jet engine in which the energy of the jet operates a turbine which in turn operates the air compressor.

TURBOPROP AIRCRAFT—An aircraft having a jet engine in which the energy of the jet operates a turbine which drives the propeller.

T-VOR/TERMINAL-VERY HIGH FREQUENCY OMNIDIRECTIONAL RANGE STATION—A very high frequency terminal omnirange station located on or near an airport and used as an approach aid. (See VOR, Navigational Aid)

TWO WAY RADIO COMMUNICATIONS FAILURE—(See Lost Communications)

ULTRAHIGH FREQUENCY/UHF—The frequency band between 300 and 3,000 MHz. The bank of radio frequencies used for military air/ground voice communications. In some instances this may go as low as 225 MHz and still be referred to as UHF.

UNABLE—Indicates inability to comply with a specific instruction, request, or clearance.

UNCONTROLLED AIRSPACE—That portion of the airspace that has not been designated as continental control area, control area, control zone, terminal control area, or transition area within which ATC has neither the authority nor the responsibility for exercising control over air traffic. (See Controlled Airspace)

UNDER THE HOOD—Indicates that the pilot is using a hood to restrict visibility outside the cockpit while simulating instrument flight. An appropriately rated pilot is required in the other control seat while this operation is being conducted. (Refer to FAR Part 91)

UNICOM—A non-government air-ground radio communication facility which may provide airport advisory service at certain airports. Locations and frequencies of UNICOMs are shown on aeronautical charts and publications. (Refer to AIM and Airport/Facility Directory)

UNPUBLISHED ROUTE—A route for which no minimum altitude is published or charted for pilot use. It may include a direct route between NAVAIDS, a radial, a radar vector, or a final approach course beyond the segments of an instrument approach procedure. (See Route, Published Route)

UPWIND LEG—(See Traffic Pattern)

VECTOR—A heading issued to an aircraft to provide navigational guidance by radar.

ICAO—RADAR VECTORING—Provision of navigational guidance to aircraft in the form of specific headings, based on the use of radar.

VERIFY—Request confirmation of information; e.g., "verify assigned altitude."

VERIFY SPECIFIC DIRECTION OF TAKEOFF (OR TURNS AFTER TAKEOFF)—Used by ATC to ascertain an aircraft's direction to takeoff and/or direction of turn after takeoff. It is normally used for IFR departures from an airport not having a control tower. When direct communication with the pilot is not possible, the request and information may be relayed through an FSS, dispatcher, or by other means. (See IFR Takeoff Minimums and Departure Procedures)

VERTICAL SEPARATION—Separation established by assignment of different altitudes or flight levels. (See Separation)

ICAO—VERTICAL SEPARATION—Separation between aircraft expressed in units of vertical distance.

VERTICAL TAKEOFF AND LANDING AIRCRAFT/VTOL AIRCRAFT—Aircraft capable of vertical climbs and/or descents and of using very short runways or small areas for takeoff and landings. These aircraft include, but are not limited to, helicopters. (See Short Takeoff and Landing Aircraft)

VERY HIGH FREQUENCY/VHR—The frequency band between 30 and 300 MHz. Portions of this band, 108 to 118 MHz, are used for certain NAVAIDS; 118 to 136 MHz are used for civil air/ground voice communications. Other frequencies in this band are used for purposes not related to air traffic control.

VERY LOW FREQUENCY/VLF—The frequency band between 3 and 30 kHz.

VFR AIRCRAFT/VFR FLIGHT—An aircraft conducting flight in accordance with visual flight rules. (See Visual Flight Rules)

VFR MILITARY TRAINING ROUTES (VR)—Routes used by the Department of Defense and associated Reserve and Air Guard units for the purpose of conducting low-altitude navigation and tactical training under VFR rules below 10,000 feet MSL at airspeeds in excess of 250 kts IAS.

VFR NOT RECOMMENDED—An advisory provided by a Flight Service Station to a pilot during a preflight or inflight weather briefing that flight under visual flight rules is not recommended. To be given when the current and/or forecasted weather conditions are at or below VFR minimums. It does not abrogate the pilot's authority to make his own decision.

VFR ON TOP/VFR CONDITIONS ON TOP—An IFR clearance term used in lieu of a specific altitude assignment upon pilot's request which authorizes the aircraft to be flown in VFR weather conditions at an appropriate VFR altitude/flight level which is not below the minimum IFR altitude. (Refer to FAR Part 91)

VFR OVER THE TOP—The operation of an aircraft over-the-top under VFR when it is not being operated on an IFR flight plan. (See VFR On Top)

VFR TOWER/NON-APPROACH CONTROL TOWER—(See Tower/Airport Traffic Control Tower)

VIDEO MAP—An electronically displayed map on the radar display that may depict data such as: airports, heliports, runway centerline extensions, hospital emergency landing areas, NAVAIDS and fixes, reporting points, airway/route centerlines, boundaries, handoff points, special use tracks, obstructions, prominent geographic features, map alignment indicators, range accuracy marks, minimum vectoring altitudes.

VISIBILITY—The ability, as determined by atmospheric conditions and expressed in units of distance, to see and identify prominent unlighted objects by day and prominent lighted objects by night. Visibility is reported as statute miles, hundreds of feet or meters. (Refer to FAR Part 91, AIM)

1. Flight Visibility—The average forward horizontal distance, from the cockpit of an aircraft in flight, at which prominent unlighted objects may be seen and identified by day and prominent lighted objects may be seen and identified by night.

ICAO—Flight Visibility—The visibility forward from the cockpit of an aircraft in flight.

2. Ground Visibility—Prevailing horizontal visibility near the earth's surface as reported by the United States National Weather Service or an accredited observer.

ICAO—Ground Visibility—The visibility at an aerodrome, as reported by an accredited observer.

3. Prevailing Visibility—The greatest horizontal visibility equaled or exceeded throughout at least half the horizon circle which need not necessarily be continuous.

4. Runway Visibility Value/RVV—The visibility determined for a particular runway by a transmissometer. A meter provides a continuous indication of the visibility (reported in miles or fractions of miles) for the runway. RVV is used in lieu of prevailing visibility in determining minimums for a particular runway.

5. Runway Visual Range/RVR—An instrumentally derived value, based on standard calibrations, that represents the horizontal distance a pilot will see down the runway from the approach end; it is based on the sighting of either high intensity runway lights or on the visual contrast of other targets whichever yields the greater visual range. RVR, in contrast to prevailing or runway visibility, is based on what a pilot in a moving aircraft should see looking down the runway. RVR is horizontal visual range, not slant visual range. It is based on the measurement of a transmissometer made near the touchdown point of the instrument runway and is reported in hundreds of feet. RVR is used in lieu of RVV and/or prevailing visibility in determining minimums for a particular runway.

   a. Touchdown RVR—The RVR visibility readout values obtained from RVR equipment serving the runway touchdown zone.

   b. MID RVR—The RVR readout values obtained from RVR equipment located midfield of the runway.

   c. Rollout RVR—The RVR readout values obtained from RVR equipment located nearest the rollout end of the runway.

ICAO—Runway Visual Range—The maximum distance in the direction of takeoff or landing at which the runway or the specified lights or markers delineating it can be seen from a position above a specified point on its centerline at a height corresponding to the average eye-level of pilots at touchdown.

VISUAL APPROACH—An approach wherein an aircraft on an IFR flight plan, operating in VFR conditions under the control of an air traffic control facility and having an air traffic control authorization, may proceed to the airport of destination in VFR conditions.
ICAO—VISUAL APPROACH—An approach by an IFR flight when either

part or all of an instrument approach procedure is not completed and the approach is executed in visual reference to terrain.

VISUAL APPROACH SLOPE INDICATOR—(See Airport Lighting)

VISUAL DESCENT POINT—A defined point on the final approach course of a nonprecision straight-in approach procedure from which normal descent from the MDA to the runway touchdown point may be commenced, provided visual reference is established.

VISUAL FLIGHT RULES/VFR—Rules that govern the procedures for conducting flight under visual conditions. The term "VFR" is also used in the United States to indicate weather conditions that are equal to or greater than minimum VFR requirements. In addition, it is used by pilots and controllers to indicate type of flight plan. (See Instrument Flight Rules, Instrument Meteorological Conditions) (Refer to FAR Part 91; AIM)

VISUAL HOLDING—The holding of aircraft at selected, prominent, geographical fixes which can be easily recognized from the air. (See Hold, Holding Fixes)

VISUAL METEOROLOGICAL CONDITIONS/VMC—Meteorological conditions expressed in terms of visibility, distance from cloud, and ceiling equal to or better than specified minima. (See Instrument Meteorological Conditions, Visual Flight Rules, Instrument Flight Rules)

VISUAL SEPARATION—A means employed by ATC to separate IFR aircraft in terminal areas. There are two ways to effect this separation:

1. The tower controller sees the aircraft involved and issues instructions, as necessary, to ensure that the aircraft avoid each other.

2. A pilot sees the other aircraft involved and upon instructions from the controller provides his own separation by maneuvering his aircraft as necessary to avoid it. This may involve following another aircraft or keeping it in sight until it is no longer a factor. (See, See and Avoid) (Refer to FAR Part 91)

VORTAC/VHR OMNIDIRECTIONAL RANGE/TACTICAL AIR NAVIGATION—A navigation aid providing VOR azimuth, TACAN azimuth, and TACAN distance measuring equipment (DME) at one site. (See VOR, Distance Measuring Equipment, TACAN, Navigational Aid) (Refer to AIM)

VORTICES/WING TIP VORTICES—Circular patterns of air created by the movement of an airfoil through the air when generating lift. As an airfoil moves through the atmosphere in sustained flight, an area of high pressure is created beneath it and an area of low pressure is created above it. The air flowing from the high pressure area to the low pressure area around and about the tips of the airfoil tends to roll up into two rapidly rotating vortices, cylindrical in shape. These vortices are the most predominant parts of aircraft wake turbulence and their rotational force is dependent upon the wing loading, gross weight, and speed of the generating aircraft. The vortices from medium to heavy aircraft can be of extremely high velocity and hazardous to smaller aircraft. (See Wake Turbulence, Aircraft Classes) (Refer to AIM)

VOR/VERY HIGH FREQUENCY OMNIDIRECTIONAL RANGE STATION—A ground-based electronic navigation aid transmitting very high frequency navigation signals, 360 degrees in azimuth, oriented from magnetic north. Used as the basis for navigation in the national airspace system. The VOR periodically identifies itself by morse code and may have an additional voice identification feature. Voice features may be used by ATC or FSS for transmitting instructions/information to pilots. (See Navigational Aid) (Refer to AIM)

VOT/VOR TEST SIGNAL—A ground facility which emits a test signal to check VOR receiver accuracy. The system is limited to ground use only. (Refer to FAR Part 91, AIM and Airport/Facility Directory)

WAKE TURBULENCE—Phenomena resulting from the passage of an aircraft through the atmosphere. The term includes vortices, thrust stream turbulence, jet blast, jet wash, propeller wash and rotor wash, both on the ground and in the air. (See Jet Blast, Aircraft Classes) (Refer to AIM Part 1)

WARNING AREA—(See Special Use Airspace)

WAYPOINT—(See Area Navigation)

WEATHER ADVISORY/INFLIGHT WEATHER ADVISORY—(See SIGMET, AIRMET)

WEATHER ADVISORY/WS/WA—In aviation weather forecast practice, an expression of hazardous weather conditions not predicted in the area forecast, as they affect the operation of air traffic and as prepared by the NWS.

WILCO—I have received your message, understand it, and will comply with it.

WIND SHEAR—A change in wind speed and/or wind direction in a short distance, resulting in a tearing or shearing effect. It can exist in a horizontal or vertical direction and occasionally in both.

WORDS TWICE—

1. As a request: "Communication is difficult. Please say every phrase twice."

2. As information: "Since communications are difficult, every phrase in this message will be spoken twice."

Abbreviations

Additional weather contractions can be found in Section 2, Weather.

ASS—Airport Advisory Service	**ACFT**—Aircraft
	ACRBT—Acrobatic
ABM—Abeam	**AD**—Airworthiness Directive
APP CON—Approach Control	

ADCUS—Advise Customs
ADF—Automatic Direction Finder
ADIZ—Air Defense Identification Zone
A&E—Airframe and Engine Mechanic
AGL—Above Ground Level
AILS—Automatic Instrument Landing System
AIM—Airman's Information Manual
AIRAD—Airmen Advisory (local only)
ALS—Approach Light System
ALSTG—Altimeter Setting
ALT—Altitude
ALTN—Alternate
AOA—At or Above
AOB—At or Below
A&P—Airframe and Powerplant Mechanic
APC—Area Positive Control
APCH—Approach
ARPT—Airport
ARSR—Air Route Surveillance Radar
ARTCC—Air Route Traffic Control Center
ASR—Airport Surveillance Radar
ATC—Air Traffic Control
ATCRBS—Air Traffic Control Radar Beacon System
ATD—Actual Time of Departure

ATIS—Automatic Terminal Information Service
AWY—Airway

BC—Back Course
BCN—Beacon
BCST—Broadcast
BFDK—Before Dark
BLN—Balloon

CAF—Cleared as Filed
CAS—Calibrated Air Speed
CAT—Clear Air Turbulence
CIRNAV—Circumnavigate
CLNC—Clearance
CPF—Complete Power Failure
CR—ATC Requests
CTC—Contact
CTLZ—Control Zone

DF—Direction Finder
DH—Decision Height
DME—Distance Measuring Equipment
DOT—Department of Transportation
DVFR—Defense Visual Flight Rules

EAC—Expected Approach Clearance Time
EFAS—Enroute Flight Advisory Service
EFC—Expect Further Clearance
ELEV—Elevation
ELT—Emergency Locator Transmitter

ETA—Estimated Time of Arrival

ETD—Estimated Time of Departure

ETE—Estimated Time Enroute

FAA—Federal Aviation Administration

FAF—Final Approach Fix

FAR—Federal Aviation Regulation

FBO—Fixed Base Operator

FIR—Flight Information Region

FL—Flight Level

FM—Fan Marker

FSS—Flight Service Station

GADO—General Aviation District Office

GMT—Greenwich Mean Time

GS—Glideslope, or Groundspeed

GWT—Gross Weight

HAA—Height Above Airport

HAT—Height Above Touchdown

HF—High Frequency

HIRL—High Intensity Runway Lighting

HZ—Hertz (cycles per second)

IAF—Initial Approach Fix

IAP—Initial Approach Procedure

IAS—Indicated Air Speed

ICAO—International Civil Aviation Organization

IDENT—Identification

IF—Intermediate Fix

IFR—Instrument Flight Rules

ILS—Instrument Landing System

INT—Intersection

INTCP—Intercept

INTST—Intensity

ISMLS—Interim Standard Microwave Landing System

J-BAR—Jet runway barrier

KHZ—KiloHertz

KT—Knots

LAT—Latitude

LCL—Local

LDA—Localizer Type Directional Aid

LF—Low Frequency

LIRL—Low Intensity Runway Lights

LMM—Locator, Middle Marker

LOC—Localizer

LOM—Locator, Outer Marker

LRCO—Limited Remote Communications Outlet

MAA—Minimum Authorized Altitude

MAG—Magnetic

MALS—Medium Intensity Approach Light System

MAP—Missed Approach Point

MCA—Minimum Crossing Altitude

MDA—Minimum Descent Altitude

MEA—Minimum Enroute Altitude, IFR

MF—Medium Frequency

MHZ—MegaHertz

MIRL—Medium Intensity Runway Edge Lights

MLS—Microwave Landing System

MM—Middle Marker, ILS

MOA—Military Operations Area

MOCA—Minimum Obstruction Clearance Altitude

MPH—Miles Per Hour

MRA—Minimum Reception Altitude

MSA—Minimum Safe Altitude

MSL—Mean Sea Level

NA—Not Authorized

NAVAID—Navigational Aid

NDB—Nondirectional Radio Beacon

NM—Nautical Miles

NOPT—No Procedure Turn Required

NTE—Not To Exceed

NOTAM—Notice To Airmen

NTSB—National Transportation Safety Board

NWS—National Weather Service

OBS—Omnibearing Selector

OCL—Obstruction Clearance Limit

OM—Outer Marker, ILS

OTS—Out of Service

PAR—Precision Approach Radar

PATWAS—Pilot's Automatic Telephone Weather Answering Service

PCPN—Precipitation

PPO—Prior Permission Only

PPR—Prior Permission Required

PWI—Proximity Warning Indicator

QDM—Bearing to Facility

QDR—Bearing from Facility

QFE—Altitude above ground based on station pressure

QNE—Altimeter setting 29.92 inches Hg.

QNH—Altitude above sea level based on station pressure

QSY—Change radio frequency now to—

QUAD—Quadrant

RADAR—Radio Detection and Ranging

RAPCON—Radar approach control (USAF)

RBN—Radio Beacon

RCLS—Runway Centerline Lights System

RCO—Remote Communications Outlet

RCV—Receive
REIL—Runway End Identifier Lights
RNAV—Area Navigation
RRP—Runway Reference Point
RSTR—Restricted
RTS—Returned to Service
RVO—Runway Visibility by Observer
RVR—Runway Visual Range
RVV—Runway Visibility Values
RWY—Runway

SALS—Short Approach Lighting System
SAR—Search and Rescue
SDF—Simplified Directional Facility
SFL—Sequence Flashing Lights
SI—Straight-in Approach
SID—Standard Instrument Departure
SIGMET—Significant Meteorological Information
SM—Statute Miles
SR—Sunrise
SS—Sunset
STAR—Standard Terminal Arrival Route
STC—Supplemental Type Certificate
STOL—Short Take-off & Landing

TABS—Telephone Automated Briefing Service
TAC—Terminal Area Chart
TACAN—UHF Tactical Air Navigation Aid
TAS—True Airspeed
TCA—Terminal Control Area
TCH—Threshold Crossing Height
TDZL—Touchdown Zone Lights
TFC—Traffic
TERPS—Terminal Instrument Procedures
TKOF—Take-off
TPA—Traffic Pattern Altitude
TRACON—Terminal Radar Approach Control
TRSA—Terminal Radar Service Area
TSMTR—Transmitter
TSO—Technical Standard Order
TVOR—Terminal VOR
TWEB—Transcribed Weather Broadcast
TWR—Tower
TWY—Taxiway

UFA—Until Further Advised
UFN—Until Further Notice
UHF—Ultra-High Frequency
UNICOM—Aeronatutical Advisory Service

VASI—Visual Approach Slope Indicator

VFR—Visual Flight Rules

VHF—Very High Frequency

VIS—Visibility

VOR—VHF Omni-Directional Radio Range

VORTAC—Combined VOR and TACAN System

VOT—VOR Test Facility

WAC—World Aeronautical Chart

WILCO—Will Comply

WP—Way Point

WS—Weather Service

WT—Weight

WX—Weather

Z—Greenwich Mean Time

ZM—VHF Station Location (Z) Marker

SECTION 2
Weather

AVIATION WEATHER KEY

Location type and time of report	Sky and Ceiling	Visibility, Weather & Obstructions to Vision	Sea Level Pressure	Temp. & Dew Point	Wind	Altimeter Setting	Runway Visual Range	Coded Pireps

MKC SA 0758 15 SCT M25 OVC 4R-K 132/58/56 /1807 /993/RO4LVR20V40/UA
OVC 55

Decoded Report: Kansas City: Record observation taken at 0758 GMT, 1,500 feet scattered clouds, measured ceiling, 2,500 feet overcast, visibility 4 miles, light rain, smoke, sea level pressure 1013.2 millibars, temperature 58°F, dew point 56°F, wind 180°, 7 knots, altimeter setting 29.93 in. Hg. Runway 04 left, visual range 2,000 ft. variable to 4,000. Pilot reports top of overcast at 5,500 ft.

Location: Three letters always used as station-location identifier.

Type and Time of Report: SA indicates a scheduled record observation, SP an unscheduled special observation indicating a significant change in one or more elements, and RS a scheduled record observation that also qualifies as a special observation. All three types of observations (SA, SP, RS) are followed by the time of observation given in 24 hour Greenwich Mean Time.

Sky and Ceiling: Sky cover contractions are in ascending order. Figures preceding contractions are heights in hundreds of feet above the station. Sky cover contractions are:

CLR Clear: Less than ¹/₁₀ sky cover

SCT Scattered: ¹/₁₀ to less than ¹/₂ sky cover

BKN Broken: ³/₅ to ⁹/₁₀ sky cover

OVC Overcast: More than ⁹/₁₀ sky cover

— Thin (when prefixed to the preceding contractions)

—X Partial obscuration: ¹/₁₀ to less than ¹⁰/₁₀ sky hidden by precipitation or obstruction to vision (bases at surface)

X Obscuration: Sky hidden completely (¹⁰/₁₀) by precipitation or obstruction to vision (bases at surface)

135

Letter preceding height of layer identifies ceiling layer and indicates how ceiling height was obtained. Thus:

E   Estimated heights
M   Measured
W   Indefinite

V Immediately following numerical value, indicates a varying ceiling

Visibility: Reported in statute miles and fractions (V = Variable). The symbol + indicates visibility greater than that being reported.

Weather and Obstructions-to-Vision Symbols:

A	Hail	**IC**	Ice crystals	**S**	Snow
BD	Blowing dust	**IF**	Ice fog	**SG**	Snow grains
BN	Blowing sand	**IP**	Ice pellets	**SP**	Snow pellets
BS	Blowing snow	**IPW**	Ice pellet showers	**SW**	Snow showers
D	Dust	**K**	Smoke	**T**	Thunderstorm
F	Fog	**L**	Drizzle	**T+**	Severe
GF	Ground fog	**R**	Rain		thunderstorm
H	Haze	**RW**	Rain showers	**ZL**	Freezing drizzle
				ZR	Freezing rain

Precipitation intensities are indicated thus:
  − light; (no sign) moderate; + heavy
The intensity indicator *follows* the precipitation symbol.

Sea Level Pressure

Station pressure in millibars, corrected to sea level. Used primarily by meteorologists, it is not normally reported to pilots. For brevity, only the final three digits of the actual pressure are reported. (See conversion table, Millibars—Inches of Mercury, Section 1.)

Temperature and Dew Point

Reported in degrees Fahrenheit. When the temperature and dew point spread is reduced to three degrees or less, the formation of fog is possible if other conditions are favorable.

Wind

Direction in tens of degrees from true north, speed in knots. 0000 indicates calm. G indicates gusty. Peak speed of gusts follows G or Q when squall is reported.

Examples: 3627—360 degrees, 27 knots.
3627G40—360 degrees, 27 knots; peak speed in gusts, 40 knots.

Altimeter Setting

The first figure of the actual altimeter setting is always omitted from the report. Reported in inches of mercury (in. Hg).

Runway Visual Range

RVR is reported from some stations. Extreme values for 10 minutes prior to observation are given in hundreds of feet. Runway identification precedes RVR report.

Coded Pireps

Pilot reports (Pireps) when available are appended to weather observations. "UA" precedes all Pireps.

Aviation Weather Forecasts

Terminal Forecasts: These forecasts contain information for specific airports on ceiling, cloud heights, cloud amounts, visibility, weather and obstructions to vision, surface wind, and a categorical forecast (whether VFR, MVFR, IFR, LIFR conditions are expected for the last six hours of each forecast). Terminal forecasts have a 24-hour valid period and are issued three times a day. Terminal forecasts use the following form:

CEILING: identified by the letter "C".

CLOUD HEIGHTS: in hundreds of feet above the station (ground).

CLOUD LAYERS: stated in ascending order of height.

VISIBILITY: in statute miles but omitted if over 6 miles.

WEATHER AND OBSTRUCTION TO VISION: standard weather and obstruction symbols are used.

SURFACE WIND: in tens of degrees and knots; omitted when less than 10.

Example of Terminal Forecasts:

DCA 222323—DCA forecasts, 22nd day of month, valid time 23Z to 23Z.

10SCT C18BKN 5SW 3415G25 OCNL C8X1SW: Scattered clouds at 1,000 ft., ceiling 1,800 ft. broken, visibility 5 miles, snow showers, surface wind 340° at 15 k. with gusts to 25 k., occasional ceiling 800 feet sky obscured, visibility 1 mile in snow showers.

12Z C50BKN 3312G22: At 12Z ceiling becoming 5,000 ft. broken clouds, surface wind 330° at 12 k. with gusts to 22 k.

17Z MVFR BCMG VFR AFT 21Z: Last six hours of forecast at 17Z marginal VFR conditions becoming VFR after 21Z.

Area Forecasts (FA): These are 18-hour forecasts plus a 12-hour categorical outlook prepared two times a day which give general details of cloud, weather and frontal conditions for an area the size of several states. Heights of cloud tops, icing and turbulence are above SEA LEVEL; ceiling heights are above GROUND LEVEL; bases of cloud layers are ASL UNLESS INDICATED. Sigmets or Airmets may amend an area forecast.

TWEB (Continuous Transcribed Weather Broadcast): Individual route forecasts covering a 25 nautical mile zone on either side of a flight route, may be obtained by requesting a specific route number. Detailed en route weather for a 12 or 18 hour period (depending on forecast issuance) plus a synopsis of the weather can be obtained.

Special Advisories:

Significant Meteorological Advisories (SIGMETs)

SIGMETs warn airmen in flight of weather potentially hazardous to all aircraft. SIGMETs will include reports of severe turbulence, severe icing, and widespread duststorms or sandstorms which lower visibilities below 3 miles. *Convective SIGMETs* will include reports associated with thunderstorms, i.e., tornadoes, hail (3/4 inch or greater), lines of thunderstorms, embedded thunderstorms, and thunderstorms in areas covering 40% or more and with radar determined intensities of level 4 or greater.

Advisories for Light Aircraft (AIRMETS)

AIRMETs concern less severe weather conditions which may be hazardous to some smaller aircraft or to relatively inexperienced pilots. They will include reports of moderate icing, moderate turbulence, sustained wind of 30 knots or more at the surface, widespread areas of ceilings below 1000 feet and/or visibility below 3 miles (1FR), and extensive mountain obscurement.

AIRMETs also serve as amendments to the Area Forecast. This means that if AIRMET Weather conditions are forecast in the Area Forecast then an AIRMET will not be issued. If a weather condition develops that had not been forecast in the Area Forecast then an AIRMET will be issued. The consequences of this is that pilots *should consult* the Area Forecast when they are briefing themselves or *should ask* the briefer for any flight precautions affecting the pilots route of flight. Both types of SIGMETs and AIRMETs may be broadcast by FAA on Navaid voice channels.

Winds (and Temperatures) Aloft Forecasts

Winds (and temperatures) aloft forecasts are 12-hour forecasts of direction (nearest 10° true N) and speed (knots) for selected flight levels. Temperatures aloft (+ or −) are given in degrees centigrade.

Example of a winds aloft forecast:

FD	/6000	/9000	/12000
DCA	2833+00	2930-03	3030-06

(At Washington National Airport the wind at 6,000 ft. is from 280° at 33 knots. The 9,000-ft. wind is from 290° at 30 knots with a −3°C temperature, etc.)

When wind velocities greater than 100 knots are forecast, they are coded by adding 50 to the first two digits (direction indicators) of the report; thus,

7608 means a wind from 260° at 108 knots (26+50=76). Light and variable winds are shown by using 9900 instead of direction and velocity.

Weather Contractions

(Also see weather-report symbols in this section)

ABNML—abnormal
ABV—above
ADVN—advance
ADVSY—advisory
AFCT—affect
AFTN—afternoon
AGL—above ground level
AHD—ahead
ALQDS—all quadrants
ALT—altitude
ALTN—alternate
AMD—amend
APH—approach
ARPT—airport
AWX—account weather

B—beginning of precipitation (followed by time in min. past the hour on wx rprt only)
BHND—behind
BINOVC—breaks in overcast
BLD—build
BLZD—blizzard
BDRY—boundary
BNTH—beneath
BOVC—base of overcast
BRAF—braking action fair
BRAG—braking action good
BRAP—braking action poor
BRAXP—braking action extremely poor
BKN—broken

C—Centigrade
CAT—clear air turbulence
CAUFN—caution advised until further notice
CAVOK (cav-oh-kay)—no clouds below 5,000 ft., visibility 6 miles or more, and no precipitation or thunderstorm

CAVU—clear or scattered clouds, visibility greater than 10 miles
CB—cumulonimbus
CIG—ceiling
CLD—cloud
CLR—clear
CTN—caution
CU—cumulus
CVR—cover

DALGT—daylight
DLA—delay
DNS—dense
DRFT—drift
DRZL—drizzle
DSIPT—dissipate
DTRT—deteriorate
DURG—during
DLVP—develop
DWPNT—dew point

E—ending of precipitation (followed by time in minutes past the hour on wx rprts only)
E—estimated (wx rprt only)
EXC—except
EXPC—expect
EXTRM—extreme
EXTN—extension
EXTV—extensive

F—Fahrenheit
FCST—forecast
FLG—falling
FLW or FOL—follow
FREQ—frequent/frequency
FRMN—formation
FROPA—frontal passage
FRST—frost
FRZ—freeze

G—gust (wx rprt only)
GNDFG—ground fog
GRAD—gradient
GRDL—gradual

HAZ—hazard
HDFRZ—hard freeze
HDWND—head wind
HGT—height
HIALS—high-intensity approach lighting system
HLSTO—hailstones
HRZN—horizon
HURCN—hurricane
HVY—heavy

ICG—icing
ICGIC—icing in clouds
ICGICIP—icing in clouds and in precipitation
ICGIP—icing in precipitation
IMT—immediate
INCL—include
INCR—increase
INDEF—indefinite
INFO—information
INST—instrument
INSTBY—instability
INTMT—intermittent
INTS—intense
INVOF—in the vicinity of
IOVC—in the overcast
IPV—improve
IR—icy runway
IVFRC—in VFR conditions

JTSTR—jet stream

KDEP—smoke layer estimated _____ft. deep
KOCTY—smoke over city
KT—knots

LCL—local
LKLY—likely
LTGCC—lightning, cloud to cloud

LTGCCCG—lightning, cloud to cloud, cloud to ground
LTGCG—lightning, cloud to ground
LTGCW—lightning, cloud to water
LTGIC—lightning in clouds
LTLCG—little change
LVL—level

M—measured ceiling
MB—millibars
MDFY—modify

M—missing (wx rprt only)
MAX—maximum
MDT—moderate
MFV—forward visibility more than _____ miles
MSL—mean sea level

NCWX—no change in weather
NGT—night
NMRS—numerous
NO or NR—number
NXT—next

OBSC—obscure
OCFNT—occluded front
OCLN—occlusion
OCNL—occasional
OCR—occur
OFSHR—off shore
ONSHR—on shore
OTLK—outlook
OVC—overcast

PBL—probable
PCPN—precipitation
PIREP—pilot report of meteorological conditions
PRES—pressure
PRESFR—pressure falling rapidly
PRESRR—pressure rising rapidly
PSBL—possible
POSN—position
PSR—packed snow on runwy
PT—point

PTCHY—patchy
PVL—prevail

Q—squall (wx rpt only)
QUAD—quadrant

R—runway (wx rpt only)
RAFL—rainfall
RAREP—radar weather report
RESTR—restrict
RGD—ragged
RH—relative humidity
RPD—rapid
RPRT—report
RSG—rising
RTE—route
RTRN—return
RVR—runway visual range

SCTD—scattered
SFC—surface
SHFT—shift
SHWR—shower
SL—sea level
SLO—slow
SLR—slush on runway
SML—small
SMTH—smooth
SNW—snow
SNWFL—snowfall
SNFLK—snowflake
SQAL—squall
SQLN—squall line
SR—sunrise
SS—sunset
STDY—steady
STM—storm
SVR—severe
SVRL—several

TAS—true airspeed
TDA—today
TEMP—temperature
THDR—thunder
THK—thick

THSD—thousand
TLWD—tail wind
TMPRY—temporary
TMW—tomorrow
TNDCY—tendency
TNGT—tonight
TOVC—top of overcast
TRML—terminal
T—thunderstorm (wx rprt only)
TROF—trough
TROP—tropopause
TRRN—terrain
TSHWR—thundershower
TSQLS—thundersqualls
TSTM—thunderstorm
TURBC—turbulence
TURBT—turbulent
TWRG—towering

U—unlimited; unrestricted
U—intensity unknown (wx rprt only)
UNKN—unknown
UNL—unlimited
UNSTBL—unstable
UNSTDY—unsteady
UPR—upper
UWNDS—upper winds

V—variable (wx rprt only)
VSBY— visibility
VLNT—violent
VRBL—variable
VSBY—visibility

WA—Airmet
WDLY—widely
WND—wind
WR—wet runway
WRM—warm
WS—Sigmet
WSHFT—wind shift
WX—weather

YDA—yesterday

Weather Fronts and Clouds

As air masses of differing properties move across the earth's surface, they come in contact with each other, creating areas of instability where they touch. These areas of contact are called frontal zones, or fronts.

Frontal weather may range from a minor wind shift, with no clouds or other visible weather activity, to severe thunderstorms accompanied by low clouds, poor visibility, hail, severe turbulence and icing conditions. In addition, the weather associated with one section of the front is frequently quite different from that in other sections of the same front.

Warm Fronts—The uplifting of warm air sliding over cold air preceding it causes a warm front to move relatively slowly and form a gentle frontal slope. It may produce a cloud system extending up to 1,000 miles ahead of the surface position of the front. Clouds are mostly stratiform and may appear in the following sequence with the approach of the front—cirrus, cirrostratus, altostratus and nimbostratus. Near the surface position of the front the cloud bases may be very low. As the warm air gradually rises along the frontal slope, cloud heights may exceed 20,000 feet, and, in some conditions, thunderstorms may develop.

Cold Fronts—Cold fronts may move faster and have a steeper slope than warm fronts. The cold fronts that move very rapidly have very steep slopes and narrow bands of clouds that are mostly ahead of the fronts. The slower moving cold fronts have less steep slopes and cloud systems that may extend far to the rear of the surface position of the fronts. When the warm air ahead of a cold front is moist and unstable, cloud types are mostly cumuliform. A line of thunderstorms (squall line) frequently develops ahead of a fast-moving cold front. If the cold air mass behind the front is moist and unstable, cumulus clouds and showers may occur for some time after frontal passage. At the surface, cold-front passage is characterized by a temperature decrease, a wind shift, and on occasion by gusty winds. Although the weather associated with cold fronts is usually in a narrower band than that associated with warm fronts, it presents more serious flying hazards.

Stationary Fronts—On occasion, both warm and cold fronts gradually lose their momentum and for a period of time have no motion. During this period they are called stationary fronts. The slope, cloud sequence and weather associated with stationary fronts may be the same as those associated with warm fronts.

Occluded Fronts—Fronts frequently have bends or waves in them and move in such a fashion that the cold air is retreating ahead of a warm front in one section, and advancing behind a cold front in an adjacent section. When the cold-front section moves faster than the warm-front section, it eventually overtakes the warm front. The warm air mass between the fronts is lifted above the surface by the two colder air masses. The resulting front is called an occluded front, or an occlusion.

CLOUDS

Types	Approx. Height of Bases	Description	Associated Weather	
			Precipitation Types	General
Cumulus	1,500 ft. to 10,000 ft.	Detached domes or towers; flat bases; brilliant white in sun, dark blue or gray in shadows.	If building, showers (rain or snow)	Good surface visibility; fair weather if not building; if building, high winds, turbulence.
Altocumulus	6,500 ft. to 16,500 ft.	White or gray layers, rolls or patches of wavy solid clouds.	Intermittent rain or snow, usually light	Turbulence likely; generally good surface visibility.
Stratocumulus	Near the surface to 6,500 ft.	Gray or blue; individual rolls or globular masses.	Light showers (rain or snow)	Strong, gusty surface winds, particularly if ahead of a cold front; turbulence.
Cumulonimbus	1,500 ft. to 10,000 ft.	Large, heavy, towering clouds; black bases; cauliflower-like or anvil-shaped tops.	Heavy showers; possibility of hail	Associated with severe weather, turbulence, high surface winds; surface visibility usually fair-to-good outside precipitation.
Stratus	Near the surface to 3,000 ft.	Low, gray, uniform, sheet-like cloud.	Light drizzle, snow grains	Poor surface visibility; air smooth.

143

CLOUDS

Types	Approx. Height of Bases	Description	Associated Weather	
			Precipitation Types	General
Altostratus	6,500 ft. to 16,500 ft.	Gray or blue veil or layer of clouds; appears fibrous; sun may show as through frosted glass.	Light, continuous precipitation	Usually poor surface visibility; air smooth, moderate surface winds.
Nimbostratus	1,500 ft. to 10,000 ft.	Dark gray, thick, shapeless cloud layer (really a low altostratus with precipitation).	Continuous precipitation	Visibility restricted by precipitation; air smooth; calm-to-light surface winds.
Cirrus	16,500 ft. to 45,000 ft.	White, thin, feathery clouds in patches or bands.	None	If cirrus clouds are arranged in bands or associated with other clouds, usually a sign of approaching bad weather.
Cirrostratus	16,500 ft. to 45,000 ft.	White, thin cloud layers; looks like sheet or veil; halo around moon or sun.	None	Often a sign of approaching bad weather; surface winds bring overcast skies.
Cirrocumulus	16,500 ft. to 45,000 ft.	Thin clouds in sheets; individual elements look like tufts of cotton.	None	Cirrocumulus clouds indicate high-level instability.

Icing Conditions

The total effect of aircraft icing is a loss of efficiency, both from an aerodynamic and a power standpoint. This loss of efficiency results in a number of adverse conditions, such as decreased lift, increased drag, higher stalling speeds, loss of power, increased fuel consumption, lower flying speeds and decreased maneuverability.

It is difficult to establish exact temperature limits wherein icing may be encountered. The most severe structural icing occurs usually between 32°F (0°C) and 14°F (−10°C), but it is not uncommon to find structural icing at temperatures as cold as −13°F (−25°C). Fast-freezing rime ice, from supercooled water droplets, may accumulate at temperatures down to −40°F (−40°C).

Structural ice may accumulate at rates varying from less than one-half inch per hour to as high as one inch per minute, for brief periods of two or three minutes. *The most dangerous icing conditions are usually associated with freezing rain or freezing drizzle; these can build hazardous amounts of ice in a few minutes.*

Carburetor icing may occur in clear air at temperatures far above freezing, when the humidity is high. Accumulations may occur at temperatures as high as 100°F (38°C) with relative humidity as low as 50 percent. The possibility of carburetor icing is greatest with a combination of ambient temperature below 70°F (21°C) and relative humidity above 80 percent. At about 14°F (−10°C) and colder, moisture becomes ice crystals, which usually pass through the induction system harmlessly. Fuel vaporization and air expansion within the carburetor cause an extreme temperature drop that will turn any moisture to ice whenever that cooling effect reaches 32°F (0°C) or colder.

IN A TYPICAL COLD
FRONT CROSS-SECTION

IN A TYPICAL WARM
FRONT CROSS-SECTION

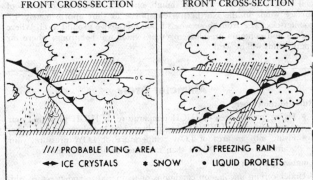

//// PROBABLE ICING AREA ⌒ FREEZING RAIN
◄► ICE CRYSTALS * SNOW • LIQUID DROPLETS

Source: USAF

The illustrations depicted on the preceding page are models, and one should keep in mind that actual situations may vary considerably from those shown here.

Weather Radar

With the use of radar, and through the combined efforts of the National Weather Service and FAA Flight Service Stations, a pilot can receive a comprehensive picture of the weather to assist him in planning a safe flight. In the conterminous United States 140 radar sites are used to collect data on precipitation areas, their intensity and movement. In Alaska, an additional 15 radar sites gather similar information. The data obtained is transmitted over weather teletype circuits for use in flight planning.

Weather radar repeaterscopes are available at selected Flight Service Stations. At these locations, FSS specialists are certified to interpret the weather pattern displayed on the radarscope as to area covered and movement. Additional technical analysis is made by the National Weather Service, which forwards this information to the FSS pilot briefer. Flight Service Stations equipped with weather radar receivers are identified in the Airport/Facility Directory published by the FAA.

Relation of Wind to Pressure

In the Northern Hemisphere winds blow clockwise around highs and counterclockwise around lows. When flying with a direct tailwind, high pressure will be to the right and low pressure to the left. The reverse is true in the Southern Hemisphere.

Isobars (lines of equal pressure on a surface chart) and contours (lines of equal altitude on a constant pressure chart) are drawn to picture pressure and height distribution. Winds above 2,000 ft. agl will generally blow in a direction parallel to these isobars and contours. Because of surface friction and coriolis force, as a rule of thumb, one may expect the direction of surface winds in the Northern Hemisphere to shift approximately 45° counter-clockwise from those winds 2,000 feet above ground level. Where isobars and contours are close together, winds will be strong; where far apart, winds will be weak.

Altimeter Errors

Rules to remember:

- Flying into an area of HIGH temperature or HIGH pressure, your aircraft will be HIGHER than indicated on the altimeter.
- Flying into an area of LOW temperature or LOW pressure, your aircraft will be LOWER than indicated on the altimeter.

Combined errors:

Under certain uncommon conditions of temperature and pressure, altimeter errors can be introduced which are greater than 1,000 feet. This may occur when a deep trough of low pressure aloft lies over a high pressure area at the surface. The compounded error occurs because the altimeter may be reset according to a reported high altimeter setting, as measured on the ground, while the aircraft is actually flying in an area of lower-than-standard pressure. The aircraft is already lower than indicated on the altimeter, and resetting for a higher pressure calls for further descent to get back "on altitude."

Constant Pressure Levels

Upper-air constant pressure charts are constructed with reference to the following constant pressure levels:

Pressure Level (millibars)	Approximate Altitude (ft. msl)	Meters
1,000	400	120
850	5,000	1,500
700	10,000	3,000
500	18,000	5,500
300	30,000	9,000
200	39,000	12,000
100	53,000	16,000

Lines used on Constant Pressure Charts depict:
Equal Altitude with solid lines (————————) called "Contour" lines
Equal Temperature with dashed lines (— — —) called "Isotherm" lines
Equal Wind Speed with dotted lines (• • • • • • • • • •) called "Isotach" lines
Jet Stream Flow with arrows (→ → → →) called "Jet Stream" lines

En Route Flight Advisory Service

Flight Watch, or more formally En Route Flight Advisory Service (EFAS), is designed to provide the pilot with timely weather information for his flight. The system is available throughout the conterminous U.S. along prominent and heavily traveled flyways. Routine weather information and pilot weather reports including current reports on the location of thunderstorms and other hazardous weather as observed and reported by pilots or observed on weather radar will be provided, but the frequency may not be used for filing flight plans, routine position reporting, or for preflight weather briefings. EFAS will normally be available seven days a week, 6 a.m. to 10 p.m. local time.

A continuous exchange of weather information between pilots in flight and Flight Watch personnel on the ground is essential to the success of this program. Pilots are encouraged to report weather encountered to the nearest Flight Watch facility or in the absence of such, to the nearest FSS.

To contact an EFAS facility call on 122.0 MHz and use the name of the controlling FSS followed by the words "FLIGHT WATCH". If the controlling FSS is unknown, simply call "FLIGHT WATCH" and give the aircraft position. Locations of controlling FSS's and remote outlets are shown on Sectional and Low Altitude En route charts. On sectional charts a Flight

Watch facility will be depicted on the FSS frequency box with filled in upper corners.

The following map shows the Flight Watch control stations. Various remote communications outlets for each station are not depicted since they are subject to change.

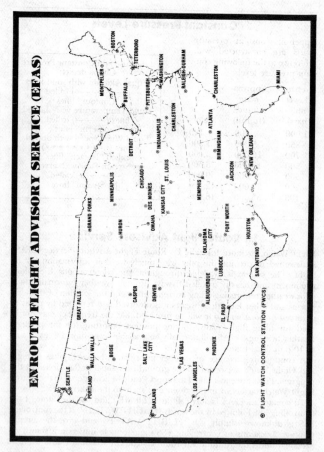

Airport Identifiers

The following is a list of the three-letter airport identifiers for those airports with weather reporting facilities in the conterminous United States. These identifiers are used as abbreviations for the respective airfields in teletyped aviation weather reports, and for some new weather disseminating programs instituted by FAA.

ALABAMA

ANB	Anniston
BHM	Birmingham
DHN	Dothan
GAD	Gadsden
HSV	Huntsville
MOB	Mobile
MGM	Montgomery—Dannelley Field Arpt.
MXF	Montgomery—Maxwell AFB Arpt.
MSL	Muscle Shoals
OZR	Ozark, Ft. Rucker
SEM	Selma
TCL	Tuscaloosa

ARIZONA

CHD	Chandler
DUG	Douglas
FLG	Flagstaff
FHU	Ft. Hauchuca/Sierra Vista
GBN	Gila Bend
LUF	Glendale
GCN	Grand Canyon
JBR	Jonesboro
IGM	Kingman
PGA	Page
PHX	Phoenix
PRC	Prescott
SAD	Safford
DMA	Tuscon—Davis Monthan AFB Arpt.
TUS	Tucson—Tucson Int'l Arpt.
INW	Winslow
YUM	Yuma

ARKANSAS

BYH	Blytheville
ELD	El Dorado
FYV	Fayetteville
FSM	Ft. Smith
HRO	Harrison
HOT	Hot Springs
LRF	Jacksonville
LIT	Little Rock
PBF	Pine Bluff
TXK	Texarkana
ARG	Walnut Ridge
AWM	West Memphis

CALIFORNIA

NGZ	Alameda
ACV	Arcota
AVX	Avalon
BFL	Bakersfield
BUO	Beaumont
BIH	Bishop
BLU	Blue Canyon
BLH	Blythe
BUR	Burbank
BNY	Burney
CZZ	Campo
CRQ	Carlsbad
CIC	Chico
CCR	Concord
CEC	Crescent City
NRC	Crows Landing
DAG	Daggett
EDW	Edwards
SUU	Fairfield
FAT	Fresno
FUL	Fullerton
HHR	Hawthorne
HWD	Hayward

IPL	Imperial	NUC	San Clemente
NRS	Imperial Beach	NZY	San Diego/Halsey Field
NID	Inyokern	NKX	San Diego/Mitscher Field
WJF	Lancaster	SAN	San Diego/San Diego
NLC	Lemoore		Int'l, Lindbergh Field
VBG	Lompoc	SEE	San Diego/Santee
LGB	Long Beach	SFO	San Francisco
NTB	Los Alamitos	SJC	San Jose
LAX	Los Angeles—	NSI	San Nicolas Island
	Los Angeles Int'l Arpt.	SRF	San Rafael
VNY	Los Angeles/Van Nuys	SDB	Sandberg
BAB	Marysville/Beale AFB	NZJ	Santa Ana/El Toro
MYV	Marysville/Yuba		MCAS Arpt.
	County Arpt.	SNA	Santa Ana/Orange
MER	Merced		County Arpt.
MOD	Modesto	SBA	Santa Barbara
SIY	Montaque	SXC	Santa Catalina
OAR	Monterey/Fort Ord	SZN	Santa Cruz Island
MRY	Monterey/Monterey	SMX	Santa Maria
	Peninsula Arpt.	SMO	Santa Monica
MHS	Mount Shasta	STS	Santa Rosa
MWS	Mount Wilson	TVL	South Lake Tahoe
NUQ	Mountain View	SCK	Stockton
APC	Napa	SVE	Susanville
EED	Needles	TRM	Thermal
OAK	Oakland	TOA	Torrance
ONT	Ontario/Ontario	UKI	Ukiah
	Int'l Arpt.	VCV	Victorville
ONO	Ontario/Ontario	VIS	Visalia
	Muni. Arpt.	L22	Yucca Valley
OXR	Oxnard		
PSP	Palm Springs		
PMD	Palmdale	**COLORADO**	
PRB	Paso Robles	AKO	Akron
NTD	Port Hueneme	ALS	Alamosa
RBL	Red Bluff	ASE	Aspen
RDD	Redding	COS	Colorado Springs/
RIV	Riverside		Colorado Springs
MHR	Sacramento/Mather AFB		Muni. Arpt.
MCC	Sacramento/	CEZ	Cortez
	McClellan AFB	BKF	Denver/Buckley
SAC	Sacramento/Sacramento		ANGB Arpt.
	Executive Arpt.	DEN	Denver/Stapleton
SMF	Sacramento/Sacramento		Int'l Arpt.
	Metro Arpt.	DRO	Durango
SNS	Salinas	EGE	Eagle
SJT	San Angelo	FCS	Fort Carson/Butts
SBD	San Bernardino		AAF Arpt.

150

FCL	Fort Collins
GJT	Grand Junction
GUC	Gunnison/Gunnison County Arpt.
2V9	Gunnison/Weather Reporting Station
HDN	Hayden
4LJ	Lamar
LHX	La Junta
LXV	Leadville
LIC	Limon
MTJ	Montrose
PUB	Pueblo
STK	Sterling
TAD	Trinidad

CONNECTICUT

BDR	Bridgeport
DXR	Danbury
GON	Groton/New London
HFD	Hartford
HVN	New Haven
NOA	New London
BDL	Windsor-Locks

DELAWARE

DOV	Dover
ILG	Wilmington

DISTRICT OF COLUMBIA

IAD	Washington/Dulles
DCA	Washington/National Arpt.

FLORIDA

AQQ	Apalachicola
AGR	Avon Park
BOW	Barton
X53	Clewiston
COF	Cocoa
CEW	Crestview
CTY	Cross City
DAB	Daytona Beach
FLL	Ft. Lauderdale

FMY	Ft. Myers
GNV	Gainesville
HST	Homestead
NZC	Jacksonville/Cecil Field NAS Arpt.
JAX	Jacksonville/Jacksonville Int'l Arpt.
NIP	Jacksonville/Jacksonville NAS Towers Field Arpt.
EYW	Key West
HRT	Mary Esther
NRB	Mayport
MLB	Melbourne
MIA	Miami/Miami Int'l Arpt.
NSE	Milton
ORL	Orlando/Herndon Arpt.
MCO	Orlando/Orlando Int'l Arpt.
PFN	Panama City/Panama City-Bay County Arpt.
PAM	Panama City/Tyndall AFB Arpt.
NPA	Pensacola/Forrest Sherman Field
PNS	Pensacola/Pensacola Regional Arpt.
SFB	Sanford
SRQ	Sarasota/Bradenton
PIE	St. Petersburg/Clearwater
TLH	Tallahassee
MCF	Tampa/MacDill AFB
TPA	Tampa/Tampa Int'l Arpt.
VPS	Valparaiso
VRB	Vero Beach
PBI	West Palm Beach

GEORGIA

ABY	Albany
AMG	Alma
AHN	Athens
FTY	Atlanta/Cahrlie Brown County Arpt.
ATL	Atlanta/The William B. Hartsfield Int'l Arpt.
AGS	Augusta
SSI	Brunswick

CSG	Columbus	CPS	East St. Louis
LSF	Ft. Benning	NBU	Glenview
LHW	Hinesville	MWA	Marion
LGC	La Grange	MTO	Mattoon-Charleston
MCN	Macon/Lewis B.	MLI	Moline
	Wilson Arpt.	MVN	Mt. Vernon
WRB	Macon/Warner Robins	PIA	Peoria
MGE	Marietta	UIN	Quincy
MGR	Moultrie	RFD	Rockford
7A9	Plains	SPI	Springfield
RMG	Rome	VLA	Van Dalia
SAV	Savannah		
VAD	Valdosta/Moody		
	AFB Arpt.	**INDIANA**	
VLD	Valdosta/Valdosta		
	Muni. Arpt.	BMG	Bloomington
		BRL	Burlington
		EVV	Evansville
IDAHO		FWA	Ft. Wayne
		IND	Indianapolis
BOI	Boise	LAF	Lafayette
BYI	Burley	MIE	Muncie
GNG	Gooding	GUS	Peru
S80	Grangeville	SBN	South Bend
SUN	Hailey	HUF	Terre Haute
IDA	Idaho Falls		
LWS	Lewiston		
MLD	Malad City	**IOWA**	
MUO	Mountain Home		
PIH	Pocatello	CID	Cedar Rapids
SMN	Salmon	DSM	Des Moines
TWF	Twin Falls	DBQ	Dubuque
		FOD	Ft. Dodge
		3OI	Lamoni
ILLINOIS		MEY	Mapleton
		MCW	Mason City
ALN	Alton	OTM	Ottumwa
BLV	Belleville	SUX	Sioux City
BMI	Bloomington/Normal	3SE	Spencer
BDF	Bradford	ALO	Waterloo
MDH	Carbondale/Murphysboro		
CMI	Champaign/Urbana		
MDW	Chicago/Chicago	**KANSAS**	
	Midway Arpt.	CNU	Chanute
CGX	Chicago/Merrill	CNK	Concordia
	C. Meigs Arpt.	DDC	Dodge City
ORD	Chicago/O'Hare	1K5	Elkhart
	Int'l Arpt.	EMP	Emporia
DPA	Chicago/West Chicago	FRI	Ft. Riley
DNV	Danville	GCK	Garden City
DEC	Decatur	GLD	Goodland

152

GBD	Great Bend
HLC	Hill City
HUT	Hutchinson
FLV	Leavenworth
LBL	Liberal
MHK	Manhattan
OJC	Olathe
RSL	Russell
SLN	Salina
FOE	Topeka/Forbes Field Arpt
TOP	Topeka/Philip Billard Muni. Arpt.
IAB	Wichita/McConnell AFB Arpt.
ICT	Wichita/Wichita Mid-Continent Arpt.

KENTUCKY

BWG	Bowling Green
FTK	Ft. Know
HOP	Hopkinsville
LEX	Lexington
LOZ	London
LOU	Louisville/Bowman Field Arpt.
SDF	Louisville/Standiford Field Arpt.
OWB	Owensboro
PAH	Paducah

LOUISIANA

AEX	Alexandria/England AFB
ESF	Alexandria/Esler Regional Arpt.
BTR	Baton Rouge
BVE	Boothville
HUM	Houma
7R4	Intracostal City
LFT	Lafayette
LCH	Lake Charles
POE	Leesville
MLU	Monroe
NBG	New Orleans/Alvin Callendar Field
NEW	New Orleans/Lakefront Arpt.

MSY	New Orleans/New Orleans Int'l Arpt.
BAD	Shreveport/Barksdale AFB
SHV	Shreveport/Shreveport Regional Arpt.

MAINE

AUG	Augusta
BGR	Bangor
BHB	Bar Harbor
NHZ	Brunswick
CAR	Caribou
6B2	Greenville
HUL	Houlton
LIZ	Limestone
MLT	Millinacket
75B	Mount Vernon
OLD	Oldtown
PWM	Portland
PQI	Presque Isle
RKD	Rockland

MARYLAND

BWI	Baltimore/Baltimore-Washington Int'l.
MTN	Baltimore/Glenn L. Martin State Arpt.
ADW	Camp Springs
FME	Ft. Meade
HGR	Hagerstown
NHK	Patuxent River
SBY	Salisbury

MASSACHUSETTS

BED	Bedford
BVY	Beverly
BOS	Boston
CEF	Chicopee Falls
GTR	Columbus
FMH	Falmouth
HYA	Hyannis
MVY	Marthas Vineyard
ACK	Nantucket
EWB	New Bedford

153

OWD	Norwood
OLV	Olive Branch
UOX	Oxford
PSF	Pittsfield
NZW	South Weymouth
BAF	Westfield
ORH	Worcester

MICHIGAN

APN	Alpena
ARB	Ann Arbor
BTL	Battle Creek
BEH	Benton Harbor
DET	Detroit/Detroit City Arpt.
DTW	Detroit/Metro Wayne County Arpt.
YIP	Detroit/Willow Run
ESC	Escanaba
FNT	Flint
GRR	Grand Rapids
SAW	Gwinn
CMX	Hancock
HTL	Houghton Lake
MT	Iron Mountain/Kingsfor
IWD	Ironwood
JXN	Jackson/Jackson County Reynolds Field
AZO	Kalamazoo
LAN	Lansing
MBL	Manistee
MQT	Marquette
MNM	Menominee
MTC	Mt. Clemens
MKG	Muskegon
OSC	Oscoda
PLN	Pellston
PTK	Pontiac
MBS	Saginaw
SSM	Sault Ste./Marie County Arpt.
INR	Sault Ste. Marie/ Kincheloe AFB Arpt.
TVC	Traverse City

MINNESOTA

| AXN | Alexandria |
| BDE | Baudette |

BJI	Bemidji
BRD	Brainerd
DLH	Duluth
FRM	Fairmont
HIB	Hibbing
INL	International Falls
MKT	Mankato
MSP	Minneapolis
RWF	Redwood Falls
RST	Rochester
STC	St. Cloud
TVF	Thief River Falls
OTG	Worthington

MISSISSIPPI

BIX	Biloxi
CBM	Columbus
GLH	Greenville
GWO	Greenwood
GPT	Gulfport
HBG	Hattiesburg
JAN	Jackson/Allen C. Thompson Field
LUL	Laurel
MCB	McComb
MEI	Meridian/Key Field
NMM	Meridian/McCain Field
HEZ	Natchez
PGL	Pascagoula
TUP	Tupelo
VKS	Vicksburg

MISSOURI

CGI	Cape Girardeau
COU	Columbia
TBN	Ft. Leonard Wood
GVW	Grandview
JEF	Jefferson City
JLN	Joplin
MKC	Kansas City/Kansas City downtown
MCI	Kansas City/Kansas City Int'l Arpt.
IRK	Kirksville
SZL	Knob Noster
VIH	Rolla/Vichy

STL	Saint Louis/Lambert St. Louis Int'l.
SUS	Saint Louis/Spirit of St. Louis
STJ	Saint Joseph
SGF	Springfield

MONTANA

BIL	Billings
BZN	Bozeman
4BQ	Broadus
BTM	Butte
CTB	Cut Bank
DLN	Dillon
3DU	Drummond
GGW	Glasgow
GDV	Glendive
GTF	Great Falls/Great Falls Int'l
GFA	Great Falls/Malmstrom AFB Arpt.
3HT	Harlowton
HVR	Havre
HLN	Helena
FCA	Kalispell
LWT	Lewistown
LVM	Livingston
MLS	Miles City
MSO	Missoula
MQM	Monida
SDY	Sidney
3TH	Thompson Falls
WYS	West Yellowstone
4HA	Whitehall
OLF	Wolf Point

NEBRASKA

ANW	Ainsworth
AIA	Alliance
BIE	Beatrice
BBW	Broken Bow
CDR	Chadron
OLU	Columbus
GRI	Grand Island
HSI	Hastings
IML	Imperial
EAR	Kearney

LNK	Lincoln
MCK	McCook
MHN	Mullen
OFK	Norfolk
LBF	North Platte
OMA	Omaha/Eppley Airfield
OFF	Omaha/Offutt AFB
ONL	O'Neill
BFF	Scottsbluff
SNY	Sidney
VTN	Valentine

NEVADA

BAM	Battle Mountain
EKO	Elko
ELY	Ely
NFL	Fallon
LAS	Las Vegas/McCarran Int'l Arpt.
LSV	Las Vegas/Nellis AFB Arpt.
LOL	Lovelock
OWY	Owyhee
RNO	Reno
TPH	Tonopah
WMC	Winnemucca
UCC	Yucca Flats

NEW HAMPSHIRE

BML	Berlin
CON	Concord
EEN	Keene
LCI	Laconia
LEB	Lebanon
MHT	Manchester
MWN	Mount Washington
PSM	Portsmouth

NEW JERSEY

ACY	Atlantic City
NEL	Lakehurst
MIV	Millville
MMU	Morristown
EWR	Newark
TEB	Teterboro
TTN	Trenton
WRI	Wrightstown

NEW MEXICO

HMN	Alamogordo
ABQ	Albuquerque
CNM	Carlsbad
CAO	Clayton
CVS	Clovis
4CR	Corona
4SL	Cuba
DMN	Deming
FMN	Farmington
GUP	Gallup
GNT	Grants
HOB	Hobbs
LRU	Las Cruces
LVS	Las Vegas
LAM	Los Alamos
4MY	Moriarty
RTN	Raton
ROW	Roswell
RUI	Ruidoso
SAF	Santa Fe
SVC	Silver City
ONM	Socorro
TCS	Truth or Consequences
TCC	Tucumcari
ZUN	Zuni Pueblo

NEW YORK

ALB	Albany
BGM	Binghamton
BUF	Buffalo
ELM	Elmira
FRG	Farmingdale
GFL	Glens Falls
ISP	Islip
ITH	Ithaca
JHW	Jamestown
MSS	Massena
MSV	Monticello
SWF	Newburgh
JFK	New York/John F. Kennedy Int'l
LAG	New York/La Guardia Arpt.
IAG	Niagara Falls
OGS	Ogdensburg
PBG	Plattsburg

POU	Poughkeepsie
ROC	Rochester
RME	Rome
SLK	Saranac Lake
SYR	Syracuse
UCA	Utica
ART	Watertown
FOK	Westhampton Beach
HPN	White Plains

NORTH CAROLINA

AVL	Asheville
CLT	Charlotte
NKT	Cherry Point
ECG	Elizabeth City
FAY	Fayetteville/Muni Arpt.
FBG	Fayetteville/Ft. Bragg
POB	Fayetteville/Pope AFB
GSB	Goldsboro
GSO	Greensboro
HAT	Hatteras
HKY	Hickory
HSS	Hot Springs
OAJ	Jacksonville/Albert J. Ellis Arpt.
NCA	Jacksonville/ New River Arpt.
ISO	Kinston
EWN	New Bern
RDU	Raleigh/Durham
RMT	Rocky Mount/ Downtown Arpt.
RWI	Rocky Mount/Rocky Mount-Wilson Arpt.
SOP	Southern Pines
ILM	Wilmington
INT	Winston-Salem

NORTH DAKOTA

BIS	Bismarck
DVL	Devils Lake
DIK	Dickinson
FAR	Fargo
RDR	Grand Forks/Grand Forks AFB
GFK	Grand Forks/Grand Forks Int'l

JMS	Jamestown
MIB	Minot/Minot AFB
MOT	Minot/Minot Int'l
ISN	Williston

OHIO

CAK	Akron
LUK	Cincinnati
BKL	Cleveland/Burke Lakefront Arpt.
CGF	Cleveland/Cuyahoga Country Arpt.
CLE	Cleveland/Cleveland Hopkins Int'l
OSU	Columbus/Ohio State University Arpt.
CMH	Columbus/Port Columbus Int'l
LCK	Columbus/Rickenbacker AFB
CVG	Covington/Cincinnati
DAY	Dayton/James M. Cox Dayton Int'l
FFO	Dayton/Wright-Patterson AFB Arpt.
FDY	Findlay
MFD	Mansfield
30I	Plain City
SGH	Springfield
TOL	Toledo
ILN	Wilmington
YNG	Youngstown
ZZV	Zanesville

OKLAHOMA

LTS	Altus
ADM	Ardmore
BVO	Bartlesville
CSM	Clinton
END	Enid
FSI	Ft. Sill
GAG	Gage
HBR	Hobart
MLC	McAlester
TIK	Oklahoma City/Tinker AFB
OKC	Oklahoma City/Will Rogers World Arpt.

PNC	Ponca City
SWO	Stillwater
TUL	Tulsa

OREGON

AST	Astoria
BKE	Baker
4BK	Brookings
4BW	Burns
CZK	Cascade Locks
LMT	Clamath Falls
CVO	Corvallis
EUG	Eugene
HIO	Hillsboro
LGD	La Grande
4LW	Lakeview
MEH	Meacham
MFR	Medford
JNW	Newport
OTH	North Bend
PDT	Pendleton
PDX	Portland
RDM	Redmond
RBG	Roseburg
SLE	Salem
SXT	Saxton Summit
DLS	The Dalles
TTD	Troutdale

PENNSYLVANIA

ABE	Allentown
BSI	Blairsville
BFD	Bradford
ERI	Erie
FKL	Franklin
CXY	Harrisburg/Capital City Arpt.
HAR	Harrisburg/Harrisburg FSS
HZL	Hazelton
JST	Johnstown
LNS	Lancaster
LBE	Latrobe
AOO	Martinsburg
MDT	Middletown
PNE	Philadelphia/North Philadelphia Arpt.

PHL	Philadelphia/ Philadelphia Int'l
PSB	Philipburg
AGC	Pittsburg/Allegheny County Arpt.
PIT	Pittsburg/Greater Pittsburgh Int'l
RDG	Reading
7TB	Tobyhanna
AVP	Wilkes-Barre/Scranton
IPT	Williamsport
NXX	Willow Grove

RHODE ISLAND

| BID | Block Island |
| PVD | Providence |

SOUTH CAROLINA

AND	Anderson
NBC	Beaufort
CHS	Charleston
CAE	Columbia/Columbia Metro Arpt.
MMT	Columbia/McEntire ANGB Arpt.
FLO	Florence
GRD	Greenwood
GSP	Greer
MYR	Myrtle Beach
CRE	North Myrtle Beach
SPA	Spartanburg
SSC	Sumter

SOUTH DAKOTA

ABR	Aberdeen
BKX	Brookings
HON	Huron
Y22	Lemmon
MHE	Mitchell
Y26	Mobridge
PHP	Philip
PIR	Pierre
RCA	Rapid City/Ellsworth AFB
RAP	Rapid City/Rapid City Regional Arpt.
FSD	Sioux Falls

| ATY | Watertown |
| YKN | Yankton |

TENNESSEE

TRI	Bristol
CHA	Chattanooga
CKV	Clarksville
CSV	Crossville
DYR	Dyersburg
MKL	Jackson
TYS	Knoxville
MEM	Memphis/Memphis Int'l Arpt.
NQA	Memphis/Memphis NAS Arpt.
MGL	Monteagle
BNA	Nashville

TEXAS

ABI	Abilene/Abilene Muni Arpt.
DYS	Abilene/Dyess AFB
ALI	Alice
AMA	Amarillo
BSM	Austin/Bergstrom AFB
AUS	Austin/Robert Mueller Muni Arpt.
BPT	Beaumont
NIR	Beeville
HCA	Big Spring/Howard County Arpt.
BGS	Big Spring/Webb AFB
BGD	Borger
BRO	Brownsville
BWD	Brownwood
CDS	Childress
CLL	College Station
CRP	Corpus Christi/Int'l Arpt.
NGP	Corpus Christi/NAS Arpt.
NBE	Dalles/Hensley Field
DAL	Dalles/Love Field
DFW	Dalles-Ft. Worth
DHT	Dalhart
DRT	Del Rio/Del Rio Int'l
DLF	Del Rio/Laughlin AFB
ELP	El Paso
FWH	Ft. Worth/Carswell AFB

FTW	Ft. Worth/Meacham Field	HIF	Ogden/Hill AFB
GLS	Galveston	OGD	Ogden/Ogden Muni
GDP	Guadalupe Pass	PUC	Price
HRL	Harlingen	SLC	Salt Lake City
EFD	Houston/Ellington AFB	VEL	Vernal
IAH	Houston/Houston Intercontinental Arpt.	ENV	Wendover
HOU	Houston/William P. Hobby Arpt.		

VERMONT

JCT	Junction	MPV	Barre-Montpelier
ERV	Kerrville	BTV	Burlington
HLR	Killeen/Hood AFB	RUT	Rutland
GRK	Killeen/Robert Gray AAF	9B2	Saint Johnsbury
LOI	Laredo/Laredo Arpt.	VSF	Springfield
LRD	Laredo/Laredo Int'l		
GGG	Longview		

VIRGINIA

LBB	Lubbock/Lubbock Int'l	BKT	Blackstone
REE	Lubbock/Reese AFB	CHO	Charlottesville
LFK	Lufkin	WAL	Chincoteague
MRF	Marfa	DAN	Danville
MFE	McAllen	PSK	Dublin
MAF	Midland	DAA	Ft. Belvoir
MWL	Mineral Wells	FAF	Ft. Eustis
PSX	Palacios	LFI	Hampton
PRX	Paris	HSP	Hot Springs
PVW	Plainview	LYH	Lynchburg
SKF	San Antonio/Kelly AFB	PHF	Newport News
RND	San Antonio/Randolph AFB	ORF	Norfolk/Norfolk Int'l Arpt.
SAT	San Antonio/San Antonio Int'l Arpt.	NGU	Norfolk/Norfolk NAS Arpt.
TPL	Temple	NTU	Oceana
TYR	Tyler	NYG	Quantico
VCT	Victoria	RIC	Richmond
ACT	Waco	ROA	Roanoke
SPS	Wichita Falls	SHD	Staunton/Waynesb/Harrisonb
INK	Wink		

UTAH

WASHINGTON

4BL	Blanding	BLI	Bellingham
BCE	Bryce Canyon	PWT	Bremerton
U17	Bullfrog	63S	Coleville
CDC	Cedar City	EPH	Ephrata
DPG	Dugway/Tooele	PAE	Everette
U20	Green River	HQM	Hoquiam
4HV	Hankesville	MWH	Moses Lake
MLF	Milford	OLM	Olympia
CNY	Moab	4OM	Omak

PSC	Pasco		SSU	White Sulphur Springs
NOW	Port Angeles/CGAS Arpt.			
CLM	Port Angeles/William R. Fairchild Int'l		**WISCONSIN**	
PUW	Pullman		VOK	Camp Douglas
UIL	Quillayute		EAU	Eau Claire
RLD	Richland		GRB	Green Bay
BFI	Seattle/Boeing Field/ King County Int'l Arpt.		JVL	Janesville
			LSE	LaCrosse
SEA	Seattle/Seattle-Tacoma Int'l Arpt.		LNR	Lone Rock
			MSN	Madison
SHN	Shelton		MTW	Manitowoc
SKA	Spokane/Fairchild AFB		MKE	Milwaukee/General Mitchell Field
SFF	Spokane/Felts Field			
GEG	Spokane/Spokane Int'l		MWC	Milwaukee/Lawrence J. Timmerman Arpt.
SMP	Stampede Pass			
GRF	Tacoma/Ft. Lewis		CWA	Mosinee
TIW	Tacoma/Industrial Arpt.		OSH	Oshkosh
TCM	Tacoma/McChord AFB		RHI	Rhinelander
TDO	Toledo		AUW	Wausau
ALW	Walla Walla			
EAT	Wenatchee		**WYOMING**	
NUW	Whidbey Island			
YKM	Yakima		BPI	Big Piney
			CPR	Casper
WEST VIRGINIA			CYS	Cheyenne
			COD	Cody
BKW	Beckley		4DG	Douglas
BLF	Bluefield		EVW	Evanston
CRW	Charleston		GCC	Gilette
CKB	Clarksburg		JAC	Jackson
EKN	Elkins		LND	Lander
HTS	Huntington		LAR	Laramie
LWB	Lewisburg		RWL	Rawlings
MRB	Martinsburg		RIW	Riverton
MGW	Morgantown		RKS	Rock Springs
PKB	Parkersburg		SHR	Sheridan
HLG	Wheeling		WRL	Worland

U.S. Weather Broadcasts

Transcribed Weather Broadcasts (TWEB)

Equipment is available at selected Flight Service Stations by which meteorological and Notice to Airmen data is recorded on tapes and broadcast continuously over low-frequency (200–415 kHz) navigational aids (L/MF range or H facility) and VORs.

Broadcasts are made from a series of individual tape recordings. The first three tapes identify the station, give general weather forecast conditions in the area, pilot reports (PIREP), radar reports when available, and winds aloft data. The remaining tapes contain weather at selected locations within a 400-mile radius of the central point. Changes, as they occur are transcribed onto the tapes.

Weather Broadcasts
Scheduled

All flight service stations having voice facilities on radio ranges (VORs) or radio beacons (NDBs) broadcast weather reports and Notice to Airmen information at 15 minutes past each hour from reporting points within approximately 150 miles from the broadcast station.

Unscheduled

These broadcasts will be made at random times and will begin with the announcement "Aviation broadcast" followed by identification of the data.

Example:

Aviation Broadcast, Special Weather Report, (Notice to Airmen, Pilot Report, etc.) (location name twice) three seven (past the hour) observation ... etc.

Automatic Weather Broadcast (AB) Facilities

ALABAMA
McDen NDB—BH/224
(Birmingham FSS); 24 hours
Montgomery VORTAC—
MGM/112.1
(Montgomery FSS); 24 hours
Muscle Shoals VORTAC—
MSL/116.5
(Muscle Shoals FSS);
0500–2200 hours
Semmes VORTAC—
SJI/115.3
(Mobile FSS); 24 hours

ALASKA
Fort Davis NDB—
FOV/239
(Nome FSS); 24 hours
Nome VORTAC—
OME/115.0
(Nome FSS); 24 hours
North River NDB—
JNR/382
(Nome FSS); 24 hours
Unalakleet VORTAC—
UNK/116.9
(Nome FSS); 24 hours

ARIZONA
Casa Grande VORTAC—
CZG/114.8
(Phoenix FSS); 0500–2200
hours
Douglas VORTAC—
DUG/108.8
(Douglas FSS); 0500–2200
hours
Papago NDB—PQO/326
(Phoenix FSS); 0500–2200
hours
Ryan NDB—RYN/338
(Tucson FSS); 0500–2200 hours

ARKANSAS
Lasky NDB—LI/353
(Little Rock FSS); 24 hours

CALIFORNIA
Arcata VOR—ACV/110.2
(Arcata FSS); 24 hours
Bakersfield VORTAC—
BFL/115.4
(Bakersfield FSS); 24 hours

Chandler NDB—FCH/344
(Fresno FSS); 24 hours
Daggett VORTAC—DAG/
113.2
(Daggett FSS); 0500–2200
hours
East Bay NDB—EZB/362
(Oakland FSS); 24 hours
Fillmore VORTAC—
FIM/112.5 (Santa
Barbara FSS); 24 hours
Fort Jones VORTAC—
FJS/109.6
(Red Bluff FSS); 24 hours
Fortuna VORTAC—FOT/
114.0
(Arcata FSS); 24 hours
Fresno VORTAC—
FAT/112.9
(Fresno FSS); 24 hours
Goffs VORTAC—GFS/
114.4
(Las Vegas FSS); 24 hours
Imperial VORTAC—IPL/
115.9
(Imperial FSS); 24 hours
Inglewood NDB—IGD/332
(Los Angeles FSS); 24 hours
Maxwell VORTAC—
MXW/110.0
(Red Bluff FSS); 0500–2200
hours
Miramar (Navy) UHF NDB—
NKX/280.4 (San
Diego FSS); 24 hours
Mission Bay VORTAC—
MZB/117.8
(San Diego FSS); 0600–2100
hours
Montague NDB—MOG/
382
(Red Bluff FSS); 24 hours
Needles VORTAC—EED/
115.2
(Las Vegas FSS); 24 hours
North Island (Navy) UHF
NDB—NZY/283.0
(San Diego FSS); 24 hours

Ontario VORTAC—ONT/
112.2
(Ontario FSS); 24 hours
Paso Robles VORTAC—
PRB/114.3
(Paso Robles FSS); 24 hours
Pomona VORTAC—
POM/110.4
(Ontario FSS); 0600–2100
hours
Proberta NDB—PBT/338
(Red Bluff FSS); 24 hours
Red Bluff VORTAC—
RBL/115.7
(Red Bluff FSS); 24 hours
Ripley NDB—RPY/251
(Blythe FSS); 24 hours
Sacramento VORTAC—
SAC/115.2
(Sacramento FSS);
0500–2200 hours
Salinas VORTAC—SNS/
117.3
(Salinas FSS); 24 hours
Santa Barbara VORTAC—
SBA/114.9
(Santa Barbara FSS); 24 hours
Santa Catalina VORTAC—
SXC/109.4
(Los Angeles FSS); 24 hours
Sausalito VORTAC—
SAU/116.2
(Oakland FSS); 24 hours
Visalia VOR/DME—
VIS/109.4
(Fresno FSS); 0800–1700
hours

COLORADO
Castle NDB—AP/260
(Denver FSS); 24 hours
Fruita NDB—FRU/396
(Grand Junction FSS); 24
hours
Grand Junction VORTAC—
GJT/112.4
(Grand Junction FSS); 24
hours

Kiowa VORTAC—IOC/
117.5 (Denver FSS); 24 hours
Trinidad NDB—TAD/329
(Trinidad FSS); 24 hours

CONNECTICUT
Brainard NDB—
AQD/329
(Windsor Locks FSS)
Rain NDB—UJW/371
(Windsor Locks FSS); 24 hours

DISTRICT OF COLUMBIA
Oxonn NDB—DC/332
(Washington FSS); 24 hours

FLORIDA
Dinns NDB—JA/344
(Jacksonville FSS); 24 hours
Ortan NDB—MF/365
(Miami FSS); 24 hours
Pickens NDB—PKZ/326
(Pensacola FSS); 24 hours
Picny NDB—AM/388
(St. Petersburg FSS); 24 hours
Vero Beach VORTAC—
VRB/117.3
(Vero Beach FSS); 24 hours
Wakul NDB—TL/379
(Tallahassee FSS); 24 hours

GEORGIA
Albany VORTAC—ABY/
116.1
(Albany FSS); 0500–2200
hours
Redan NDB—BR/266
(Atlanta FSS); 24 hours

IDAHO
Boise VORTAC—
BOI/113.3
(Boise FSS); 24 hours
Burley VORTAC—BYI/
114.1
(Burley FSS); 0500–2200
hours
Dubois VORTAC—
DBS/116.9
(Idaho Falls FSS); 24 hours

Idaho Falls VOR—IDA/109.0
(Idaho Falls FSS); 24 hours
Lewiston VOR—LWS/108.2
(Walla Walla FSS); 0500–2200
McCall VORTAC—MYL/
116.2 (Boise FSS); 24 hours
Mullan Pass VORTAC—
MLP/117.8
(Spokane FSS); 24 hours
Pocatello VORTAC—
PIH/112.6
(Burley FSS); 0500–2200
hours
Salmon VOR/DME—
LKT/113.5
(Idaho Falls FSS); 24 hours
Sweden NDB—SWU/350
(Idaho Falls FSS); 24 hours
Twin Falls, VORTAC—
TWF/115.8
(Burley FSS); 0500–2200
hours
Ustik NDB—BO/359
(Boise FSS); 24 hours

ILLINOIS
Deana NDB—ME/350
(Chicago FSS); 24 hours
Decatur VORTAC—DEC/
117.2
(Decatur FSS); 0500–2200
hours
Dupage VOR/DME—
DPA/108.4
(Chicago FSS); 24 hours
Quincy VORTAC—UIN/113.1
(Quincy FSS); 0500–2200
hours

INDIANA
Pully NDB—IN/266
(Indianapolis FSS); 24 hours
Shelbyville VORTAC—
SHB/112.0
(Indianapolis FSS); 24 hours
South Bend VORTAC—
SBN/115.4
(South Bend FSS); 24 hours

IOWA

Cody NDB—BBC/
224 (Cedar Rapids FSS); 24
hours

Des Moines VORTAC—
DSM/114.1
(Des Moines FSS); 0600–2400
hours

Mason City VORTAC—
MCW/114.9
(Mason City FSS); 0500–2200
hours

KANSAS

Anthony VORTAC—ANY/
112.9 (Wichita FSS); 24 hours

Goodland VORTAC—
GLD/115.1
(Goodland FSS); 24 hours

Hill City VORTAC—
HLC/113.7
(Goodland FSS); 24 hours

Holcomb NDB—HMB/257
(Garden City FSS); 24 hours

Piche NDB—IC/332
(Wichita FSS); 24 hours

Salina VORTAC—
SLN/115.3
(Salina FSS); 24 hours

LOUISIANA

Alexandria VORTAC—
AEX/116.1 (Lake Charles
FSS); 24 hours

Crakk NDB—SH/230
(Shreveport FSS); 24 hours

Grand Isle NDB—GNI/236
(New Orleans FSS); 24 hours

Lake Charles VORTAC—
LCH/113.4 (Lake Charles
FSS); 24 hours

MAINE

Sterns NDB—SRX/344
(Bangor FSS); 24 hours

MASSACHUSETTS

Hyannis VORTAC—HYA/
114.7
(Boston FSS); 24 hours

Lyndy NDB—LQ/382
(Boston FSS); 24 hours

Nantucket NDB—TUK/194
(Boston FSS); 24 hours

MICHIGAN

Calumet NDB—CUT/227
(Houghton FSS); 24 hours

Chippewa NDB—CPW/400
(Traverse City FSS); 24 hours

Marquette VOR/DME
MQT/109.0
(Marquette FSS); 24 hours

Revup NDB—DT/388
(Detroit FSS); 24 hours

Saginaw VORTAC—MBS/
112.9
(Saginaw FSS); 24 hours

Salem VORTAC—SVM/
114.3 (Detroit FSS); 24 hours

Traverse City NDB—TV/
365 (Traverse City FSS); 24
hours

Traverse City VORTAC—
TVC/114.6
(Traverse City FSS); 24 hours

MINNESOTA

Flying Cloud VOR/DME—
FCM/111.8
(Minneapolis FSS); 0500–2200
hours

Hibbing VORTAC—
HIB/110.8
(Hibbing FSS); 24 hours

Narco NDB—MS/266
(Minneapolis FSS); 0500–2200
hours

Orr NDB—ORB/341
(Hibbing FSS); 24 hours

Pykla NDB—DL/379
(Hibbing FSS); 24 hours

Raize NDB—IN/353
(Hibbing FSS); 24 hours

MISSISSIPPI

Hawkins NDB—HKS/260
(Jackson FSS); 24 hours

MISSOURI
Cape Girardeau VOR—
CGI/112.9
(Cape Girardeau FSS); 24
hours
Columbia VOR—CBI/111.2
(Columbia FSS); 24 hours
Foristell VORTAC—FTZ/
110.8 (St. Louis FSS); 24 hours
Limestone NDB—LM/338
(St. Louis FSS); 24 hours
Napoleon VORTAC—ANX/
114.8
(Kansas City FSS); 24 hours
Springfield VOR—SGF/
116.8 (Springfield FSS); 0600-
2300 hours
Willard NDB—ILJ/254
(Springfield FSS); 24 hours
Wyandotte NDB—DO/359
(Kansas City FSS);24 hours

MONTANA
Amsterdam NDB—AMD/
329
(Bozeman FSS); 24 hours
Desmet NDB—DST/308
(Missoula FSS); 24 hours
Great Falls VORTAC—
GTF/115.1
(Great Falls FSS); 24 hours
Horton NDB—HTN/320
(Miles City FSS); 24 hours
Lockwood NDB—LKO/400
(Billings FSS); 24 hours
Truly NDB—GT/371
(Great Falls FSS); 24 hours

NEBRASKA
Bignell NDB—BGN/224
(North Platte FSS); 24 hours
Gerfi NDB—OM/320
(Omaha FSS); 24 hours
Grand Island VORTAC—
GRI/112.0
(Grand Island FSS); 0500-2200
hours

Scottsbluff VORTAC—
BFF/112.6
(Scottsbluff FSS); 0500-2300
hours

NEVADA
Beatty VORTAC—BTY/114.7
(Las Vegas FSS); 24 hours
Blackjack NDB—BKJ/206
(Las Vegas FSS); 24 hours
Boulder City VORTAC—
BLD/116.7 (Las Vegas
FSS); 24 hours
Reno VORTAC—RNO/
117.9 (Reno FSS); 24 hours
Sparks NDB—SPK/254
(Reno FSS); 24 hours

NEW JERSEY
Progress NDB—GKO/379
(Teterboro FSS); 24 hours

NEW MEXICO
Gallup VORTAC—GUP/
115.1 (Gallup FSS); 24 hours
Isleta NDB—ILT/230
(Albuquerque FSS); 24 hours
Walker NDB—AKH/305
(Roswell FSS); 24 hours

NEW YORK
Albany VORTAC—
ALB/117.8
(Albany FSS); 0600-2300
hours
Elmira NDB—ELM/375
(Elmira FSS); 24 hours
Kingston VORTAC—IGN/
117.6
(Poughkeepsie FSS); 24 hours
Riverhead VORTAC—
RVH/117.2
(New York FSS); 24 hours
Utica VORTAC—UCA/
108.6
(Utica FSS); 24 hours

NORTH CAROLINA
Barretts Mtn. VOR/DME—
BZM/110.8
(Hickory FSS); 0600-2200
hours
Leevy NDB—LE/350
(Raleigh FSS); 0500-2200
hours
New Bern VOR—EWN/
113.6 (New Bern FSS); 0600-
2200 hours

NORTH DAKOTA
Colij NDB—BI/230
(Minot FSS); 24 hours
Grand Forks VORTAC—
GFK/109.4
(Grand Forks FSS); 0600-2200
hours
Harwood NDB—HAW/365
(Jamestown FSS); 24 hours
Minot VORTAC—
MOT/117.1
(Minot FSS); 24 hours

OHIO
Appleton VORTAC—
APE/116.7
(Columus FSS); 0500-2200
hours
Cincinnati NDB—LUK/335
(Cincinnati FSS); 24 hours
Columbus NDB—CMH/391
(Columbus FSS); 24 hours
Findlay VORTAC—
FDY/108.2
(Findlay FSS); 0500-2200
hours
Harri NDB—CL/344
(Cleveland FSS); 24 hours

OKLAHOMA
McAlester VORTAC—
MLC/112.0
(McAlester FSS); 24 hours
Oklahoma City NDB—
OKC/350
(Oklahoma City FSS); 24
hours

Tulsa NDB—DW/375
(Tulsa FSS); 24 hours

OREGON
Corvallis VOR—CVO/
108.4
(Portland FSS); 24 hours
Emire NDB—OT/379
(North Bend FSS); 24 hours
Eugene VORTAC—EUG/
112.9
(Portland FSS); 24 hours
Klamath Falls VORTAC—
LMT/115.9
(Redmond FSS); 24 hours
Medford NDB—MFR/263
(Redmond FSS); 24 hours
Medford VORTAC—
MFR/113.6
(North Bend FSS); 24 hours
Newberg VORTAC—
UBG/117.4
(Portland FSS); 24 hours
Newport VORTAC—
ONP/117.1
(North Bend FSS); 24 hours
North Bend VORTAC—
OTH/112.1
(North Bend FSS); 24 hours
Pendleton NDB—PDT/341
(Walla Walla FSS); 0500-2200
hours
Pendleton VORTAC—
PDT/114.7
(Walla Walla FSS); 0500-2200
hours
Portland VORTAC—
PDX/116.6
(Portland FSS); 24 hours
Redmond VORTAC—
RDM/117.6
(Redmond FSS); 24 hours
Roberts NDB—OBT/368
(Redmond FSS); 24 hours
Rome VORTAC—
REO/112.5
(Boise FSS); 24 hours
Roseberg VOR—RBG/108.2
(North Bend FSS); 24 hours

Sauvies Island NDB—
  SVY/332
  (Portland FSS); 24 hours
The Dalles VORTAC
  DLS/112.3
  (Portland FSS); 24 hours

PENNSYLVANIA
  Cecil NDB—CCZ/254
    (Pittsburgh FSS); 24 hours
  Clarion VORTAC—
    CIP/112.9
    (Du Bois FSS); 24 hours
  Pottstown VORTAC—
    PTW/116.5
    (Philadelphia FSS); 24 hours
  Ravine VORTAC—RAV/
    114.6 (Harrisburg FSS); 24
    hours
  Wilkes-Barre VORTAC—
    AVP/112.4
    (Wilkes-Barre FSS); 24 hours

SOUTH CAROLINA
  Ashley NDB—CH/329
    (Charleston FSS); 24 hours
  Fairmont NDB—FRT/248
    (Greer FSS); 2200-0500 hours
  Florence VORTAC—FLO/
    115.2
    (Florence FSS); 24 hours

SOUTH DAKOTA
  Huron VORTAC—
    HON/117.6
    (Huron FSS); 24 hours
  Pierre VORTAC—
    PIR/112.5
    (Pierre FSS); 24 hours
  Rapid City NDB—RAP/
    254
    (Rapid City FSS); 24 hours
  Rokky NDB—FS/245
    (Huron FSS); 24 hours

TENNESSEE
  Davidson NDB—BN/304
    (Nashville FSS); 0500-2200
    hours
  Elvis NDB—TE/371
    (Memphis FSS); 24 hours

Singleton NDB—SGK/281
  (Knoxville FSS); 0500-2200
  hours

TEXAS
  Abilene VORTAC—ABI/
    113.7 (Abilene FSS); 24 hours
  Amarillo NDB—AM/251
    (Amarillo FSS); 24 hours
  Austin VORTAC—AUS/
    114.6
    (Austin FSS); 0500-2200 hours
  Fort Worth NDB—FT/365
    (Ft. Worth FSS); 24 hours
  Galveston NDB—
    GLS/206
    (Houston FSS); 24 hours
  Lubbock VORTAC—LBB/
    110.8
    (Lubbock FSS); 24 hours
  Midland NDB—MA/326
    (Midland FSS); 24 hours
  San Antonio VORTAC—
    SAT/116.8 (San
    Antonio FSS); 0600-2200
    hours
  Valtr NDB—EL/242
    (El Paso FSS); 24 hours
  Wichita Falls VORTAC—
    SPS/112.7
    (Wichita Falls FSS); 24 hours

UTAH
  Ogden NDB—OGD/263
    (Salt Lake City FSS); 24 hours
  Ogden VORTAC—OGD/
    115.7
    (Salt Lake City FSS); 24 hours
  Salt Lake City VORTAC—
    SLC/116.8
    (Salt Lake City FSS); 24 hours

VIRGINIA
  Hopewell VORTAC—
    HPW/112.0
    (Washington FSS); 24 hours
  Roanoke NDB—ROA/371
    (Roanoke FSS); 0500-2200
    hours

WASHINGTON
  Ellensburg VORTAC—
    ELN/117.9
    (Seattle FSS); 24 hours
  Marshall NDB—MZS/365
    (Spokane FSS); 0500-2200
    hours
  Olympia VORTAC—
    OLM/113.4
    (Seattle FSS); 0500-2200 hours
  Paine VOR—PAE/114.2
    (Seattle FSS); 24 hours
  Pasco VOR/DME—PSC/
    108.4 (Walla Walla FSS); 0500-
    2200 hours
  Port Angeles VOR—
    CLM/108.4
    (Seattle FSS); 0500-2200 hours
  Pullman VOR—PUW/109.0
    (Walla Walla FSS); 0500-2200
    hours
  Seattle NDB—SEA/362
    (Seattle FSS); 24 hours
  Seattle VORTAC—
    SEA/116.8
    (Seattle FSS); 0500-2200 hours
  Spokane VORTAC—GEG/
    115.5
    (Spokane FSS); 24 hours
  Tatoosh VORTAC—
    TOU/112.2 (Seattle
    FSS); 24 hours
  Walla Walla VOR—ALW/
    116.4 (Walla Walla FSS);
    0500-2200 hours

  Wenatchee VOR—EAT/111.0
    (Wenatchee FSS); 24 hours
WEST VIRGINIA
  Martinsburg VORTAC—
    MRB/112.1
    (Martinsburg FSS); 24 hours
  Rainelle VOR—RNL/116.6
    (Charleston FSS); 24 hours
WISCONSIN
  Badger VORTAC—BAE/
    116.4 (Milwaukee FSS); 24
    hours
  Green Bay VORTAC—
    GRB/117.0
    (Green Bay FSS); 24 hours
  La Crosse VOR—
    LSE/108.4 (La Crosse
    FSS); 24 hours
  Teels NDB—GM/242
    (Milwaukee FSS); 24 hours
WYOMING
  Antelope NDB—AOP/290
    (Rock Springs FSS); 0500-2200
    hours
  Casper VORTAC—CPR/
    116.2
    (Casper FSS); 24 hours
  Harford NDB—HAD/269
    (Casper FSS); 24 hours
  Jackson VOR—JAC/108.4
    (Idaho Falls FSS); 24 hours
  Rock Springs VORTAC—
    RKS/114.7
    (Rock Springs FSS); 24 hours

Weather and Flight Information Telephone Numbers

Weather and flight information necessary to the general aviation pilot is available by phone through the resources of the National Weather Service and the Federal Aviation Administration. Flight Service Stations (FSSs) and Combined Station/Towers (CS/Ts) provide information on airport conditions, radio aids, and other facilities, and process flight plans. CS/T personnel are not certified pilot weather briefers; however, they provide factual data from weather reports and forecasts. Airport Advisory Service is provided at the pilot's request on 123.6 by FSSs located at airports where there are no control towers in operation.

The telephone area code is shown in parentheses in the following listing. (Where one area code applies throughout the state, the area code number will appear just once, at the beginning of the listing for that particular state.) Each number given is the preferred telephone number to obtain flight weather information. Automatic answering devices are sometimes used on listed lines to give general local weather information during peak workloads. To avoid getting the recorded general weather announcement, use the selected telephone number listed. See the Airman's Information Manual, Basic Flight Information, and ATC Procedures for further information. Also, be sure to check in the Airport/Facility Directory for updated FSS numbers.

Fast File Flight Plan System

Some Flight Service Stations have inaugurated this system for pilots who desire to file IFR/VFR flight plans. Pilots may call the discrete telephone numbers listed and file flight plans in accordance with prerecorded taped instructions. IFR flight plans will be extracted from the recorder and subsequently entered into the appropriate ARTCC computer. VFR flights will be transcribed; and both IFR/VFR flight plans will be filed in the FSS. This equipment is designed to automatically disconnect after 8 seconds of no transmission, so pilots are instructed to speak at a normal speech rate without lenghty pauses between flight plan elements. Pilots are urged to file flight plans into this system at least 30 minutes in advance of proposed departure. The system may be used to close and cancel flight plans.

Preflight weather briefing services remain available through regular telephone numbers.

LEGEND

WS—Weather Service

FSS—Flight Service Station

IFSS—International Flight Service Station

CS/T—Combined Station/Tower

　　#—Indicates Pilot's Automatic Telephone Weather Answering Service (PATWAS) or telephone connected to Transcribed Weather Broadcast (TWEB) providing transcribed aviation weather information.

　　*—Indicates a restricted number; used for aviation weather information.

　　@—Call FSS for "one call" FSS/WS briefing service.

　　+—Automatic Aviation Weather Service (AAWS).

　　¢—Indicates fast file telephone number for prerecorded and transcribed flight plan filing only.

ALABAMA

(Area Code—205)
Anniston FSS 831-2303.
Birmingham FSS 254-1387 @; 595-2101 #; (N.W. Route) 595-5416+; (S.E. Route) 595-6452+; (N.E. Route) 595-7957+;(S.W. Route) 595-7896+.
Dothan FSS 983-3551.
Huntsville WS 772-3521*.
Mobile FSS 344-3610 @.
Montgomery FSS 832-7516 @.
Muscle Shoals FSS 383-6541; 381-2500 #.
Tuscaloosa FSS 758-3628.

ALASKA

(Area Code—907)
Anchorage FSS 279-8491; 279-3376 #;**IFSS** 272-6823.
Barrow FSS 852-2511; **WS** 852-6484.
Bethel FSS 543-2231.
Bettles FSS 692-5222.
Big Delta FSS 895-4511.
Cold Bay FSS 532-2453 @; **WS** 532-2448.
Cordova FSS 424-3254.
Deadhorse FSS 659-2401.
Dilingham FSS 842-5275.
Fairbanks FSS 452-7137@.
Gulkana FSS 822-3236.
Homer FSS 235-8588.
Iliamna FSS 571-1240.
Juneau FSS 789-7380.
Kenai FSS 283-7211; 283-4332 #; 486-5550.
Ketchikan FSS 225-5800; 225-5923.
King Salmon FSS 246-3313 @.
Kotzebue FSS 442-3103.
McGrath FSS 524-3611 @.
Nome FSS 443-2291 @.
Northway FSS 778-6611.
Palmer FSS 745-3269.
Sitka FSS 966-2222.
Talkeetna FSS 733-2277.
Tanana FSS 366-7945.

170

Yakutat FSS 784-3314; **WS** 784-3322.

ARIZONA

(Area Code—602)
Douglas FSS 364-8458.
Flagstaff WS 774-2851; 774-1424; 774-0475.
Phoenix FSS 275-4121 @; (Eastbound) 244-8331 +; (Westbound) 244-8341 +.
Prescott FSS 445-2160. **Grand Canyon:** 638-2943. **Kingman:** 753-5659.
Tuscon FSS 889-9638 +; 889-8549 #, (1300-0600Z); (Eastbound) 889-9588 +; (Westbound) 889-9638 +.
Winslow WS 289-3592.
Yuma FSS 726-2601 @.

ARKANSAS

(Area Code—501)
El Dorado FSS 363-5128.
Fayetteville FSS 442-8277.
Ft. Smith WS 646-7885*.
Harrison FSS 741-3433.
Jonesboro FSS 935-3471 (1200-0400Z; other hrs Little Rock FSS (Toll free) 1-800-482-1159)
Little Rock FSS 376-0721; (IFR Flight Plans Only) 371-0060¢; (50 NM Radius) 376-9894 #.
Elsewhere in Arkansas (call Toll Free) 1-800-482-9974 ¢

CALIFORNIA

Arcata FSS (707) 839-1545.
Bakersfield FSS (805) 399-1787 @ (no wea bcst avbl 0700-1300Z).
Bishop WS (714) 873-3213 (1345-0300Z).
Blythe FSS (714) 922-6151.
Cresent City FSS (707) 464-2514 (1400-0600Z, other hrs Arcata).
Dagget FSS (714) 254-2958; (714) 254-2959; (800) 634-6474 @.
Eureka WS (707) 442-2171*.

Fresno FSS (209) 251-8269 @; (209) 251-7597 #. **Visalia:** (209) 734-7475 #.

Imperial FSS (714) 352-8740.

Lancaster FSS (805) 948-5385.

Long Beach WS (213) 429-0337.

Los Angeles FSS (213) 776-2727 @ (North of LAX) (213) 466-4116 ¢; (South of LAX) (213) 263-6776 ¢, 670-1000 @; (LAX Basin Forecast) (213) 776-8803 #; (Route Forecast) (213) 776-1640 #. **Van Nuys:** (213) 781-5213 @; (LAX Basin Forecast) (213) 787-6580 #; (Route Forecast) (213) 787-4911 #. **Burbank:** (213) 841-3904 @; (LAX Basin Forecast) (213) 843-6911 #; (Route Forecast) (213) 841-0034 #. **Long Beach:** (213) 639-2618 @; WS (213) 429-0337; (LAX Basin Forecast) (213) 639-4200 #; (Route Forecast) (213) 639-2647 #. **John Wayne Airport/Orange County:** (714) 542-3585 @; (LAX Basin Forecast) (714) 546-1610 #; (Route Forecast) (714) 546-0595 #. **El Monte:** (213) 728-9957 @; (LAX Basin Forecast) (213) 442-3113 #; (Route Forecast) (213) 442-7800 #.

Marysville FSS (916) 742-8852.

Montague FSS (916) 459-3003 (1415-0545Z, other hrs Red Bluff).

Mt. Shasta WS (916) 926-2227 (1430-2300Z).

Needles FSS (800) 634-6474. **Oakland:** (415) 527-4481 @. **Napa:** (707) 252-7688 @. **Halfmoon Bay:** (415) 726-7611 @. **Hayward:** (415) 829-2270 @. **San Jose:** (408) 248-8912 @. **Fremont:** (415) 656-5093 @. **Palo Alto:** (415) 326-2941 @. **San Mateo:** (415) 342-8627 @. **San Rafael:** (415) 459-1062 @. **Concord:** (415) 687-1456 @. **San Francisco:** (415) 668-1455 @.

South San Francisco: (415) 692-2876 @. **Danville:** (415) 829-2271 @. **Petaluma:** (707) 795-1449 @.

Oakland FSS: (415) 527-4481; (415) 638-5773 ¢; (Bay Area Forecast) (415) 568-7956 #; (Route Forecast) (415) 632-8827 #. **San Jose:** (408) 295-6611; (Bay Area Forecast) (408) 295-9750 #; (Route Forecast) (408) 295-9800 #. **San Francisco:** (Bay Area Forecast) (415) 876-0115 #; (Route Forecast) (415) 876-0111 #. **Fremont/Newark:** (Bay Area Forecast) (415) 797-8056 #; (Route Forecast) (415) 796-3632 #. **San Rafael:** (Bay Area Forecast) (415) 457-1990 #; (Route Forecast) (415) 457-6630 #. **Redwood City:** (Bay Area Forecast) (415) 366-3871 #; (Route Forecast) (415) 366-8254 #. **Belvedere:** (Bay Area Forecast) (415) 435-0904 #; (Route Forecast) (415) 435-3886 #. **Concord:** (Bay Area Forecast) (415) 798-0652 #; (Route Forecast) (415) 798-5363. **Napa:** (707) 253-8900 ¢; (Bay Area Forecast) (707) 224-6501 #; (Route Forecast) (707) 252-7931 #. **San Mateo:** (415) 692-2870 ¢. **Palo Alto:** (415) 326-5791 ¢, (415) 321-1888 #. **Walnut Creek:** (415) 933-1088 ¢.

Ontario FSS (714) 983-2618; (LAX Basin Forecast) (714) 988-6401 #; (Route Forecast) (714) 988-6536 #. **Colton:** (714) 825-0749 (LAX Basin Forecast) (714) 825-7590 #; (Route Forecast) (714) 825-4611 #. **Corona:** (714) 734-0280 (LAX Basin Forecast) (714) 734-6300 #; (Route Forecast) (714) 734-7160 #. **El Monte:** (213) 444-5720. **Hemet:** (714) 925-9230. **Montebello:** (213) 728-9957. **Santa Ana:** (714) 836-0776.

171

Paso Robles FSS (805) 238-2448.
Paso Robles San Luis Obispo-Arroyo Grand Route: (805) 544-6323.
Red Bluff FSS (916) 527-0242 @.
Redding Muni (916) 246-1556 # (1300-0600Z).
Sacramento FSS (916) 428-6500 @; (916) 428-4027 #.
Salinas FSS (408) 422-4723.
San Diego FSS (714) 291-6381 @; (714) 291-0750 # (1400-0600Z) for East County and North County. For **Carlsbad, Fallbrook, Oceanside, Vista** (714) 728-4333 @; for **Encinitas, La Costa, Vista** (714) 722-2097 @; for **Escondido, Pauma Valley, Poway, Ramona, Rancho Santa Fe, Vista** (714) 746-0028 @.
San Francisco (see Oakland FSS).
Santa Barbara FSS (805) 967-2305; (805) 967-3869 #. **Oxnard, Ventura, Camarillo, San Paula;** (805) 486-3031. **Oxnard CS/T** (805) 486-6117 #.
Santa Maria WS (805) 925-0246 (1400-0600Z).
Santa Rosa WS (707) 545-3724.
Stockton FSS (209) 982-4284 @ (1130-0330Z).
Thermal FSS (714) 399-5155; (714) 345-1612.
Ukiah FSS (707) 462-8877.

COLORADO

(Area Code—303)
Akron FSS 345-2271.
Alamosa WS 589-2547.
Colorado Springs 837-3276 (Denver FSS)
Denver FSS 321-0031 @; 388-3653 # (0500-2200). **Denver-Cheyenne-N. Platte-Akron area:** 398-3967. **Denver-Colo. Springs-Pueblo-La Junta area:** 398-3967. **Denver-Grand Junction route:** 398-5391. **Denver-Salt Lake City:**
398-5392. **Denver-Billings route:** 398-5393. **Denver-Kansas City:** 398-5394. **Denver-Albuquerque:** 321-0564. **Denver-Dallas:** 321-0676. **Denver-Phoenix:** 321-0685.
Eagle FSS 328-6575.
Grand Junction FSS 242-1801 @.
La Junta FSS 384-4311.
Pueblo WS 948-3368*.
Trinidad FSS 846-2623.

CONNECTICUT

(Area Code—203)
Bridgeport FSS 378-2344.
Danbury FSS 743-9424; 792-3977/8 ¢; 792-4696 #.
Windsor Locks FSS 623-2416 @.

DELAWARE

(Area Code 302)
Wilmington WS 323-2284*; 652-1653 #; 652-3088 ¢. **Millville FSS** 652-3479.

DISTRICT OF COLUMBIA

Washington Dulles Intl. (toll) WS (703) 661-8526*. (For Int'l flt. briefing).
Washington National FSS (202) 347-4040. **Washington:** (Local) (202) 347-4950 #, (301) 766-0757 #; (North) (202) 920-4000 #, (301) 768-6510 #; (South) (202) 920-3603 #, (301) 768-6650 #; (IFR Flight Plans only) (202) 521-7333, (301) 521-7333.
Charlottesville FSS (800) 572-6000.
Richmond FSS (Local) (800) 572-6000; (Central Virginia) (800) 572-6001 #, (800) 573-6003 ¢.

FLORIDA

Apalachicola WS (904) 654-9318 (1100-2300Z, Monday-Friday).
Crestview FSS (904) 682-2795.
Daytona Beach WS (904) 253-6131.
Ft. Myers FSS (813) 936-1857 @; **WS** (813) 322-4220 (1300-2100Z

Monday-Friday).

Gainesville FSS (904) 376-7515/6.

Jacksonville FSS (904) 641-8333 @; (904) 641-8055 #. (North) (904) 641-2424; (South) (904) 641-2433; (Southwest) (904) 641-2450; (West) (904) 641-2468.

Key West FSS (305) 296-2042; **WS** (305) 296-2741.

Lakeland WS (813) 682-4221 (1100-0500Z, Nov 15—Mar 15; 1300-2400Z, Mar 16—Nov 14).

Melbourne FSS (305) 723-6151; (305) 783-8833; (305) 269-2022.

Miami IFSS (305) 233-2600 @; (305) 526-2642; (305) 238-1337 ¢; (305) 238-1338 ¢; (from Ft. Lauderdale) (305) 524-0233 @; 467-6490 ¢. (from West Palm Beach) (305) 655-3897, 3948 ¢; (305) 655-3725. **Miami local area** (60 NM radius); (305) 233-2616/7 +; (305) 238-1337. **Miami-Palm Beach-Daytona Beach route:** (305) 238-0703/4 + **Miami-Ft. Myers-Tampa route:** (305) 238-1107/8 +. **Miami-Bimini-Nassau Bahamas route:** (305) 238-0694/5 +. **Miami-Orlando route:** (305) 238-0821/2 +. **Miami-Key West route:** (305) 238-1435 +. **Miami-Freeport Bahamas route:** (305) 238-1496 + (from Ft. Lauderdale). **Ft. Lauderdale local area** (60 NM radius); (305) 463-2402 +.

Orlando FSS (305) 894-0861.

Pensacola FSS (904) 438-1450; (904) 438-1459; **WS** (904) 453-2488; INWATS FL: (800) 342-3229.

St. Petersburg FSS (813) 531-1495/6/7; (Toll free) (1-800) 282-5921; (N/NE Route Forecast) (813) 531-5896 #; (E/SE Route Forecast) (813) 531-7714 #; (local) (813) 536-7817.

Sarasota WS (813) 365-0980 #.

Tallahassee FSS (904) 576-3141; **WS** (904) 576-1811*; (904) 576-6318.

INWATS (1-800) 342-3177.

Tampa WS (813) 223-2758 #; (813) 879-3907*.

Vero Beach FSS (305) 562-2321/2; (305) 464-1817.

W. Palm Beach WS (305) 683-3032 #.

GEORGIA

Albany FSS (912) 435-6201.

Alma FSS (912) 632-4422 (1100-0300Z, other hrs Brunswick).

Athens WS (404) 548-7318*.

Atlanta FSS (404) 691-2240 @; (404) 691-0282 ¢; (from Columbus, GA) (404) 322-6573/4 @; (from Athens, GA) (404) 548-7318; (Toll free) (1-800) 282-8074 @. **Atlanta local area:** (404) 755-6608 +. **Atlanta-Knoxville Rt:** (404) 691-0611 +. **Atlanta-Anderson, S.C.-Charlotte, N.C. Rt:** (404) 691-1244 +. **Atlanta-Jacksonville-Miami,Fla. Rt.:** (404) 691-0801 +. **Atlanta-Birmingham, Ala.-Meridian, Miss. Rt.:** (404) 691-0956 +; (from Columbus, GA. Columbus, GA. local area) (404) 327-6549 +.

Augusta WS (404) 793-6610*.

Brunswick FSS (912) 638-8641.

Columbus WS (404) 327-1153* (1130-2345Z).

Macon FSS (912) 788-5064 @; INWATS GA: (1-800) 342-7284.

Rome WS (912) 232-6801 (1145-1945Z, Mon-Fri).

Savannah FSS (912) 964-7730 @; INWATS GA: (1-800) 342-2137.

Valdosta FSS (912) 244-2361.

IDAHO

(Area Code—208)

Boise FSS 343-2525 @; 345-6163/4 #.

Burley FSS 678-8361/2.

Idaho Falls FSS 522-9024.

Lewiston **WS** 743-3841 (1130-0330Z).

Pocatello **WS** 232-0143* (1200-0400Z).

ILLINOIS

Chicago FSS (312) 626-8266; (312) 584-5830 #; (312) 626-8629 #; (312) 584-5010; (312) 379-1522 ¢; **St. Charles** (312) 584-7182 ¢; **Wheeling** (312) 541-2113 ¢; **WS** (312) 686-2155*.

Decatur FSS (217) 429-2311.

Moline FSS (319) 762-5528; (local area) (309) 762-7338 #; (route forecast) (309) 762-0394 #. (VFR/IFR Flight Plans) (309) 762-7724. **WS** (319) 326-1322.

Quincy FSS (217) 885-3251.

Rockford FSS (815) 965-6758 @.

Springfield WS (217) 525-4252.

INDIANA

Columbus FSS (812) 372-5195

Evansville WS (812) 426-2987*.

Ft. Wayne FSS (219) 747-3139.

Indianapolis FSS (317) 244-3316 @; (317) 247-2593 #.

Lafayette FSS (317) 743-1802/3.

Muncie FSS (317) 288-8961/2.

South Bend FSS (219) 232-5858.

Terre Haute FSS (812) 877-2571.

IOWA

Burlington FSS (319) 753-1626.

Cedar Rapids FSS (319) 364-7127; (local) (319) 364-0237 #; (Route Forecast) (319) 365-0597 #; (VFR/IFR Flight Plans) (319) 365-1940.

Clinton FSS (319) 243-2290.

Davenport (via Moline, Ill.) WS (319) 326-1322.

Des Moines FSS (515) 285-4640 @; (local area) (50 NM radius) (515) 285-3280 #; (East) (515) 285-1793 #; (West) (515) 285-4793 #.

Ames: (local area) (50 NM radius): (515) 233-3651 #; (East) (515) 233-3668 #. (West) (515) 233-3670 #.

Dubuque FSS (319) 556-4488; **WS** (319) 582-3171) (0545-2105Z).

Iowa City FSS (319) 338-9852; (local area) (319) 354-4980 #; (Route Forecast) (319) 354-4981 #.

Mason City FSS (515) 423-7512.

Muscatine FSS (319) 264-2090.

Ottumwa FSS (515) 682-3492.

Sioux City WS (712) 255-3944*; **FSS,** (local area) (50 NM radius) (712) 255-0617 #; Omaha (712) 258-4593 @; (Route Forecast) (712) 255-0620 #.

Waterloo FSS (319) 234-5711; **WS** (319) 234-1602*; (local area) (319) 232-8431 #.

KANSAS

Chanute FSS (316) 431-4450.

Concordia WS (913) 243-3141.

Dodge City FSS (316) 225-0218/9 @.

Emporia FSS (316) 342-7475.

Garden City FSS (316) 275-9208.

Goodland FSS (913) 899-7154 @.

Hill City FSS (913) 674-5642 (0600-2200, other hrs Goodland).

Manhattan FSS (913) 539-4606 (0600-2200, other hrs Salina).

Russell FSS (913) 483-2165.

Salina FSS (913) 825-0506/7.

Wichita FSS (316) 942-4131 @; (IFR Flight Plans only) (316) 945-9326 ¢; (50 NM Radius) (316) 945-0235 #. Hutchinson: (316) 663-2833 #; Newton: (316) 283-7400; Winfield: (316) 221-1370 #; (North) Wichita area: (316) 945-9346 #; Hutchison: (316) 663-3052 #; Winfield: (316) 221-1470 #. (South) Wichita area: (316) 945-9381; Hutchinson: (316) 663-3001 #; Winfield: (316) 221-1540 #.

KENTUCKY

Bowling Green FSS (502) 843-1152.
Erlanger WS (606) 371-6681*.
London FSS (606) 878-6122; (606) 254-2743; (Lexington Exchange) (606) 252-4708 #; (606) 252-4715 ¢.
Louisville FSS (502) 451-5344; (800) 752-6078/9. **WS** (502) 451-5344 @.
Paducah FSS (502) 442-6828.

LOUISIANA

Alexandria FSS (318) 445-3663 @.
Lafayette FSS (318) 233-4952.
Lake Charles FSS (318) 477-1784 @.
Monroe FSS (318) 322-3157.
New Orleans FSS (504) 241-2935 @; (504) 241-2352 #.
Shreveport FSS (318) 221-2211 @; **WS** (318) 635-7769 #.

MAINE

(Area Code—207)
Augusta FSS 622-6491.
Bangor FSS 947-4028.
Caribou WS 492-0161*.
Houlton FSS 532-2475.
Portland WS 775-3071*.

MARYLAND

(Area Code—301)
Baltimore WS 787-7257*; **Washington FSS:** 766-0757 #; 766-3420.
Salisbury FSS 742-8719.

MASSACHUSETTS

(Area Code—617)
Boston FSS 223-6447 @; 567-7420 @; 569-1773 #. **Boston area:** 569-6520 ¢. **Beverly area:** 927-7166 ¢. **Great Barrington:** (1-800) 833-4509 @. **North Adams:** (1-800) 833-4505 #. **Pittsfield:** (1-800) 833-4505 #; 833-4509 @; (Airport only, direct line) (1-800) 833-4509 @.

MICHIGAN

Alpena WS (517) 354-8733*.
Detroit FSS (313) 372-3737; (313) 371-1005/9 #; **Ann Arbor:** (313) 482-7210 #; **Pontiac:** (313) 338-8750 #; **Ypsilanti:** (313) 482-7210 #; **WS** (313) 729-2111*.
Flint WS (313) 234-3987*.
Grand Rapids WS (616) 949-2580 #; (50 NM radius, 1100-0500Z) (616) 949-2580; **WS** (616) 456-2268.
Houghton FSS (906) 482-0380.
Houghton Lake WS (517) 366-5392.
Jackson FSS (517) 782-0355.
Lansing FSS (517) 371-1150.
Marquette FSS (906) 475-4197; **WS** (1000-0200Z) (906) 226-8642*.
Muskgeon WS (616) 798-1380.
Pellston FSS (616) 539-8401.
Saginaw FSS (517) 695-2511.
Saulte Ste Marie FSS (1500-2300Z) (906) 635-1551; **Traverse City:** (2300-1500Z) (906) 635-1381; **WS** (906) 632-7751.
Traverse City FSS (616) 947-5056.
Ypsilanti WS (313) 729-2111*.

MINNESOTA

Alexandria FSS (612) 763-6593.
Duluth WS (218) 722-7982*; 772-1737 #.
Hibbing FSS (218) 262-3826; (218) 263-8981 #. **Benidji:** (218) 751-6815 #; **Ely:** (218) 365-5206 #; **Eveleth:** (218) 741-7243 #; **Grand Rapids:** (218) 326-1941 #, (218) 263-8981 #.
International Falls WS (218) 285-5151; (612) 283-8425*; (612) 283-9471 #.
Minneapolis FSS (612) 726-1130 @; (50 NM radius) (612) 726-1104.
Redwood Falls FSS (507) 637-5771.
Rochester FSS (507) 288-7576 @.
St. Cloud WS (0400–2200). (612) 251-3213.
Winona—See LaCrosse, Wi.

MISSISSIPPI

(Area Code—601)
Greenwood FSS 453-2631.
Jackson FSS 939-5212 @; 939-2046
#.
McComb FSS 684-7070.
Meridian FSS 482-5556; **WS** 483-5270*.

MISSOURI

Cape Girardeau FSS (314) 334-2803.
Columbia FSS (314) 449-3836 @.
Joplin FSS (417) 623-6868.
Kansas City FSS (816) 471-7565;
    (IFR Flight Plans only) (816) 421-1270 ¢. (50 NM radius) **Metro area:** (816) 421-3288 #; **TOP area:** (913) 233-5115 #; **STJ area:** (816) 279-0141 #. (East Route) **Metro area:** (816) 421-7747 #; **TOP area:** (913) 233-5116 #; STJ area: (816) 279-0170 #. (West Route) **Metro area:** (816) 421-7492 #; **TOP area:** (913) 233-5117 #; **STJ area:** (816) 279-0370 #.
St. Louis FSS (314) 532-1011 @.
    (IFR Flight Plans only) (314) 532-1321. (50 NM radius) **Metro area:** (314) 576-1108 #; **Alton:** (618) 465-0861 #; **East St. Louis:** (618) 874-2670 #; **St. Charles:** (314) 724-5577 #. (East) **Metro area:** (314) 576-1503 #; **Alton:** (618) 465-0623 #; **East St. Louis:** (618) 874-2713 #; **St. Charles:** (314) 724-5897 #. (West) **Metro area:** (314) 576-1556 #; **East St. Louis:** (618) 874-2732 #; **Alton:** (618) 465-0529 #; **St. Charles:** (314) 724-7534 #.
Springfield FSS (417) 862-3588 @.
    Springfield area: (417) 831-1503 #. **Joplin area:** (417) 624-1011 @.
Vichy FSS (314) 299-4291.

MONTANA

(Area Code—406)
Billings FSS 259-4545 @.
Bozeman FSS 388-4242.
Butte FSS 494-3004.
Cut Bank FSS 873-4522.
Glasgow WS 228-4042.
Great Falls FSS 761-7110 @.
Havre WS 265-6424.
Helena CS/T 442-9902; **WS** 442-7312.
Kalispell WS 756-4829.
Lewiston FSS 538-3639.
Livingston FSS 222-2411.
Miles City FSS 232-1503.
Missoula FSS 542-2230 @.

NEBRASKA

Chadron FSS (308) 432-3153.
Grand Island FSS (308) 382-5196
    @.
Lincoln FSS (402) 477-3929 @.
North Platte FSS (308) 532-4034 @.
Omaha FSS (402) 422-6866 @; (IFR
    Flight Plans only) (402) 422-1063
    ¢. (Route Forecast) (402) 422-1052
    #. (50 NM radius) (402) 422-1067
    #.
Scottsbluff FSS (308) 635-2615 @.
Sidney FSS (308) 254-3130.
Valentine WS (402) 376-3442.

NEVADA

(Area Code—702)
Elko FSS 738-7222.
Ely FSS 289-3051 @ (1300, other
    hrs Las Vegas)
Las Vegas FSS 736-7011/2/3/4 @;
    736-6108 #. **Los Angeles route:**
    739-7863 #; (800) 634-6474 @.
Lovelock FSS 273-2448.
Reno FSS 323-0485/6/7.
State of Nevada: (800) 492-6557.
    WATS Adjacent States: (800) 634-6474.
Tonopah FSS 482-6421.
Winnemuca WS 623-2203.

NEW HAMPSHIRE

Concord FSS (603) 224-7474 @;
    N.H. area: (1-800) 852-3427 @;

Manchester/Nashua: (603) 424-2123 @.
Lebanon FSS (603) 298-8360; **N.H. area:** (1-800) 562-1117; **Springfield, Vt. area:** (802) 885-4373; **Rutland, Vt. area:** (802) 775-2220.

NEW JERSEY

Atlantic City WS (609) 645-2345*.
Lakewood (Toms River) FSS (Philadelphia) (201) 364-6921; (201) 364-4011 #.
Millville FSS (609) 825-1173; (609) 825-1983; (609) 825-2182 #; (609) 327-1255 ¢; (800) 582-7030 @. **Dover:** (302) 653-8274; (302) 674-8605 #. **Hammonton:** (609) 561-6060; (609) 561-6599 #; (609) 561-7079 ¢. **Pittman:** (609) 589-2586 ¢. **S. Jersey Shore:** (609) 399-8096; (609) 398-6565 #; (609) 398-1162 ¢. **Wilmington:** (302) 652-3470; (302) 652-1653 #; (302) 652-3088 ¢.
Mt. Holly (Burlington Co.) FSS (Philadelphia) (609) 267-0910; (609) 267-5102 #.
Newark FSS (201) 543-5933, 543-5934; (201) 624-0068, 624-0069 #. (Local) (201) 624-5008 #. (South) (201) 624-5048 #. (West) (201) 624-5031 #; [WS (201) 624-8118*.]
Teterboro FSS (201) 288-3208, 288-3209; (201) 288-5018, 288-5019 #. (Local)(201) 288-6280 #. (South) (201) 288-6298 #. (West) (201) 288-6297 #, 288-6436 ¢. **Morristown area:** (201) 538-8087; (Local) (201) 539-8489 #; (South) (201) 539-8499 #; (West) (201) 539-8498 #. **Caldwell area:** (201) 226-6358. **Somerville area:** (201) 722-2340; (201) 526-7829 #; (Local) (201) 722-1630 #; (South) (201) 722-1610 #; (West) (201) 722-3323 #. **Monmouth area:** (201) 531-2189. **Spring Valley area:** (914) 352-0710, 352-3388. (Local) (914) 352-1307 #; (South) (914) 352-0711 #; (914) 352-1297 #.
Trenton FSS (Philadelphia) (609) 882-1590; (609) 883-3882 #; (609) 883-3885 #; (IFR Flight Plans Only) (609) 771-0363 ¢.

NEW MEXICO

(Area Code—505)
Albuquerque FSS 243-7831 @; (North) 247-4057; (South) 247-4143; (East) 247-4231; (West) 247-4329.
Carlsbad FSS 885-2042.
Clayton WS (1130-0630Z, Mon-Fri; 1130-0430Z Sat) 374-9511.
Deming FSS 546-2726.
Farmington CS/T 327-4479 (answered in Gallup).
Gallup FSS 722-4308.
Las Vegas FSS 425-7411.
Roswell FSS 347-5400 @.
Truth or Consequences FSS 894-3277.
Tucumcari FSS 461-2900.

NEW YORK

Albany FSS (518) 869-9225 @; (518) 869-0237 #. **New York State FSS** (1-800) 342-4527 #; (1-800) 342-4524 @.
Binghamton WS (607) 797-0784*.
Buffalo FSS (716) 631-9830/1 @; (716) 632-5042/3 #; (716) 846-4801/3.
Elmira FSS (607) 739-2471.
Glens Falls FSS (518) 793-2593.
La Guardia FSS (212) 898-2323 ¢; (212) 898-2339 ¢; (516) 656-5988 ¢. (From Long Island) (516) 737-3535/6/7; (516) 737-3595/6. (From New York City) (212) 995-8657/8. (From Westchester County) (914) 723-4330/4. (International Flight Planning from New York City) (212) 656-8558;

177

(212) 995-8659.

Massena FSS (315) 769-2033.

New York FSS/IFSS (516) 737-3535/6/7; **FSS** (914) 723-4330; (212) 995-8657.

Poughkeepsie FSS (914) 462-3400; (IFR Flight Plans only) (914) 462-7680/1 ¢; (Local Area) (914) 462-7690/1 #; (914) 778-7423; (914) 794-6602.

Rochester FSS (716) 325-3320/1 @; (716) 325-6250/1 #. **WS** (716) 328-7361*.

Syracuse WS (315) 455-1214*.

Utica FSS (315) 736-9023. (East) (1-800) 342-4527 #. **Rome:** (315) 337-0115. **Syracuse:** (315) 475-9904/5. **Other:** (315) 962-5667.

Watertown FSS (315) 639-6228.

Other areas of New York State: (1-800) 462-7776 @.

NORTH CAROLINA

Asheville WS (704) 684-3787*.

Cape Hatteras WS (919) 995-2321.

Charlotte FSS (704) 332-6125; (704) 334-0886 #; **WS** (704) 399-6000*. **Gastonia:** (704) 864-9213. **Salisbury:** (704) 633-4904. **Statesville:** (704) 873-0709. **N. Wilkesboro:** (704) 667-3291. **Winston-Salem:** (919) 722-0383; (919) 724-7961 #. INWATS, N.C.: (800) 222-5743.

Elizabeth City FSS (919) 338-3808 (1200-0300Z, other hrs New Bern).

Greensboro WS (919) 294-4800*; (919) 668-0789*.

Hickory FSS (704) 328-5656; (704) 322-3994 #.

High Point WS (919) 454-1776*.

New Bern FSS (919) 638-3133. INWATS. N.C.: (800) 682-2649.

Raleigh-Durham FSS (919) 755-4306 @; (919) 596-2446 @. (Local area) (919) 787-3665 #. (Northeast) (919) 787-3681 #. (Northwest) (919) 787-3683 #. (South-

west) (919) 787-3675 #. (South) (919) 787-3668; (919) 781-1510 ¢. (Greensboro) (919) 273-8660.

Rocky Mount FSS (919) 977-1815/6. **Wilson:** (919) 237-1559.

Wilmington WS (919) 763-8331.

Winston Salem WS (919) 725-6882/3*.

NORTH DAKOTA

(Area Code—701)

Bismarck WS 223-0920*.

Dickinson FSS 225-2989.

Fargo WS 232-1584*.

Grand Forks FSS 772-7201.

Jamestown FSS 252-4350.

Minot FSS 852-3696.

Williston WS 572-3198*.

OHIO

Akron WS (216) 896-2246*.

Cincinnati FSS (513) 871-8220. (Local area 50 NM radius) (513) 871-6200 #; **WS** (606) 371-6681*.

Cleveland FSS (216) 267-3700 @. (Local area 50 NM radius) (216) 579-0220 #. **Akron:** (50 NM radius): (216) 535-6153*.

Columbus FSS (614) 237-7461 @; (614) 236-8555 #. **Mansfield:** (419) 526-2132, 526-2920 #.

Dayton FSS (513) 898-3692 @; (513) 898-1033 #.

Findlay FSS (419) 422-6176/7.

Mansfield WS (1100-2300Z) (419) 522-7070.

Toledo WS (419) 865-8859*.

Youngstown FSS (216) 539-5121; (216) 759-2117; (216) 856-1993; **WS** (216) 545-5796.

Zanesville FSS (614) 453-0649.

OKLAHOMA

Gage FSS (405) 923-2601.

Hobart FSS (405) 726-5234.

McAlester FSS (918) 423-4091.

Oklahoma City FSS (405) 787-9323 @; (405) 787-9060/1 #.

Ponca City FSS (405) 765-5485.
Tulsa FSS (918) 836-3505 @; (918)
835-2364 #; (918) 836-7761 ¢.
INWATS OK (1-800) 722-4988.

OREGON

Astoria WS (503) 861-2722.
Baker FSS (503) 523-2961.
Eugene WS (503) 687-6407*.
Klamath Falls WS (503) (1545-
2345Z) 882-9474.
Medford WS (503) 773-1525*.
North Bend FSS (503) 756-4916.
Portland FSS (503) 222-1699 @;
(505) 282-2285/6 #. Hillsboro:
(503) 648-2111 @.
Redmond FSS (503) 548-2522.
Salem WS (503) 363-9829.
The Dalles FSS (509) 767-1187.

PENNSYLVANIA

Allentown WS (215) 264-1944.
Altoona FSS (814) 793-3113.
Bradford FSS (814) 362-8860.
Du Bois FSS (814) 328-2231.
Erie FSS (814) 833-1345 (1100-
0300Z, other hrs Du Bois) WS
(814) 838-1010*.
Harrisburg FSS (717) 782-3777; WS
(717) 774-3626 #; (717) 774-1818
¢.
Johnstown FSS (814) 535-3088.
Philadelphia FSS (215) 673-8020;
(215) 677-9070 #; (215) 464-6699
#; (IFR Flight Plans only) (215)
673-5657 ¢. Collegeville: (215)
489-4080; (215) 489-6122 #. Dublin: (215) 249-3000; (215) 249-
0131. West Chester: (215) 692-
6710; (215) 692-7017 #.
(From other locations in the 215
and 717 area codes 1-800-822-
3750.)
Philipsburg FSS (814) 342-0830.
Pittsburgh FSS (412) 462-3707;
(412) 462-5585/6 #; (412) 462-
5307 #; (412) 462-5334 #; (412)
462-5558/9 ¢. WS (412) 644-

2887*. Butler: (412) 282-6520 #;
(412) 282-2974 ¢. Hookstown:
(412) 573-9112 #; (412) 573-9166
¢. Washington: (412) 228-8090 #.
Wilkes-Barre FSS (717) 346-4512;
(717) 982-4301; WS (717) 457-
5650* (toll call).
Williamsport FSS (717) 368-8547
(Sunbury Exchange); (717) 286-
2770; WS (717) 368-1866*.
Toll free: (800) 932-0402 @ for:
Annville, Carlisle, Gettysburg.
(800) 692-7471 # for: Annville,
Bethel, Broque, Carlisle, Cham-
bersburg, Columbia, Fredericks-
burg, Gettysburg, Hanover, Her-
shey, Kutztown, Lancaster,
Lebannon, Middletown, Miners-
ville, Mountsville, Mt. Joy, Myers-
town, Oxford, Palmyra, Pine
Grove, Pottsville, Quarryville,
Reading, Tower City, Wellsville,
York. (800) 692-7403 ¢ for: Ann-
ville, Bethel, Broque, Carlisle,
Chambersburg, Columbia, Fred-
ericksburg, Gettysburg, Hanover,
Hershey, Kutztown, Lancaster,
Middletown, Minersville, Mounts-
ville, Mt. Joy, Myerstown, Oxford,
Palmyra, Pine Grove, Pottsville,
Quarryville, Reading, Shippen-
burg, Tower City, Wellsville, York.

RHODE ISLAND

Providence WS (401) 737-3171*.

SOUTH CAROLINA

(Area Code—803)
Anderson FSS 224-2573/4 (1100-
0300Z, other times Greer).
Charleston FSS 747-5293 @; 747-
5778 #.
Columbia WS 794-2593*; 796-
8710/11 #; FSS (803) 256-4663 ¢.
Florence FSS 662-8197. (Local area)
665-5992 #. (North) 665-5993 #.
(South) 665-5994 #. (West) 665-
5995 #. Columbia: 256-1506/7.

179

Lumberton: (919) 739-3000. (Flight Plans only) 662-5382 ¢.

Greer FSS 271-8930 @.

Strand FSS 272-6903 (1200-0200Z, other hrs Florence).

INWATS SC (1-800) 922-1816, 922-5111.

SOUTH DAKOTA

(Area Code—605)

Aberdeen FSS 225-5264 @ (0600-2200, other hrs Huron).

Huron FSS 352-3806 @.

Pierre FSS 224-5894.

Rapid City FSS 342-2302 @.

Watertown FSS 886-4581.

TENNESSEE

Chattanooga WS (615) 892-6302*.

Crossville FSS (615) 484-9541.

Dyersburg FSS (901) 285-4842 (1200-0400Z, other hrs Jackson).

Jackson FSS (901) 423-0252.

Knoxville FSS (615) 577-6651 @; (from Merryville) (615) 983-4000.

Memphis FSS (901) 345-1510 @. **Memphis** (50 NM radius): (901) 345-0590 #. **North-Cape Girardeau-St. Louis:** (901) 345-0971 #. **East-Nashville:** (901) 345-1131 #. **South-Jackson:** (901) 345-0749 #. **West-Little Rock:** (901) 345-1151 #. (IFR Flight Plans only) (901) 345-1044 ¢. INWATS TN (800) 542-6901/02.

Nashville FSS (615) 749-5378; (615) 361-0737 #; (from Nashville) (615) 367-2757/8 ¢. (Northeast) (615) 367-2990/1 #. (Southeast) (615) 367-0808/9 #. (Southwest) (615) 367-1040/1 #. (Northwest) (615) 367-2857/8 #.

Tri City FSS (1100-0300Z) (615) 323-6204.

TEXAS

Abilene FSS (915) 677-4336/7.

Alice FSS (512) 664-0184.

Amarillo FSS (806) 335-1608 @.

Austin FSS (512) 478-6695 @.

Beaumont FSS (713) 722-0288; **WS** (1230-0330Z) (713) 722-7011*.

Brownsville CS/T (512) 546-6421; (512) 425-1115 (Harlingen Exchange); **WS** (512) 542-8231*.

Childress FSS (817) 937-3892.

College Station FSS (713) 846-8784/5.

Corpus Christi WS (512) 888-8061*.

Cotulla FSS (512) 879-2417.

Dalhart FSS (806) 249-2006.

Dallas FSS (214) 350-3311 @. (Routes West and North) (214) 357-4343 #. (Routes East and South) (214) 357-4344 #.

Del Rio WS (512) 775-1045*.

El Paso FSS (915) 778-6448 @; (915) 778-4487 #.

Fort Worth FSS (817) 624-8471 @; (817) 626-3071/2 #.

Galveston FSS (713) 744-3255 (0600-2200, other hrs Houston); **WS** (713) 765-5448*.

Gregg County CS/T (214) 643-2266/7.

Houston FSS (713) 644-8361; (713) 644-8676 ¢. (Local area:) (713) 641-3000 #. **Houston-New Orleans:** (713) 641-3001 #. **Houston-Dallas:** (713) 641-3002 #. **Houston-Midland** (713) 641-3003 #. **Houston-Brownsville:** (713) 641-3004/5.

Lubbock FSS (806) 762-0511.

Lufkin FSS (713) 634-3319.

McAllen FSS (512) 682-2878/9.

Midland FSS (915) 563-2611 @.

Mineral Wells FSS (817) 325-5922.

Palacios FSS (512) 972-2559.

Port Arthur WS (713) 722-0476*.

San Angelo WS (915) 949-3646*.

San Antonio FSS (512) 826-9561 @.

Victoria WS (512) 575-3182*.

Waco WS (817) 754-3126*.

Wichita Falls FSS (817) 855-5574 @.

Wink FSS (915) 527-3351

UTAH

(Area Code—801)
Bryce Canyon FSS 834-5311.
Cedar City FSS 586-3806.
Salt Lake City FSS 328-4251 @; 364-5571 #.

VERMONT

(Area Code—802)
Bennington FSS (1-800) 833-4505 #; (1-800) 833-4509 @.
Burlington FSS 878-3393, 863-6548 #. WS 862-9883*.
Montpelier FSS 223-2376. Vt. area: (1-800) 642-3192.

VIRGINIA

Blacksburg FSS (703) 552-6170.
Bristol WS (615) 323-8242*.
Danville FSS (804) 793-1163 (1100-0300Z, other hrs Roanoke); (804) 793-7131 #.
Lynchburg WS (0600-1930) (804) 239-5811*; FSS (804) 846-6566 #.
Newport News FSS (804) 877-0209 @; (800) 582-1013.
Norfolk WS (804) 855-3029 @.
Roanoke FSS (703) 362-1668 @; (703) 563-4901 #.
Elsewhere in Virginia (call toll free) (800) 572-6000/1/2/3/4.

WASHINGTON

Bellingham FSS (206) 734-6400.
Ephrata FSS (509) 754-2361.
Hoquiam FSS (206) 533-3432.
Olympia WS (206) 357-6169*.
Seattle FSS (206) 767-2726 @; (206) 767-4002 #.
Spokane FSS (509) 456-4546 @.
Toledo FSS (206) 864-2371 (1700-0100Z, other hrs Seattle).
Walla Walla FSS (509) 529-1413; (509) 525-6531 #. Pasco: (509) 545-9403 #. Pendleton: (503) 276-8889 #. Spokane: (509) 534-3154 #.
Wenatchee FSS (509) 884-6656.
Yakima WS (509) 453-8975.

WEST VIRGINIA

(Area Code—304)
Beckley WS 252-3171*.
Bluefield FSS 325-6521.
Charleston FSS 343-8919 @.
Elkins FSS 636-0810 @.
Huntington FSS 453-3951 @.
Martinsburg FSS 263-9353.
Morgantown FSS 292-9489.
Parkersburg FSS 464-4360.
Wheeling CS/T 277-1252.

WISCONSIN

Eau Claire FSS (2300-1500Z) (715) 835-2269.
Green Bay FSS (414) 494-7417 @.
La Crosse FSS (608) 784-3170. Winona, Mn: (507) 452-1046.
Lone Rock FSS (608) 583-2661 (1400-2200Z, other hrs LaCrosse or (608) 583-5011).
Milwaukee FSS (414) 481-1060 @; (414) 482-4601 #.
Wausau FSS (715) 845-7396.

WYOMING

(Area Code—307)
Casper FSS 235-1555 @.
Cheyenne WS 638-6437*.
Denver FSS 635-4187.
Lander WS 332-2718.
Laramie FSS 745-4845.
Rawlins FSS 324-3241.
Rock Springs FSS 362-2121.
Sheridan FSS 674-7426 @.
Worland FSS 347-4122.

PACIFIC REGION

Guam IFSS 355-5814. Terminal weather on request. SSB receiving capacity available on all HF frequencies.
Hilo FSS 935-4555; WS 935-5533. Surface weather reports for Gen-

eral Lyman, Waimea-Kohala, and Keahole available on request via air/ground voice communications frequency.

Honolulu, Oahu FSS 836-1538; 836-1968 #; **WS** 836-2102. Scheduled weather broadcast service available 1500-0800Z. Other times surface weather reports avilable on request via air/ground voice communications frequency.

Enterprise, Outer Islands: (Dial operator and ask for the enterprise number) **Kauai:** 5408; 7115 #.

Maui: 5407; 7116 #. **Lanai:** 7119; 7121 #. **Molokai:** 7118; 7120 #. **Hawaii:** 7117 #. **Lihue WS:** 245-3711

Maui FSS 877-5172; 877-3045 (1600-0800Z); **WS** 877-6825. Surface weather reports for Maui, Upolu, and Lanai are available on request via air/ground voice communications frequency.

PUERTO RICO

San Juan IFSS (809) 791-1780; **WS** (809) 791-0376.

Toll-free FSS Telephone Numbers

The FAA has embarked on a program to provide toll-free phone service to certain flight service stations. Pilots should use the numbers only when calling from within the FSS area of responsibility. **The FAA warns that abuse of toll-free calling may result in termination of the service.** Current toll-free lines are listed below.

New England Region:

Augusta, ME	(800) 452-8787
Bangor, ME	1-(800) 432-7365
Boston, MA	(800) 962-3550/3551
Bradley, CT	(800) 862-7642/7683
Concord, NH	(800) 562-3123/3125
Houlton, ME	(800) 432-7995
Lebanon, NH	1-(800) 562-1117
Montpelier, VT	(800) 642-3192

Eastern Region:

Altoona, PA	(800) 252-3887
Bradford, PA	1-(800) 652-0561
Buffalo, NY	(800) 462-7776
DuBois, PA	(800) 262-8956
Gary, PA	(800) 352-0022
Harrisburg, PA	(800) 932-0402
Newport News, VA	(800) 582-1013
Philadelphia, PA	(800) 822-3750
Pittsburgh, PA	(800) 242-8941/8954
Utica, NY	(800) 962-5667
Washington, DC	(800) 572-6000
Wilkes-Barre, Scranton, PA	(800) 432-8028

Southern Region:

Albany, GA	(800) 342-6650
Atlanta, GA	(800) 282-8074
Bowling Green, KY	(800) 452-5995
Charleston, SC	(800) 922-4503
Crossville, TN	(800) 262-6787
Florence, SC	(800) 922-5111
Fort Myers, FL	(800) 282-0808
Gainesville, FL	(800) 342-3405
Greer, SC	(800) 922-1816
Hickory, NC	(800) 222-5743
Jackson, TN	(800) 372-8220
Jacksonville, FL	(800) 342-1432
Knoxville, TN	(800) 362-9800
Lewisville, KY	(800) 752-6078
London, KY	(800) 442-7883
Macon, GA	(800) 342-7284
Melbourne, FL	(800) 432-6281
Memphis, TN	(800) 552-5002 (within area code 901)
Miami, FL	(800) 432-4716
Nashville, TN	(800) 342-1654
New Bern, NC	(800) 682-2649
Orlando, FL	(800) 432-0344
Paducah, KY	(800) 592-5415
Pensacola, FL	(800) 432-3229
Raleigh, NC	(800) 662-7272
Savannah, GA	(800) 342-2137
St. Petersburg, FL	(800) 282-5921
Tallahassee, FL	(800) 342-3177
Vero Beach, FL	(800) 432-8240

Central Region:

Mason City, IA	(800) 392-6690
North Platte, NE	(800) 662-2930
Springfield, MO	1-(800) 492-7621

Rocky Mountain Region:

Cedar City, UT	(800) 662-1610
Denver, CO	(800) 332-1854
Salt Lake City, UT	(800) 662-9038
Trinidad, CO	(800) 332-3644

Western Region:

Las Vegas, NV	(800) 492-6557, 634-6474
Red Bluff, CA	(800) 822-9636

183

Little Rock, AR	(800) 482-1159
Oklahoma City, OK	(800) 522-3325
Tulsa, OK	(800) 722-4988

At the present time, the Great Lakes region does not have FSS toll-free telephone lines.

The ICAO Standard Atmosphere Table

ALTITUDE (Ft.)	TEMPERATURE		SPEED OF SOUND (Knots)	PRESSURE (In. Hg)
	(°C)	(°F)		
0	15	59.0	661.7	29.92
1,000	13.019	55.4	659.5	28.86
2,000	11.037	51.9	657.2	27.82
3,000	9.056	48.3	654.9	26.82
4,000	7,075	44.7	652.6	25.84
5,000	5.094	41.2	650.3	24.90
6,000	3.113	37.6	647.9	23.98
7,000	1.132	34.0	645.6	23.09
8,000	—.850	30.5	643.3	22.22
9,000	—2.831	26.9	640.9	21.39
10,000	—4.812	23.3	638.6	20.58
11,000	—6.794	19.8	636.2	19.79
12,000	—8.775	16.2	633.9	19.03
13,000	—10.756	12.6	631.5	18.29
14,000	—12.737	9.1	629.1	17.58
15,000	—14.718	5.5	626.7	16.89
20,000	—24.624	—12.3	614.6	13.75
25,000	—34.530	—30.2	602.2	11.10
30,000	—44.436	—48.0	589.5	8.89
35,000	—54.34	—65.8	576.7	7.04
40,000	—56.500	—69.7	573.	5.54

Note: Temperatures and speed of sound become constant in the standard atmosphere at 37,000 ft. msl.

Rule of thumb for estimating standard atmospheric temperatures up to 35,000 ft: (1) Double the altitude. (2) Subtract 15. (3) Change the sign. In lower altitudes the temperature is a positive (+) value. The result will be temp. in degrees centigrade.

SECTION 3

In Flight

VOR Reception—Altitudes and Distance

CLASS OF NAVAID	ALTITUDES	DISTANCE (Nautical Miles)
T (terminal)	to 12,000 feet	25
L (low altitude)	to 18,000 feet	40
H (high altitude)	to 18,000 feet	40
H (high altitude)	14,500 – 17,999 feet	100*
H (high altitude)	18,000 – FL 450	130
H (high altitude)	Above FL 450	100

*Applicable only within the conterminous 48 states

VORs operate within the 108.0-117.95 MHz Very High Frequency (VHF) band. They are subject to line-of-sight reception.

Altitude (Feet)	Line of Sight (Statute Miles)
500	30
1,000	45
2,000	65
3,000	80
5,000	100
7,000	120
10,000	140
15,000	175

Note: Lack of sufficient altitude is often a cause of communications difficulties when the location of remoted ATC transmitter-receiver sites is unknown.

Keep in mind, the only positive method of identifying a VOR is by its Morse Code identification or by the recorded automatic voice identification, which is always indicated by use of the word "VOR" following the Navaid's name.

Radio Frequency Utilization

Low/Medium/High Frequencies
(Low—30–300 kHz; Medium—300–3,000 kHz; High—3,000–30,000 kHz)
200–415 and 510–535 kHz—Transmitting frequencies of L/MF radio ranges,

aeronautical and marine radio beacons, and ILS compass locators.

535–1605 kHz—Radio broadcasting stations (AM) that are extensively used for aircraft homing.

500 kHz—International distress frequency for ships and aircraft over the seas.

Very High Frequencies
(30-300 MHz/30,000–300,000 kHz)

VHF frequencies that are not specified below as transmitting on guarding frequencies are normally used for both purposes.

Navigation Aids
75 MHz—Transmitting frequencies of fan markers, Z markers and ILS markers.

108.0 MHz—Used for VOR test facilities.

108.1–111.9 MHz—ILS localizers with or without voice. Operated on odd tenths.

108.2–111.8 MHz—Transmitting frequencies of terminal VORs. Operated on even tenths (nav and voice). Also used for VOR test facilities (VOT).

112.0–117.9 MHz—Transmitting frequencies of VORs (nav and voice).

Use of Frequencies in Voice Communications

In any communications with FSS or tower where the reply is expected on a different frequency from the calling frequency, the frequency on which reply is expected should be specified in the initial call.

The receive-only channel of 122.5 MHz is provided only at towers where service history warrants its continued use.

At airports where a full-time Flight Service Station is also located with a part-time tower, the tower frequency will be used by the FSS for airport advisory service during hours the tower is closed. At non-tower airports with an FSS, 123.6 MHz is the airport advisory frequency.

Standard FSS channeling includes 122.1 MHz for receive-only at VOR sites, 122.2 MHz as the common en route frequency, with additional channels as traffic warrants. 122.0 MHz is available for En route Flight Advisory Service (EFAS or Flight Watch).

Military facilities (USAF or Navy) where voice is available do not guard FSS frequencies or provide en route services; however, some military facilities guard 126.2 MHz for civil aircraft.

At non-tower airports the frequency to use to advise others of your location and intentions (flight or ground) is 123.6 MHz at airports with an FSS. At airports with Unicom, 122.7, 122.8, or 123.0 MHz as appropriate. At airports with neither an FSS nor Unicom, 122.9 MHz is used.

Voice Communication Frequencies
118.0–121.4 MHz—Air Traffic Control

121.5 MHz—Emergency Frequency, ELT signals

121.6–121.9 MHz—Airport Ground Control (ELT Test on 121.6)

121.95 MHz—Flight Schools

121.975 MHz—Private Aircraft Advisory (FSS)

122.0 MHz—FSS En route Flight Advisory Service ("Flight Watch")

122.025–122.075 MHz—FSS
122.1 MHz—FSS receive only with VOR or FSS Simplex
122.125–122.175 MHz—FSS
122.2 MHz—FSS Common En Route Simplex
122.225–122.675 MHz—FSS
122.7 MHz—Unicom, uncontrolled airports
122.725 MHz—Unicom, private airports not open to the public
122.75 MHz—Unicom, private airports not open to the public and Air-to-Air Communications
122.775 MHz—Future Unicom or Multicom
122.8 MHz—Unicom, uncontrolled airports
122.825 MHz—Future Unicom or Multicom
122.85 MHz—Multicom
122.875 MHz—Future Unicom or Multicom
122.9 MHz—Multicom
122.925 MHz—Multicom—Natural Resources
122.950 MHz—Unicom controlled airports
122.975 MHz—Unicom—high altitude
123.0 MHz—Unicom, uncontrolled airports
123.025 MHz—Future Unicom or Multicom
123.05 & 123.075 MHz—Unicom, heliports
123.1 MHz—Search and Rescue, temporary control towers
123.15–123.575 MHz—Flight Test
123.3 & 123.5 MHz—Flight Schools
123.6–123.65 MHz—FSS or Air Traffic Control
123.675–128.8 MHz—Air Traffic Control
128.825–132.0 MHz—Aeronautical En Route (ARINC)
132.05–135.95 MHz—Air Traffic Control

En Route Flight Service

All FSSs are ready to provide pilots with en route flight information or assistance at any time. You may call any FAA Radio for latest weather reports, upper wind velocities, airport conditions and other flight information. If you become lost or uncertain of your position, call any FAA Radio. Personnel at these stations are trained to assist pilots in establishing position by any of the following methods: (a) visual reference to terrain features; (b) VHF direction-finding methods; (c) VOR triangulations.

Additionally, En Route Flight Advisory Service (EFAS or "Flight Watch") is now available throughout the conterminous U.S. along prominent and heavily traveled flyways. For a more detailed description of EFAS and its weather reporting functions, see Section 2 of this Handbook.

Radio Phraseology

It is important that every pilot know and understand the proper terminology used in pilot/controller communications. Use of the proper terms in the correct context enhances safety by eliminating misunderstandings. The Pilot/Controller Glossary, found in Section 1 of this Handbook, was developed by the FAA for just this purpose. Refer to it for the standard terms and phrases used in the National Airspace System.

Aircraft Call Signs
During initial contact with a ground station, pilots should state the aircraft type, model, or manufacturer's name with the digits/letters of the aircraft registration. Example: *Comanche four three two one Papa*. Abbreviated call signs including aircraft type and the last three characters of the N-number may be used only after communications are established.

Ground Station Call Signs
Use the location name followed by the facility type. Examples:
Miami Approach—Miami Approach Control
Houston Center—Houston Air Traffic Control Center
Washington Clearance Delivery—IFR clearances at Washington National Airport
Teterboro Tower—airport traffic control tower at Teterboro
St. Louis Departure—departure control at St. Louis
Morrisville Ground—ground controller at Morrisville
Florence Radio—Flight Service Station at Florence
Oakland Flight Watch—En route FLight Advisory Service from FSS

Time
Use the 24-hour clock and speak each digit separately. Example: *Zero Eight Two Five*—0825. (Keep in mind that for operational purposes the FAA uses Greenwich Mean Time. See Section 1 for time conversions.)

Flight Altitudes
Up to, but not including, 18,000 ft. msl, state the separate digits of the thousands, plus the hundreds, if appropriate. Examples: *One Zero Thousand*—10,000; *One Four Thousand Five Hundred*—14,500. At and above 18,000 ft., state the words "flight level," followed by the separate digits of the flight level. Examples: *Flight Level Two Zero Zero*—20,000 ft.; *Flight Level Two Three Five*—23,500 ft.

Directions
Use three digits for magnetic course, bearing, heading or wind direction. The word "true" must be added when it applies. Examples: *Zero Five Zero True*—050 degree true course; *Three Six Zero*—360 degree magnetic bearing.

Speeds
Use the separate digits of the speed followed by "knots" or "miles per hour." Examples: *One Three Zero Knots* or *One Zero Five Miles Per Hour*. Note: controllers always use "Knots."

Microphone Technique
Keep contacts brief. Do not read back altimeter setting, taxi instructions, or wind and runway information to control towers except for verification or clarification of instructions.

Avoid calling Flight Service Stations at 15 minutes past the hour, which interferes with scheduled weather broadcasts.

Before transmitting, make certain that the receiver volume is turned up and that someone else is not already transmitting on the frequency. When using a hand microphone, hold it upright and directly in front of the mouth before transmitting. Speak clearly.

Remember that low altitude can often be a factor when there is poor reception from a ground facility. Repeated call-ups when no one answers probably mean that your transmissions are blocking the frequency for other users who are in a more advantageous position with respect to the ground antenna site. If necessary, ask another aircraft to relay your message.

Determining Time and Distance to a Radio Facility

Formulas:

$$\frac{\text{time in seconds between bearings}}{\text{degrees of bearing change}} = \text{minutes to the station}$$

$$\frac{\text{TAS}^* \times \text{time in minutes between bearings}}{\text{degrees of bearing change}} = \text{miles to the station}$$

*If known, ground speed should be substituted for TAS.

Procedure:

Turn aircraft to a magnetic heading that places the radio facility at a wingtip position. Start timing and fly an accurate heading until radio compass instruments indicate a measurable bearing change from the station. A bearing change of 10° is most commonly used because it greatly simplifies the mental computations.

Example

If it requires 2 minutes to fly a 10° bearing change, the aircraft is 12 minutes from the station.

$$\frac{120 \text{ seconds}}{10°} = 12 \text{ minutes from station}$$

If the true airspeed (preferably ground speed) is known to be 150 mph, then the distance to the station will be very close to 30 miles.

$$\frac{150 \text{ mph} \times 2 \text{ min}}{10°} = 30 \text{ statute miles from station}$$

Note: When flying cross-country, off airways, this procedure is a convenient way of double-checking aircraft position by utilizing any available radio facility as the aircraft comes abeam of it.

Lighted Navigation Aids

Aeronautical Light Beacons

The light beacon is a visual navaid which flashes white and/or colored light, that is used to indicate the location of airports, landmarks, certain points of the Federal airways in mountainous terrain, and to mark hazards.

Colors

The colors and color combinations of airport rotating beacons and supplementary lights are:

White and green	.Lighted land airport
*Green alone	.Lighted land airport
White and yellow	.Lighted water airport
*Yellow alone	.Lighted water airport
White and red	.Landmark or navigational point
White alone (rare)	.Unlighted land airport
Red alone	.Hazard
White	.Hazard
Green, Yellow, and White	.Lighted heliport

*Green or yellow alone is used only in connection with a not-far-distant white-and-green or white-and-yellow beacon.

Hazards

Red flashes only, from a rotating beacon or a code beacon, mean the presence of an obstruction or an area on the ground used for purposes hazardous to air navigation. (Steady-burning red lights are employed near airports to mark obstructions and are also used to supplement flashing lights in marking en route obstructions.)

Obstruction Lighting

High-intensity flashing white lights are being used to identify some supporting structures of overhead transmission lines located across rivers, canyons, and gorges. These lights flash in a middle-to-lower sequence at approximately 60 flashes per minute. The uppermost light is normally installed near the top of the supporting structure, while the lowest light indicates the approximate lower portion of the wire span. The lights are beamed toward the companion structure and identify the area of the wire span.

High-intensity flashing white lights are now being used in some locations to identify tall structures, such as smokestacks and towers, as obstructions to air navigation. These lights provide a 360° coverage about the structure and consist of from one to seven levels of lights, depending upon the height of the structure. They flash at a rate of 40 flashes per minute and when more than one level of lights is used, the vertical banks flash simultaneously.

Military Airports

Military airport beacons flash alternately white and green, but are differentiated from civil beacons by two quick white flashes (called split-beacon) between the green flashes.

Daylight Beacon Operation

Operation of an airport rotating beacon during the hours of daylight may indicate that the ground visibility in the control zone is less than 3 miles and/or the ceiling is less than 1,000 feet and that a traffic clearance is required for landings, takeoffs and flight in the traffic pattern.

Fuel Saving While Flying

Use economy cruise power settings, normally in the 50 to 65 percent power range. Such settings may be used with safety and increased fuel economy except with new or rebuilt engines during the first 100 hours of operation. Consult your aircraft manual for specifics.

Plan ground activity to reduce taxiing and on-the-ground running of engine.

Keep plane clean since mud, bird dropping, and dirt increase drag, reduce speed and raise fuel consumption.

Correct improper rigging, which may be evidenced by the need to hold aileron or rudder during level cruise. An out-of-rig plane is slower and wastes fuel.

Fly direct courses in VFR weather, rather than flying from VOR to VOR. Pay strict attention to navigation, staying on course and correcting drift using visual check points. The shorter distance saves fuel.

File IFR only when necessary due to bad weather. IFR procedures require more fuel and more time in the air, often as much as 20% more.

Use intersection takeoffs at large airports, if possible, saving taxi time and holdups at the end of a runway.

Proper spacing in the traffic pattern will reduce go-arounds which use extra fuel.

Leaning Techniques

Proper leaning at cruise power is both practical and economical. Leaning reduces the cost of fuel, provides for a smoother operating engine with less vibration, extends the range of the aircraft, reduces the possibility of spark plug fouling, establishes more normal engine temperatures (particularly in cold weather), and will provide the fastest airspeed for the power setting.

Damage to an engine by leaning is usually done at takeoff or climb. Leaning the typical general aviation piston engine at medium cruise power or less rarely damages an engine as long as the cylinder head and oil temperatures are not excessive and the engine operates smoothly.

Manufacturers of small four- and six-cylinder normally aspirated engines recommend that during climb the pilot maintain his mixture full rich until he is beyond 5,000 feet in order to prevent overheating and detonation in the engine. If climb continues above 5,000 feet, then this type of powerplant may be leaned somewhat, but only for engine smoothness and efficiency, since the climb configuration is not a fuel economy one. Climb above 5,000 feet permits some leaning because the available horsepower on the normally aspirated engine has been reduced to the point where leaning will not damage the engine. Furthermore, this type of engine would be running too rich.

Although 5,000 feet is a basic climb reference point for the normally aspirated engine, leaning these powerplants at cruise below 5,000 is a simple matter, too. With a direct-drive normally aspirated engine, leaning at cruise (75% power or less) may be accomplished at any altitude providing the pilot follows the limitations provided in the aircraft manual if the plane has a manual mixture control. For example, suppose a pilot wishes to fly cross-country over flat terrain at 2,000 feet. As long as he does not exceed the cruise power recommendation by the manufacturer, he may lean his engine at that cruise power wherever he desires as long as temperatures are not excessive and the engine operates smoothly.

Some geared and supercharged engines with manual mixture control permit similar leaning, but it should be done at cruise power (65% power or less) in order to avoid detonation and possible engine damage.

Flights from high elevation airports (5,000 feet or higher) require leaning on the ground prior to takeoff for efficient engine performance. Carburetors and fuel injectors are set by the factory on the rich side to protect the engine. In the thinner air at 5,000 feet or above, the fuel metering device will be too rich in most cases and will not perform efficiently. Furthermore, due to the less dense air the engine horsepower has deteriorated so that normally aspirated engines can only produce in the vicinity of 75% power. Thus, with normally aspirated engines and with a fixed-pitch prop, run engine up to cruise rpm and lean mixture until engine is smooth, then take off with mixture in that position. For other models, consult the airplane owner's manual.

A good rule of thumb for a satisfactory compromise between best power and best economy for all aircraft engines with an exhaust gas temperature gauge (EGT) is: at medium cruise power, lean to peak, then enrichen until the temperature drops 50° (50° on the rich side of peak). However, it is best to check the engine manufacturer's recommendation for your specific powerplant.

Cruising Altitudes – Flight Levels

Altimeter Setting

Below 18,000 feet msl, set the altimeter to the current setting reported by a station that is within 100 nautical miles, if possible. Set the altimeter to the elevation of the departure airport if the aircraft is not equipped with a radio.

At or above 18,000 feet msl, set the altimeter to standard setting of 29.92 inches Hg. From this point upward, flight levels are used to express altitude. For instance, Flight Level 195 is an altimeter indication of 19,500 feet. The lowest usable flight level may be a figure numerically greater than 180, depending upon atmospheric conditions. For example, when the actual atmospheric pressure is 27.92 inches Hg, an aircraft at Flight Level 200 will be at an actual height of 18,000 feet msl and will be at the lowest usable flight level.

Direction of Flight

Visual Flight Rules—When operating VFR above 3,000 feet and higher than 3,000 feet above the surface, in level cruising flight, you must operate at the altitude or flight level appropriate to your direction of flight, as indicated as follows (see FAR 91.109).

VFR Altitudes and Flight Levels—
Controlled and Uncontrolled Airspace

Magnetic Course	Above 3000' AGL Below 18,000' MSL	Above 18,000' MSL to FL 290 (except in PCA)	Above FL 290 (except in PCA)
0° to 179°	Odd thousands MSL plus 500'	Odd Flight Levels plus 500'	Fly 4000' intervals beginning at FL 300
180° to 359°	Even thousands MSL plus 500'	Even Flight Levels plus 500'	Fly 4000' intervals beginning at FL 320

Instrument Flight Rules—In controlled airspace, the altitude or flight level to be flown is the one assigned by air traffic control. In uncontrolled airspace, when operating IFR in level cruising flight, you must operate at the altitude or flight level appropriate to your direction of flight, as indicated below (see FAR 91.121).

IFR Altitudes and Flight Levels—
Controlled Airspace

Magnetic Course	Below 18,000' MSL	At or above 18,000' MSL but below FL 290	At or above FL 290
0° to 179°	Odd thousands MSL	Odd Flight Levels	Fly 4000' intervals beginning at FL 290
180° to 359°	Even thousands MSL	Even Flight Levels	Fly 4000' intervals beginning at FL 310

VFR WEATHER MINIMUMS

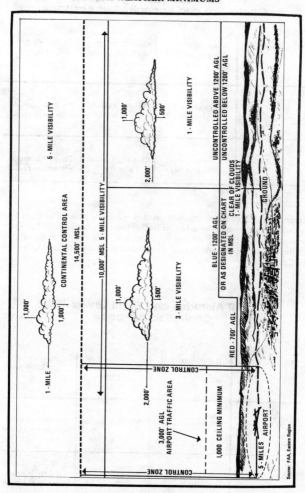

194

Mountain Flying

The following suggestions come from the most experienced mountain pilots in the Rocky Mountain area. It is recommended that flights be planned for early morning or late afternoon, since heavy turbulence is often encountered in the early afternoon, especially in the summer. Attempt flight with as little weight as possible. Stay out of canyons; fly the ridges. Know your winds at all times. Dual instruction on mountain flying with an experienced mountain pilot is VERY helpful.

General Preflight and Flight Technique Advice

1. File a flight plan, if possible. If not, fill in a "cross-country log," which mountain-state airport operators maintain.

2. Study sectionals for altitudes over route and obvious checkpoints. Prominent peaks make excellent checkpoints.

3. Plan the flight so the intended route covers populated areas and well-known mountain passes.

4. Don't hesitate to phone for weather information at your destination in case of doubt.

5. A weather check is essential for mountain flying. Ask specifically about winds aloft even when the weather is good. Expect winds above 10,000 feet to be prevailing westerlies in the mountain states.

6. If winds aloft at your proposed altitude are above 35 mph, don't fly.

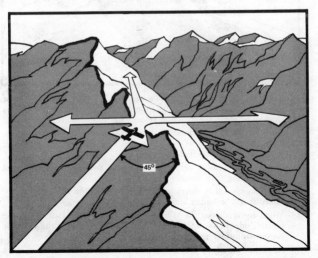

Winds will be of much greater velocity over passes than reported at stations a few miles away.

7. Don't fly in doubtful or bad weather such as thunderstorms in summer, and snowstorms with high winds in colder weather.

8. Frost, ice or snow adhering to aircraft surfaces interferes with lift and should be removed before attempting takeoff.

9. Maintain sufficient altitude en route to permit gliding to a reasonably safe landing area.

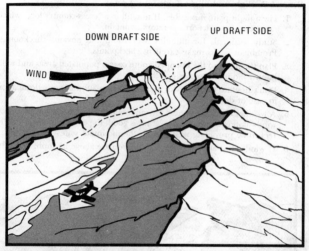

10. Know the wind direction at all times, and compare it to water as it flows up, over, and down the mountain ranges. Watch for abrupt changes of wind direction and velocity in mountain areas.

11. Keep in mind that the actual horizon is near the base of the mountain. Using summit peaks as a horizon will result in the aircraft being placed in a constant climb attitude.

12. If you have a radio, keep it tuned to the nearest FSS for current weather along your route.

13. Your engine will be developing less horsepower at higher altitudes. Takeoffs will be longer and climb angle reduced.

14. When flying through a valley or canyon, the best path is on the updraft side. If low level flight is necessary, fly through the valley or canyon from high end to low end.

15. Approach mountain passes with all the excess altitude possible, since

downdrafts may be expected on the downwind side. Approaching the pass over a ridge will lessen this effect a great deal. Two thousand feet or more of clearance is preferred on windy days.

16. Approach passes and ridges at a 45° angle so that you will be able to turn approximately 90° into a valley or lower terrain in case you encounter severe downdrafts.

17. If you encounter a downdraft, don't be alarmed. Keep your nose down and maintain normal airspeed. If you have altitude, continue through it and expect a compensating updraft. If in doubt, turn back and try crossing again at a different location and if possible at a higher altitude.

18. Don't fly up the middle of a canyon. Fly on the downwind side in order to take advantage of upcurrents and to provide room to execute a turn-around. Don't be suckered into a blind canyon climbing out of a valley.

19. Don't fly closer than necessary to terrain such as cliffs or rugged areas. Dangerous turbulence may be expected, especially with high winds.

20. Remember to file a flight plan and make position reports with Flight Service, or: LET SOMEONE KNOW AT POINT OF TAKEOFF THE ROUTE YOU INTEND TO FLY, WHEN YOU WILL TAKE OFF, AND YOUR ETA AT DESTINATION.

Airspeed Indicator Markings

Red Radial Line—Never-exceed speed (Vne)

Yellow Arc—Caution range between maximum structural cruise speed (Vno) and Vne

Green Arc—Normal operating range, upper limit is maximum structural cruise speed (Vno), lower limit is power off stall speed flaps and landing gear retracted (Vs₁)

White Arc—Flap operating range; upper limit is maximum full flaps extended speed (Vfe); lower limit is power off full flaps and landing gear extended stall speed (Vso)

For Twins

Blue Radial Line—One-engine inoperative best rate of climb speed (Vyse)

Red Radial Line—Minimum control speed one engine inoperative (Vmc)

Normally Used Transponder Codes

VFR (all altitudes) 1200
IFR .... as assigned by ATC
Hijack Code 7500
Radio Failure Code .... 7700 for 1 min., then 7600
Emergency Code 7700

Terminal Radar Programs

Stage I Service (Radar Advisory Service for VFR aircraft)

In addition to using radar for the control of IFR aircraft, Stage I facilities provide traffic information and limited vectoring to VFR aircraft on a workload permitting basis. Vectoring service may be provided when requested by the pilot or with pilot agreement when suggested by ATC.

Stage II Service (Radar Advisory and Sequencing for VFR aircraft)

Stage II facilities provide traffic information on a workload permitting basis and radar vectors to sequence IFR and participating VFR traffic into the traffic pattern. If requested by the pilot, radar traffic information may also be provided to departing VFR aircraft.

After radar contact is established, the pilot may navigate on his own into the traffic pattern or, depending on traffic conditions, he may be directed to fly specified headings to position the flight behind a preceding aircraft in the approach sequence. When a flight is positioned behind the preceding aircraft and the pilot reports having that aircraft in sight, he will be instructed to follow it.

Standard radar separation will be provided between IFR aircraft until being sequenced and the pilot sees the traffic that is to be followed. Standard radar separation between VFR or between VFR and IFR traffic will not be provided.

If arriving or departing aircraft does not want Stage II service, the pilot should state "negative Stage II" or a similar comment, on initial contact with either approach control or ground control respectively.

Stage III Service (Radar Sequencing and Separation Service for VFR aircraft)

Stage III service provides sequencing and separation between all participating VFR aircraft and all IFR aircraft operating within the airspace defined as the Terminal Radar Service Area (TRSA). The locations of TRSAs are listed and graphically depicted in the publication Graphic Notices and Supplemental Data.

There is no requirement for pilots to contact an approach facility when flying inside a designated TRSA. According to the FAA, "pilot participation is urged, but is not mandatory." A VFR aircraft entering a TRSA is assumed to be "participating" unless approach control or ground control is notified by the pilot on initial contact that he does not wish Stage III service.

Pilots operating VFR in a TRSA (1) Must maintain an altitude when assigned by ATC. ATC may assign altitudes for separation that do not conform to FAR 91.109. When the altitude assignment is no longer required, the instruction "resume appropriate VFR altitudes," will be broadcast. Pilots must then return to an altitude that conforms for FAR 91.109 as soon as practicable.

(2) When not assigned an altitude pilots should coordinate with ATC prior to any altitude change.

(3) Within the TRSA, traffic information on observed but unidentified targets will, to the extent possible, be provided all IFR and participating VFR aircraft. At the request of the pilot, he will be vectored to avoid the

observed traffic, insofar as possible, provided the aircraft to be vectored is within the airspace under the jurisdiction of the controller.

(4) Departing aircraft should inform ATC of their intended destination and/or route of flight and proposed cruising altitude, if they wish to receive Stage III service.

Note: The Terminal Radar Service Programs are not to be interpreted as relieving pilots of their responsibilities to see and avoid other traffic operating in basic VFR weather conditions, to maintain appropriate terrain and obstruction clearance, or to remain in weather conditions equal to or better than required by FAR 91.105. Whenever compliance with an assigned route, heading and/or altitude is likely to compromise the pilot's responsibility respecting terrain and obstruction clearance and weather minima, approach control should be so advised and a revised clearance or instruction obtained.

Terminal Control Areas

Special operating rules are now in effect at 21 major air-hub locations. These Terminal Control Areas consist of controlled airspace extending upward from the surface, or from specific base altitudes, to specified higher altitudes. Within this airspace all aircraft are subject to certain pilot and equipment requirements and operating rules. Details of TCA rules can be found in FAR 91.70 (c) and 91.90 and TCAs are described in Part 71 of the FARs. See Section 6 of this Handbook.

TCAs are charted by the National Ocean Survey in their VFR Terminal Area Charts series.

Group I TCAs:

Atlanta, Boston, Chicago, Dallas, Los Angeles, Miami, New York, San Francisco, Washington, DC.

Group II TCAs:

Cleveland, Denver, Detroit, Houston, Kansas City, Las Vegas, Minneapolis, New Orleans, Philadelphia, Pittsburgh, St. Louis, Seattle.

Air Traffic Guidance at Noncontrolled Airports

Pilots should look for a segmented circle normally located on the airport that is visible from the air or the ground. The segmented circle has several components. These are:

Wind Direction Indicator—A wind cone near the center of the circle is used to indicate wind direction and velocity.

Landing Direction Indicator—A tetrahedron may be installed, when conditions warrant, at the center of the circle to indicate the direction to use for landings and takeoffs. It may be free-swinging or stationary.

Landing Strip Indicators—Installed in pairs around the outside of the circle to show the alignment of the landing strips.

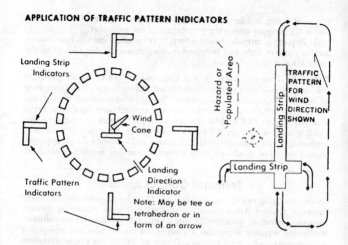

Traffic Pattern Indicators—Used in conjunction with the landing strip indicators to show the direction of traffic pattern turns **when there is a variation from the normal left traffic pattern.** (When no segmented circle is installed, right traffic pattern indicators may be found near the ends of runways.)

Flashing Amber Light—Located near center of segmented circle (or in a prominent location) to indicate that a right traffic pattern is in effect.

Recommended Standard Traffic Pattern

The FAA suggests the use of the traffic pattern outlined on the following page at uncontrolled airports. For right traffic, the flow should be reversed.

1. Enter pattern in level flight, abeam the midpoint of the runway, at pattern altitude (1,000 feet AGL recommended unless otherwise established).

2. Maintain pattern altitude until abeam approach end of the landing runway, on downwind leg.

3. Complete turn to final at least ¼ mile from runway.

4. Continue straight ahead until beyond departure end of runway.

5. If remaining in the traffic pattern, commence turn to crosswind leg beyond the departure end of the runway, within 300 feet of pattern altitude.

6. If departing the traffic pattern, continue straight out, or exit with a 45° left turn beyond the departure end of the runway, after reaching pattern altitude.

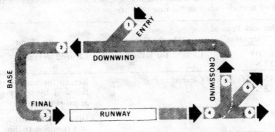

Visual Approach Slope Indicator (VASI)

The VASI gives visual descent guidance information during the landing approach to a runway. The standard two-bar VASI consists of downwind and upwind light bars that provide a visual glide path indication of safe obstruction clearance within the approach zone. When a pilot is on the proper glide path, he will see the downwind (nearer) bars as white and the upwind (farther) bars as red. If he is below the glide path, all light bars will appear red. If he is above the glide path, all light bars will appear white.

Some airports serving long-bodied jets have three-bar VASIs that provide two visual glide paths to the same runway. The second glide path is about ¼ of the degree higher than the first. When one is on the higher glide path of a three-bar VASI, the nearer two light bars will appear white and the farthest will appear red. When one is on the lower glide path of a three-bar VASI, the nearest light bar will appear white; the farther two red.

Basically, when using a VASI, remember that all-white light bars mean "too high"; all-red light bars mean "too low." Red above and white below mean you are on a safe approach path.

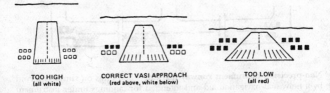

Light Signals

Air traffic control towers will use light signals (red, white, or green) to control aircraft whenever radio contact cannot be established, either because of the lack of aircraft radios or because they are inoperative.

Color and Type of Signal	On the Ground	In Flight
STEADY GREEN	Cleared for takeoff	Cleared to land
FLASHING GREEN	Cleared to taxi	Return for landing (to be followed by steady green at proper time)
STEADY RED	Stop	Give way to other aircraft and continue circling
FLASHING RED	Taxi clear of landing area (runway) in use	Airport unsafe—do not land
FLASHING WHITE	Return to starting point on airport	
ALTERNATING RED & GREEN	General warning signal—exercise extreme caution	

- Between sunset and sunrise, a pilot wishing to attract the attention of the air traffic control tower operator should turn on a landing light and taxi the aircraft in position so that light is visible to the tower operator. The landing light should remain on until appropriate signals are received from the tower.

- Pilots should acknowledge light signals by moving the ailerons or rudder during the hours of daylight or by blinking the landing or navigation lights during the hours of darkness.

Airport Runway Markings

Basic runway marking—Markings used for operations under VFR: center-line marking and runway direction numbers.

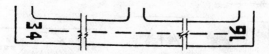

Non-precision instrument runway marking—Markings on runways served by a nonvisual navigation aid and intended for landings under instrument weather conditions: basic runway markings plus threshold marking.

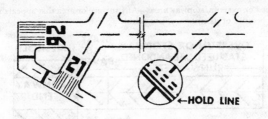

Precision instrument runway markings—Markings on runways served by nonvisual precision approach aids and on runways having special operational requirements: nonprecision instrument runway marking, touchdown zone marking, fixed-distance marking, plus side stripes.

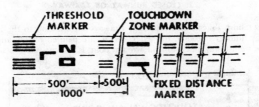

Displaced threshold—A threshold that is not at the beginning of the full-strength runway pavement.

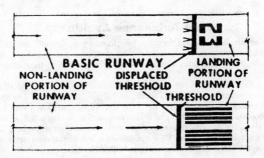

Closed or overrun/stopway areas—Any surface or area that appears usable but, because of its structure, is unusable.

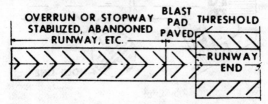

1. OVERRUN/STOPWAY AND BLAST PAD AREA

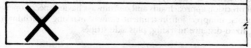

2. CLOSED RUNWAY OR TAXIWAY

STOL (Short Takeoff and Landing) runway—In addition to the normal runway number marking, the letters STOL are painted on the approach end of the runway and a touchdown aim point is shown.

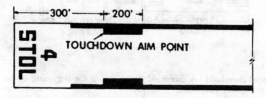

Wake Turbulence Avoidance

When lift is generated by any size fixed-wing aircraft, the pressure differential between the lower pressure over the wing and the higher pressure under it creates a roll-up wake effect of the airflow behind the wingtips.

This wake consists of two counter rotating vortices, the strength of which are determined by the weight, speed, and shape of the wing. The greatest vortex strength is present when the aircraft is HEAVY, SLOW AND CLEAN.

Helicopters in forward flight also create sizable vortices and should be given the same amount of concern as fixed-wing aircraft in flight.

Vortex avoidance during VFR operations is left to the pilot, who should exercise the same degree of caution as with collision avoidance.

Vortex movement in ground effect—no wind

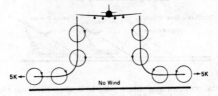

When vortices sink close to the ground in a no wind environment, they often move laterally over the ground at around 5 knots.

Vortex sink characteristics

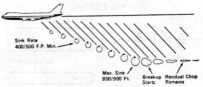

Sink Rate
400/500 F.P. Min.

Max. Sink
800/900 Ft.

Breakup
Starts

Residual Chop
Remains

Pilots should fly at or above the heavy jet's flight path. Avoid the area behind and below generating aircraft.

Landing behind a heavy jet—same runway

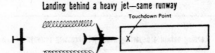

Touchdown Point

Stay at or above the heavy jet's final approach path. Note his touchdown point and land beyond it.

Landing behind a departing heavy jet—same runway

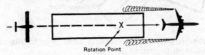

Rotation Point

Note heavy jet's rotation point, and land well prior to it.

Departing behind a heavy jet

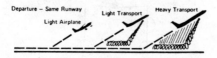

Note jet's rotation point and rotate prior to it, then continue climb above jet path until turning clear of his wake.

Landing behind heavy jet, when parallel runway is closer than 2,500 feet

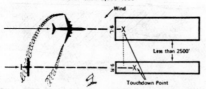

Note wind for possible vortex drift to your runway. Request upwind runway if practical. If not, stay above heavy jet's final approach path. Note his touchdown point and land beyond a point abeam his touchdown spot.

Landing behind a departing heavy jet—crossing runways

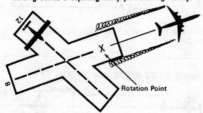

If jet rotation point is past the intersection, land prior to intersection. Do not approach under a departing jet's path.

Section 4
Emergency Procedures

STOP—THINK—COLLECT YOUR WITS. These five words may prove invaluable to the pilot faced with an emergency situation. Few flight emergencies occur that do not permit a thorough evaluation of the emergency situation by the pilot prior to initiating corrective action. Excessive haste often leads to faulty decisions and actions.

A pilot in any emergency should do three things to obtain assistance:

1. If the aircraft is equipped with a radar beacon transponder, switch to code 7700.

2. Contact an ATC facility and give the nature of distress and pilot's intentions (Contact should be made on the last frequency being used. If unable to make contact, then attempt contact using the following emergency frequencies.)

3. Comply with instructions received. Do not shift frequency or shift to another ground station unless absolutely necessary.

Transmit as much of the following as possible:

a. MAYDAY, MAYDAY, MAYDAY (if distress), or PAN, PAN, PAN (if uncertainty or alert). If CW transmission (Morse Code), use SOS (distress) or XXX (uncertainty or alert).

b. Aircraft identification repeated three times.

c. Type of aircraft.

d. Position or estimated position (stating which).

e. Heading—true or magnetic (stating which).

f. True airspeed or estimated true airspeed (stating which).

g. Altitude.

h. Fuel remaining in hours and minutes.

i. Nature of distress.

j. Pilot's intentions (bailout, ditch, crash landing, etc.).

k. Assistance desired (fix, steer, bearing, escort, etc.).

l. Two 10-second dashes with mike button (voice) or key (CW) followed by aircraft identification (once) and OVER (voice) or K (CW).

m. If crash is imminent and aircraft is equipped with an emergency locator transmitter, activate the emergency signal.

Emergency Radio Frequencies

Contact should be attempted on these frequencies if no contact can be established on normal frequencies with ground controlling agencies:

Frequency	Emission	Effective Range in Nautical Miles	Guarded By
121.5 MHz	Voice	Generally limited to radio line-of-sight	All military towers, most civil towers, VHF direction finding stations, radar facilities, Flight Service Stations.
243.0 MHz	Voice	Generally limited to radio line-of-sight	All military towers, most civil towers, UHF direction finding stations, radar facilities, Flight Service Station.
2182 kHz	Voice	Generally less than 300 miles for average aircraft installations	Some ships and boats, Coast Guard stations, most commercial coast stations
500 kHz	CW	Generally less than 100 miles for average aircraft installations	Most large ships, most Coast Guard radio stations, most commercial coast stations
8364 kHz	CW	Up to several thousand miles, depending upon propagation conditions. Subject to "skip"	U.S.N. Direction Finding Stations, most Coast Guard radio stations and some FAA International Flight Service Stations (IFSS)

Note:—ARTCC emergency frequency capability normally does not extend to radar coverage limits. If the ARTCC does not respond to transmission on emergency frequency 121.5 MHz or 243.0 MHz, pilots should initiate a call to the nearest Flight Service Station or airport traffic control tower.

International Distress Calls

MAYDAY — Immediate danger exists to equipment and personnel.
PAN — Potential danger exists to equipment and personnel.

Airports With Continuous Power

In the event of a commercial power failure, certain airports have been equipped with an independent power capability that will provide a basic ATC system, including approach and lighting aids. Each airport so designated will have a runway with an ILS and associated approach, runway and taxiway lighting, plus ceiling and wind-measuring capability.

The following facilities have been designated as "Continuous Power Airports."

Albuquerque; Andrews AFB; Atlanta; Baltimore; Bismarck; Boise; Boston; Chicago-O'Hare; Chicago-Midway; Charlotte; Cincinnati; Cleveland; Dallas-Fort Worth; Denver; Des Moines; Detroit Metro; El Paso; Great Falls; Houston; Indianapolis; Jacksonville; Kansas City; Los Angeles; Memphis; Miami; Milwaukee; Minneapolis; Nashville; Newark; New Orleans; New York-J.F. Kennedy; New York-LaGuardia; Oklahoma City; Omaha; Ontario, Calif.; Philadelphia; Phoenix; Pittsburgh; Reno; Salt Lake City; San Antonio; San Diego; San Francisco; St. Louis; Seattle; Tampa; Tulsa; Washington National; Washington-Dulles; Wichita.

Radio Failure While Operating IFR

If the radio failure occurs under VFR conditions, or if VFR conditions are encountered en route, the pilot will maintain VFR conditions and land as soon as practicable. Notify ATC after landing.

If failure occurs under IFR conditions and VFR conditions are not encountered en route, the pilot shall continue the flight according to the following:

Route

1. By the route assigned in the last ATC clearance received.
2. If on a radar vector, by the direct route from the point of failure to the fix, route or airway specified in the vector clearance.
3. In the absence of an assigned route, by the route ATC has advised may be expected in a further clearance.
4. In the absence of either an assigned route or a route that ATC has advised may be expected in a further clearance, by the route filed in the flight plan.

Altitude—At the highest of the following altitudes:

1. The altitude assigned in the last ATC clearance received, except that the altitude in b. shall apply for only the segment(s) of the route where the minimum altitude is higher than the ATC assigned altitude.
2. The minimum altitude for IFR operations, or
3. The altitude ATC has advised may be expected in a further clearance.

Leave Holding Fix—If holding instructions have been received, leave the holding fix at the expect further clearance time received, or, if an expected approach clearance time has been received, leave the holding fix in order to arrive over the fix from which the approach begins as close as possible to the expected approach clearance time. If holding instructions have *not* been received and the aircraft is ahead of its ETA, the pilot is expected to hold at the fix from which the approach begins. If more than one approach fix is available, it is pilot choice, and ATC protects airspace at all of them.

Descent for Approach—Begin descent from the en route altitude upon reaching the fix from which the approach begins, but not before:

1. The expect approach clearance time (if received); or

2. If no expect approach clearance time has been received, at the ETA, shown on the flight plan, as amended with ATC.

In the event of a two-way radio failure, ATC service will be provided on the basis that the pilot is operating in accordance with FAR 91.127. Pilots who have radio failure are urged to transmit their intentions in the blind and listen on any operational radio receiver for ATC information, since controllers have the capability of transmitting on most navigational facilities.

Emergency Locator Transmitters (ELT)

Under Federal law, emergency locator transmitters are now mandatory equipment on practically all general aviation aircraft, except helicopters and agricultural aircraft. These battery-powered electronic signaling devices transmit a distinctive downswept audio tone on either 121.5 MHz or 243.0 MHz, or both (243.0 MHz is the UHF emergency frequency used by military aircraft). Search-and-rescue aircraft can home in on this signal to locate a downed aircraft. ELTs may or may not have voice transmission capability. To be effective, an ELT should be capable of 24 to 48 hours of continuous operation over a very wide temperature range. ELT details are in Federal Aviation Regulation 91.52.

Forced Landing

1. Immediately establish a glide at the best glide speed for your aircraft. If glide speed is unknown, use power-off stall speed times 1.4.

2. Select a landing site before making restart attempts. Three primary considerations in their order of importance are:

   a. Available altitude.

   b. Terrain.

   c. Wind direction and velocity.

   (Should engine failure occur at low altitude shortly after takeoff, there is usually less risk in landing straight ahead than in attempting to return to the airport.)

3. Fly a planned, definite traffic pattern, altitude permitting, to assure putting your aircraft on the selected landing site.

4. It is impossible to "stretch" a glide. Attempting to do so will increase the rate of sink and cause an aircraft to land short of the desired point.

Spiral Approach to a Forced Landing:

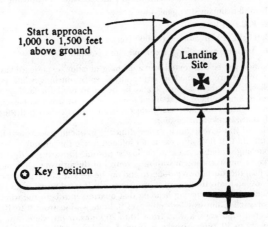

Note: Forced landing procedures should be periodically reviewed in flight with an instructor and again with every change of aircraft.

VFR Pilot in IFR Conditions

A person without instrument knowledge *and experience* simply cannot fly an airplane once he has lost all outside references; therefore, no written words or checklist can satisfactorily cover such situations. Immediately contact an FAA air traffic control facility for assistance and follow the controller's instructions.

The best possible insurance against such a situation for the VFR pilot is the AOPA 360° Rating Course. A course syllabus kit from AOPA is available, at a nominal fee, to your local flight instructor.

Write:
AOPA Air Safety Foundation, Air Rights Bldg., 7315 Wisconsin Ave., Bethesda, Md. 20014.

Ditching

Ditching situations for general aviation aircraft vary greatly, depending upon the type of aircraft. A ten-year study of ditching in general aviation aircraft has shown a 98% success rate. However, regardless of the specific situation, any ditching must be considered hazardous and to be avoided if at all possible. Primary considerations against the possibility of ditching include:

1. Well-maintained engine(s).
2. Full fuel load.
3. Flight at high altitude (10,000 feet or above).
4. Accurate navigational techniques and equipment.

Should you be confronted with a ditching situation, experience has shown best results are obtained in larger airplanes by ditching while power is available. In lighter aircraft it may be better to head for land or shallow water as long as there is a spark of life in the engine. Instruct passengers to remove glasses and take sharp objects from pockets, then pad themselves with coats, blankets or cushions.

Should you have to ditch, expect difficulty in opening doors and hatches. Be careful that flotation gear is not inflated inside the aircraft.

Ditching should be made at the lowest possible forward speed, at time of surface contact, consistent with safe control of the airplane. On a moderate sea, plan the touchdown parallel to and on the lee side of the primary swells. Do not land into the face of a primary swell. If wind speed is 25 knots or greater, choose a ditching heading that quarters into both the wind and a major swell. Calm seas with no waves indicate a wind from 0 to 10 knots; scattered white caps, a wind from 10 to 20 knots; many white caps, a wind from 20 to 30 knots; streaks of foam, a wind from 30 to 40 knots; spray from the wave crest, a wind of 40 to 50 knots or greater.

With smooth surface conditions it is easy to misjudge altitude above water by 50 feet or more. If possible, throw out a seat cushion for better surface reference.

Best ditching configuration: for retractable-gear aircraft, gear up; for high-wing aircraft, full flaps. For low-wing aircraft, an NTSB special study, "Emergency Landing Techniques in Small, Fixed-Wing Aircraft," recommends using no more than intermediate flaps, since water resistance of fully extended flaps could result in asymmetrical flap failure and slewing of the aircraft. Use any available power to touch down in a nose-high altitude.

At night or in weather, make an instrument letdown, maintaining a vertical speed of 100 feet per minute or less.

Equipment advisable for overwater flight includes:

1. Flotation equipment—both inflatable raft and inflatable life jackets.
2. Location aids—signal mirror, signal flares, dye marker, emergency radio and crash locator beacon, if possible.
3. Survival equipment—fishing gear, water, sun protection equipment.

Before any overwater flight: **FILE A FLIGHT PLAN.**
If trouble develops: **COMMUNICATE YOUR DISTRESS EARLY.**

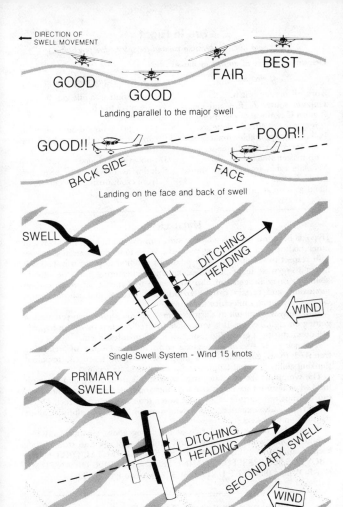

DIRECTION OF SWELL MOVEMENT

GOOD GOOD FAIR BEST

Landing parallel to the major swell

GOOD!! POOR!!

BACK SIDE FACE

Landing on the face and back of swell

SWELL DITCHING HEADING WIND

Single Swell System - Wind 15 knots

PRIMARY SWELL DITCHING HEADING SECONDARY SWELL WIND

Double Swell System - Wind 30 knots

Fire in Flight

(Check your aircraft operating manual for specific fire procedures.)

Determine source of smoke or flame!

If electrical:

Turn off master switch.

Pinpoint source of fire and extinguish if removal of electrical current has not already done so.

Pull or trip applicable circuit breakers for affected equipment. Turn on master switch.

Ventilate cabin to eliminate smoke and fumes.

Land as soon as practicable.

If from engine compartment:

Mixture control to idle cutoff.

Fuel control to off.

Retard throttle.

(This procedure should burn all combustible fuels ahead of the firewall.)

Do not restart engine.

Sideslip as necessary to keep fire from cabin during descent.

Hypoxia

Hypoxia in simple terms is a lack of sufficient oxygen to keep the brain and other body tissues functioning properly. Wide individual variation occurs with respect to susceptibility to hypoxia. In addition to progressively insufficient oxygen at higher altitudes, anything interfering with the blood's ability to carry oxygen can also contribute to hypoxia (anemias, carbon monoxide, and certain drugs.) In addition, alcohol and various drugs decrease the brain's tolerance to hypoxia.

Your body has no built in alarm system to let you know when you are not getting enough oxygen. It is impossible to predict when or where hypoxia will occur during a given flight, or how it will manifest itself.

A major early system of hypoxia is an increased sense of well-being (referred to as euphoria). This progresses to slow reactions, impaired thinking ability, unusual fatigue, and a dull headache feeling.

The symptoms are slow but progressive, insidious in onset, and are most marked at altitudes starting above ten thousand feet. Night vision, however, can be impaired starting at altitudes lower than ten thousand feet. Heavy smokers may also experience early symptoms of hypoxia at altitudes lower than for non-smokers.

If you observe the general rule of not flying above ten thousand feet without supplemental oxygen you will probably not get into trouble, but keep in mind that PILOTS MUST USE SUPPLEMENTAL OXYGEN IF ABOVE 12,500 FEET FOR 30 MINUTES OR LONGER, OR ANYTIME IF ABOVE 14,000 FEET UNPRESSURIZED. (See FAR 91.32)

Emergency Resuscitation Procedures

When heartbeat and breathing stop, a person will be clinically and biologically dead within 4 to 6 minutes, unless emergency resuscitation procedures are started. Keep in mind that proper resuscitation efforts can keep victims alive indefinitely, but attempts to restore breathing without also restoring the heartbeat cannot succeed.

1. If the victim is unconscious and not breathing, lay him on his back and open his air passage by:
   a. Clearing mouth of mucus and foreign objects, then
   b. Raise neck with one hand and tilt head as far back as possible to keep victim's tongue from blocking airway.

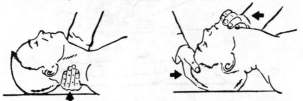

2. If the victim is still not breathing, begin artificial breathing for him:
   a. Close victim's nostrils with fingers, and keeping victim's head tilted back;

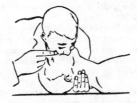

   b. Place your mouth completely over victim's mouth, then;
   c. Exhale into victim's mouth and watch chest expand. Give four quick, full breaths.
   d. If the airway is blocked, try back blows, abdominal or chest thrusts, and/or finger probes until airway is open.
3. Feel for carotid pulse on either side of victim's adam's apple.
4. If pulse is absent, begin artificial circulation by:
   a. Placing heel of hand over lower half of breastbone and cover with other hand, then;
   b. Press down firmly and quickly, 1½ to 2 inches and release. (For ONE RESCUER, use 15 external heart compressions at the rate of 80 per minute, followed by two quick breaths. For TWO RESCUERS (where one performs external heart massage and the other breathing) give

five external heart compressions at the rate of one per second, and inflate the victim's lungs after every fifth compression.) Continue without interruption until advanced life support equipment is available.

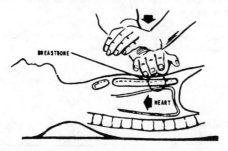

Survival on Land

Immediate Action

• Stay away from the airplane until the engine(s) has cooled and spilled gas has evaporated.

• Check injuries. Give first aid. Be careful when removing injured persons from the airplane, particularly those with possible injured backs or fractures.

• Get out of the wind and rain. Construct a temporary shelter. If fire is needed, start it at once. In cold weather, make hot drinks.

• Get signaling equipment ready, then rest until you are over the shock of the crash.

• Do not leave the airplane unless you know that you are within easy walking distance of help. If you travel, leave a note giving planned route. Stick to that route.

• Staying near the airplane, organize your camp. Improve the temporary shelter for protection from the elements. Collect all possible fuel. Look for a water supply. Look for animal and plant food.

• Prepare signals so that you will be recognized from the air.

• Help search parties to find you, and follow their instructions when they sight you. They can use all the help you can give. Don't take chances that might result in injury. You will be easier to rescue if you stay in one piece.

Arctic

Protection from cold is the most immediate and constant problem. Keep dry. Avoid snow blindness. Check for frostbite. Immediately warm possible frostbite area using body heat or warm (105°F) water.

Keep snow out of boots, gloves and clothing. Avoid open water. Overexertion causes perspiration, which will freeze inside clothing, decreasing

216

effective insulation. Always work or move with outer clothing removed. Use outer garments when you stop, to avoid chilling.

Collect wood, gasoline, oil, heather, brush or peat for fuel. Build fire at a safe distance from the shelter. Get under shelter. Aircraft engine oil must be drained quickly, before it can congeal from the cold, if it is to be used as fuel for heat.

In summer, protect exposed parts of body from insects. Keep dry.

Desert

Water will be the biggest problem. Do not waste it. Keep head and back of neck covered, and get into shade as soon as possible to reduce sweating and loss of body water. Travel only if you are sure you can walk to assistance easily, and if you are certain you have enough water. If you decide to travel, travel only at night. Digging 18 to 24 inches into sand, one may find the surface temperature reduced by as much as 30°F. Temperature may be reduced a like amount at 12 inches above the ground.

The only way to conserve your water is to control your sweating. Drink water as you need it, but keep heat out of your body by keeping clothes on. Clothing helps control sweating by not letting perspiration evaporate so fast that you get only part of its cooling effect.

Drs. R. D. Jackson and C. van Bavel, of the U.S. Water Conservation Laboratory, have developed a simple solar still that may generate usable amounts of water in desert terrain.

Hot sunshine is what makes the still work at peak efficiency. Components are a small container and a 6-foot-square sheet of clear plastic, one mil thick, such as "Tedlar." Build the still as shown in the illustration, *making certain that the cone formed by the weighted plastic sheet does not touch the sides of the pit at any point,* since this would cause water loss. If possible, line the pit with pulp from desert plants to increase water production. Water will condense on the underside of the plastic sheet, flow toward the weighted center, and drop into the container. A small plastic drinking tube can be used to obtain water from the container without dismantling the still.

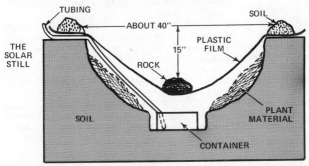

Tropics

Take shelter from rain, sun, and insects. Insect pests are the immediate dangers of the tropics. Protect yourself against bites.

Set up fires and other signals in natural clearings and along edges of streams. Signals under dense jungle growth won't be seen.

Food, shelter and water are more available in the tropics, a fact that makes travel from the crash site a more feasible consideration than in any other climate area.

Most stories about the animals, snakes, spiders and nameless terrors of the jungle are pure bunk. You probably will never see a poisonous snake or a large animal. What may scare you most are the howls, screams and crashing sounds made by noisy monkeys, birds, night insects and falling trees. The real dangers of the tropics are the insects, which may pass on diseases and parasites.

Survival at Sea

Stay clear of the airplane, out of gas-saturated waters, until the airplane sinks.

Salvage floating equipment; stow and secure all items in rafts.

Bail water out of raft and take precautions not to snag raft with shoes or sharp objects.

Rig a windbreak, spray shield and canopy, as protection from chilling winds. Exercise regularly. Prepare signaling devices for instant use.

Keep compasses, watches, matches and lighters dry. Place them in water-proof containers.

In warm oceans, rig sun shade. Keep skin covered. Use sunburn cream and chapstick if available.

Save water and food by saving energy. Keep calm.

Suggested Items For Compact 2-Pound Survival Kit

First Aid:	Bandaids—roll of half-inch adhesive tape—pack of X-acto knife blades—tube of antiseptic ointment—aspirin—water purification tablets—ammonia inhalers—triangle bandages.
Food:	Concentrated soup mixes—bouillon cubes—dehydrated coffee and milk—sugar—salt—hard candy—vitamin capsules. Wrap in several layers of heavy-duty aluminum foil, which can later be formed into cooking utensils.
Fish and Game:	50 feet of high-strength fishing line—six fish hooks—small gill net—light wire for snares.
Tools:	Scout knife and pocket whetstone—waterproof match container—waterproof matches—heat tablets—needles—safety pins—a file—plastic canteen—signal mirror—button compass—penlight flashlight (keep batteries separate, out of flashlight).

—FAA

Wind Chill Factors

This chart illustrates why it may feel a great deal colder, on a windy day, than the reported temperature. When planning your flight, dress appropriately for existing conditions. Remember that clothing that feels comfortable in the cockpit could prove less than adequate in the event of a forced landing.

Cooling Power of Wind on Exposed Flesh Expressed as an Equivalent Temperature

Estimated wind speed (in mph)	Actual Thermometer reading (F.)											
	50	40	30	20	10	0	-10	-20	-30	-40	-50	-60
	EQUIVALENT TEMPERATURE (F.)											
calm	50	40	30	20	10	0	-10	-20	-30	-40	-50	-60
5	48	37	27	16	6	-5	-15	-26	-36	-47	-57	-68
10	40	28	16	4	-9	-24	-33	-46	-58	-70	-83	-95
15	36	22	9	-5	-18	-32	-45	-58	-72	-85	-99	-112
20	32	18	4	-10	-25	-39	-53	-67	-82	-96	-110	-124
25	30	16	0	-15	-29	-44	-59	-74	-88	-104	-118	-133
30	28	13	-2	-18	-33	-48	-63	-79	-94	-109	-125	-140
35	27	11	-4	-20	-35	-51	-67	-82	-98	-113	-129	-145
40	26	10	-6	-21	-37	-53	-69	-85	-100	-116	-132	-148

Wind speeds greater than 40 mph have little added effect.

LITTLE DANGER (for properly clothed person) Maximum danger of false sense of security.

INCREASING DANGER Danger from freezing of exposed flesh.

GREAT DANGER

Source: NAVMED Bulletin 5052-29

Food

Take stock of available food and water. Allow two-thirds of your food for the first half of estimated time before rescue and save remainder for the second half.

Traveling requires about twice as much food to remain in the same physical shape as if one had stayed with the aircraft.

Eating increases thirst. If you have less than a quart of water daily, avoid dry, starchy and highly flavored foods and meat. Best foods are those such as hard candy and fruit bars.

The less work you do, the less food and water you will need.

If water is plentiful, drink more than your normal amount to keep fit. You can live many days without food if you have water.

Eat off the land whenever you can, saving your rations for emergencies. Don't nibble. Plan one good meal daily and make a feast of it. Two meals a day are preferable, especially if one meal can be hot.

The body needs 2 quarts of water a day to maintain efficiency. Don't drink urine or seawater.

Health and Hygiene

Save your strength. Get lots of sleep and take it easy. If you are doing hard work or walking, rest 10 minutes of each hour.

Take care of your feet. If your feet hurt, stop and care for them. Apply adhesive tape to skin where shoes rub and blisters develop.

Guard against skin infection. Use an antiseptic on even the smallest scratch, cut or insect bite.

Guard against intestinal sickness. Cook your food and purify your water.

Keep your body, your clothing and your camp clean. Adherence to basic sanitation measures may prevent illness.

Signaling

Mirror

Practice signaling with a mirror, a pocket mirror, or any bright piece of metal. If possible, punch a hole in the center of the metal piece for sighting. On hazy days, an aircraft can see the flash of the mirror before the survivors can see the aircraft, so flash the mirror in the direction of a plane when you hear it, even when you cannot see it. When the airplane is sighted, keep signaling.

Pyrotechnics

Use smoke signals in the daytime and red signals at night. Keep signal flares dry; don't waste them. Be very careful of fire hazard when using flares.

Sea Marker

Use sea marker during daytime. Except in very rough sea, these spots of dye remain conspicious for about 3 hours. Conserve by rewrapping when not in use. Also excellent for use on snow.

Lights

At night, use flashlights, red flares or any available light. Light can be seen over water for several miles.

On land, use smoke by day, bright flame by night. Add engine oil, rags soaked in oil, or pieces of rubber to make black smoke. Green leaves, moss, or a little water will send up billows of white smoke.

Signal Size

The larger the signal, the more easily it can be spotted from the air. Do everything you can to disturb the "natural" look of the ground. Use reflective cowling and parts from the aircraft.

Emergency Body Signals

Need medical
assistance, URGENT

Negative (no)

Affirmative (yes)

Land here (point in
direction of landing)

Do not attempt
to land here

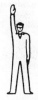

All OK, do not wait

Our receiver
is operating

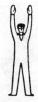

Pick us up—
plane abandoned

Can proceed shortly, wait if practicable

Use drop message

Need mechanical help or parts—long delay

Ground-Air Visual Code

Require doctor, serious injuries	**I**	Indicate direction to proceed	**K**
Require medical supplies	**II**	Not understood	**⅃L**
Unable to proceed	**X**	Am proceeding in this direction	**↑**
Require food and water	**F**	Will attempt takeoff	**▷**
Require firearms and ammunition	**⋁**	Aircraft seriously damaged	**⌐⌐**
Require map and compass	**□**	Probably safe to land here	**△**
Require signal lamp with battery, and radio	**|**	Require fuel and oil	**L**

All well .... **LL**	Yes .... **Y**
No .... **N**	Require mechanic .... **W**

IF IN DOUBT, USE INTERNATIONAL SYMBOL .... **SOS**

Standard Aircraft Acknowledgments

Message received and understood by aircraft:

    Day or moonlight — Rocking wings
    Night   — Green flashes from signal lamp

Message received and NOT understood by aircraft:

    Day or moonlight — Making a complete right-hand circle
    Nigth   — Red flashes from signal lamp

Affirmative reply from aircraft: Dip nose of aircraft several times

Negative reply from aircraft: Fishtail aircraft

Aircraft Accident Reporting

An operator of an aircraft must immediately notify (by telephone, telegraph, or notification to FAA for relay) the nearest National Transportation Safety Board (NTSB) field office when there is an accident resulting in fatal or serious injury to any person, or in which any aircraft receives substantial damage, or if aircraft collide in flight, or if certain in-flight hazards are experienced, such as fire, rapid decompression requiring emergency action, unwanted or asymmetrical thrust reversal, flight control system malfunction or failure, inability of any required flight crewmember to perform his normal flight duties as a result of injury or illness, or if an aircraft is overdue and believed to have been involved in an accident.

Fatal injury is defined as any injury that results in death within seven days. Serious injury means any injury that: 1. requires hospitalization for more than 48 hours, commencing within seven days from the date the injury was received; 2. results in a fracture of any bone (except simple fractures of the fingers, toes or nose); 3. involves lacerations that cause severe hemorrhages or nerve, muscle or tendon damage; 4. involves injury to any internal organ; or 5. involves second- or third-degree burns, or any burns affecting more than 5% of the body surface. Substantial damage means damage or structural failure that adversely affects the structural strength, performance or flight characteristics of the aircraft, and that would normally require major repair or replacement of the affected component. (Engine failure; damage limited to an engine; bent fairings or cowling; dented skin; small puncture holes in the skin of fabric; ground damage to rotor or propeller blades; damage to landing gear, wheels, tires, flaps, engine accessories, brakes, or wingtips are not considered "substantial damage.")

In addition to the requirement for immediate notification, an operator must also file a report, within 10 days, of an accident involving a fatal or serious injury, substantial damage or a midair collision. Specified in-flight hazards, though subject to immediate notification, do not require a written report. The necessary forms are available from NTSB field offices (see Section 5); the National Transportation Safety Board, Washington, DC 20594; and FAA Flight Standards District Offices. (General aviation accidents also may be reported to the FAA General Aviation District Offices—see Section 5.)

SECTION 5

Addresses and Services

NATIONAL OPERATIONS

AIRCRAFT OWNERS AND PILOTS ASSOCIATION (AOPA)

7315 Wisconsin Ave., Bethesda, MD, 20014
Mail: P.O. Box 5800, Washington, DC, 20014
Phone (301) 654-0500
(301) 654-7895 (after-hours telephone recording service)
TWX: (710) 824-0095
Cable address: AOPA, Washington, D.C.
Offices open Monday through Friday,
8:30 a.m.–5 p.m. (Eastern Time)
Closed on New Year's Day, Washington's Birthday*, Memorial Day*, Independence Day, Labor Day, Veterans Day, Thanksgiving and Christmas. (*Monday holiday law.)

AOPA Board of Trustees

J. B. Hartranft, Jr., Chairman	R. Anderson Pew, Vice Chairman
Elaine Harrison	John J. Serrell
Paul C. Heintz	Philip T. Sharples (emeritus)
Fitzgerald S. Hudson	Alfred L. Wolf
D. Charles Merriwether	John S. Yodice

AOPA Officers

John L. Baker, President
William S. Brassel, Senior Vice President—Fiscal and Internal Operations
Victor J. Kayne, Senior Vice President—Policy and Technical Planning
Ralph F. Nelson, Senior Vice President—Operations
Harmon O. Pritchard, Jr., Senior Vice President—Marketing
Robert M. Butler, Vice President—Printing and Mail Service
Catherine V. Howser, Vice President—Flight Planning
Robert E. Monroe, Vice President—Data Research
Laurel A. Smith, Vice President—Marketing Services
Charles Spence, Vice President—Public Relations
Edward G. Tripp, Vice President—Publications
John J. Serrell, Treasurer
Lawrence E. Peters, Comptroller
Alfred L. Wolf, Secretary and General Counsel

225

John S. Yodice, Assistant Secretary and Washington Counsel
Russell S. Lawton, Assistant Vice President—Operations and Safety
Ann M. Lennon, Assistant Vice President—Manager, Oklahoma City office
William J. Orchard, Assistant Vice President—Business/Production—Publications
Katherine W. Post, Assistant Vice President—Membership Processing/Servicing
David D. Salmon, Jr., Assistant Vice President—Congressional Affairs
Arthur H. Sanfelici, Assistant Vice President—Publications
Robert T. Warner, Assistant Vice President—Policy and Technical Planning

AOPA Services

- Aircraft financing assistance
- Legal assistance
- Aircraft title search and related services
- Liaison with legislative bodies
- Airport development and problem solving
- Pilot services—help with aircraft and airmen's problems
- Chart subscriptions and related services
- Publications—AOPA PILOT, Newsletter, AOPA Airport Report, Airports U.S.A., Handbook for Pilots
- Flight education and safety
- Public relations activities
- Insurance—pilot and aircraft
- Regulatory and federal agency relations
- International support of general aviation

AOPA Telephone Numbers

AOPA General Information	(301) 654-0500
Address Changes	(301) 951-3814
	(301) 951-3886
After Hours (record your message)	(301) 654-7895
Aircraft Title Search	(405) 682-2511
	(301) 951-3855
Airport Report	(301) 951-3819
Airports U.S.A.	(301) 951-3823
Air Safety Education and Foundation Courses	(301) 951-3959
	(800) 638-0853 (toll free)

AOPA PILOT editorial offices .... (301) 951-3826
Chart Service .... (301) 951-3855
Federal Legislative Affairs .... (301) 951-3934
Flight Planning (24 hour number) .... (301) 951-3844
Insurance .... (301) 951-3861
International Aviation
  Theft Bureau .... (301) 951-3866
Membership/Renewal Questions .... (301) 951-3987
Newsletter .... (301) 951-3819
Personal Pilot Service
  Operations and Safety .... (301) 951-3910
  Service and Reference .... (301) 951-3914
  Medical and Technical Assistance .... (301) 951-3912
Public Relations .... (301) 951-3818
Destinations Unlimited Inc. .... (301) 951-3954
AOPA Office hours: 8:30 a.m. to 5:00 p.m., eastern time.

AOPA Title Search

Aircraft Owners and Pilots Association

Box 19244, South Station

Oklahoma City, OK 73144

Phone (405) 682-2511

TELEX 747-265

(Services include title search, complete chain of title, present registered owner, filing of documents, pilot certificate status, medical data, copies of documents. One-day service, report by airmail; faster rush service with collect phone, wire or Telex report if desired. Preferential member rates.)

AOPA Air Safety Foundation

7315 Wisconsin Ave., Bethesda, MD, 20014

Mail: P.O. Box 5800, Washington, DC, 20014

Phone: (301) 654-0500, or (800) 638-0853 (toll free)

AOPA Air Safety Foundation Officers

J. B. Hartranft, Jr., Chairman of the Board
John L. Baker, President
William R. Stanberry, Executive Vice President
Richard D. Gless, Vice President
William S. Brassel, Vice President
J. J. Serrell, Treasurer
Alfred L. Wolf, Secretary and General Counsel
John S. Yodice, Washington Counsel
Lawrence E. Peters, Comptroller

(Contributions to the AOPA Air Safety Foundation are deductible under Code Sec. 170, Reg. 1.170-2, as provided for tax-exempt nonprofit organizations.)

AOPA Service Corporation (ASCO)
5100 Wisconsin Ave., Washington, DC, 20016
Phone (202) 244-6440/1
Richard F. Busch, Jr., Executive Vice President
Ferrele Garling, Vice President
(*Insurance and Aircraft Financing*)

DEPARTMENT OF TRANSPORTATION

400 Seventh St., S.W.
Washington, DC, 20591

Listed below are those DOT offices which may be of particular interest to general aviation:

Secretary, Neil Goldschmidt
Deputy Secretary, Linda H. Kamm (acting)
Assistant Secretary for Policy Plans and International Affairs, Charles Swinburn (acting)
Assistant Secretary for Governmental and Public Affairs, Susan J. Williams (acting)
General Counsel, Linda H. Kamm
Assistant Secretary for Administration, Edward W. Scott, Jr.
Director, Public Affairs, Robert Holland
Director, Consumer Affairs, Lee Gray (acting)

FEDERAL AVIATION ADMINISTRATION

800 Independence Ave., S.W.
Washington, DC, 20591
Phone (202) 426-4000, 655-4000

Listed below are those FAA offices which may be of particular interest to general aviation:

Administrator, Langhorne M. Bond
Deputy Administrator, Quentin S. Taylor
Chief Counsel, Clark H. Onstad
Associate Administrator for Engineering & Development, A. P. Albrecht
Associate Administrator for Air Traffic & Airway Facilities, William M. Flener
Director of Aviation Safety, John Harrison
Office of International Aviation Affairs, Norman H. Plummer, Acting Director
Office of Aviation Medicine, H. L. Reighard, MD, Federal Air Surgeon
Office of Public Affairs, Jerome H. Doolittle, Assistant Administrator
Air Traffic Service, Richard L. Failor, Director
Flight Standards Service, J. A. Ferrarese (Acting)
Civil Aviation Security, Richard F. Lally, Director

FAA Aeronautical Center—

The following offices at the FAA Monroney Aeronautical Center (P.O. Box 25082, Oklahoma City, OK 73125; Phone (405) 686-2011) should be contacted for the services indicated:

Aircraft Registration Branch (405-686-2116)—Registering aircraft ($5 application fee); recording aircraft titles and security documents ($5 fee for each document); requesting duplicate of lost aircraft registration certificates ($2 each duplicate); requesting special "N" number ($10); request to reserve, change or reassign an "N" number ($10 fee); request for dealer's registration ($10 fee). Address communication to P.O. Box 25504, Oklahoma City, OK, 73125.

Airmen Certification Branch (405-686-2261)—Notification of change in permanent mailing address (must be given in writing within 30 days) or change of name (must furnish legal proof of change); requesting duplicate of lost pilot certificate (must furnish full name, date of birth, place of birth, Social Security number, and $2 fee).

Aeromedical Certification Branch (405-686-4821)—Requesting duplicate of lost medical certificate ($2 fee); requesting information on medical certification problems, if not being handled by Regional Flight Surgeon.

DOMESTIC FAA REGIONAL OFFICES

Alaskan Region—Anchorage
Governing Alaska and Aleutian Islands

Robert L. Faith, Director; 701 C St., Anchorage, AK, 99501; phone (907) 271-5645; Duty Officer (907) 271-5936

Areas and Area Coordinators

Anchorage—Frank Babiak, Coordinator; 4510 International Airport Road, Anchorage AK, 99502; phone (907) 272-1020

Fairbanks Central Sector—Paul Gallagher, Coordinator; 5460 Airport Way, Fairbanks, AK, 99701; phone (907) 456-4600

Fairbanks North Sector—Thor Weatherby, Coordinator; 5460 Airport Way, Fairbanks, AK, 99701; phone (907) 452-1257

Juneau—Lyndol Pruitt, Coordinator; P.O. Box 1647, Juneau, AK, 99801; phone (907) 586-7245

King Salmon—Carl Fundeen, Coordinator; P.O. Box 67, King Salmon, AK, 99613; phone (907) 246-3321

Central Region—Kansas City
Governing Iowa, Kansas, Missouri, Nebraska

C. R. Melugin, Director; 601 East 12th St., Kansas City, MO, 64106; phone (816) 374-5626; Duty Officer (816) 374-3246; Duty Hours 7:30–4:00 (8:30–5:00 EST)

Eastern Region—New York
Governing Delaware, District of Columbia, Maryland, New Jersey, New York, Pennsylvania, Virginia, West Virginia

Murray Smith, Director; John F. Kennedy Intl. Airport, Jamaica, NY, 11430; phone (212) 995-2801; Duty Officer (212) 995-8555; Duty hours 8: 00-4:30 EST (Daylight Saving Time from last Sunday in April through last Sunday in October)

Great Lakes Region—Chicago

Governing Illinois, Indiana, Minnesota, Michigan,
Ohio, Wisconsin

Wayne J. Barlow, Acting Director; 2300 E. Devon Ave., Des Plaines, IL, 60018; phone (312) 694-4500; Duty Officer (312) 694-4401

New England Region—Boston

Governing Connecticut, Maine, Massachusetts,
New Hampshire, Rhode Island, Vermont
Robert E. Whittington, Director; 12 New England Executive Park, Burlington, MA, 01803; phone Director (617) 273-7244; Duty Officer (617) 273-7000

Northwest Region—Seattle

Governing Idaho, Oregon, Washington

C. B. Walk, Jr., Director; FAA Building, Boeing Field, (King County Int'l.), Seattle, WA, 98108; phone (206) 767-2780; Duty Officer (206) 767-2600

Pacific Region—Honolulu

Governing Hawaii, Western Pacific

Robert O. Ziegler, Director; P.O. Box 50109, Honolulu, HI, 96850; phone (808) 546-8641; Duty Officer (808) 546-7544

Rocky Mountain Region—Denver

Governing Colorado, Montana, North Dakota,
South Dakota, Utah, Wyoming

Mervyn Martin, Director; 10455 East 25th Ave., Aurora, CO, 80010; phone (303) 837-3646; Duty Officer (303) 837-4677

Southern Region—Atlanta

Governing Alabama, Florida, Georgia, Mississippi, North Carolina,
South Carolina, Tennessee, Kentucky, Puerto Rico, U.S. Virgin Isl.,
Canal Zone

Phillip M. Swatek, Director; P.O. Box 20636, Atlanta, GA, 30320; phone (404) 763-7222; Duty Officer (404) 763-7541; Duty hours 8:30–5 EST.

Southwest Region—Fort Worth

Governing Arkansas, Louisiana, New Mexico,
Oklahoma, Texas

C. R. (Tex) Melugin, Jr., Director; P.O. Box 1689, Fort Worth, TX, 76101; phone (817) 624-4911 ext. 200; Duty Officer (817) 624-4911 ext. 321; Duty hours 8:30–5 (9:30–6 EST)

Western Region—Los Angeles

Governing Arizona, California, Nevada

Leon C. Daugherty, Director; P.O. Box 92007, World Way Postal Center, Los Angeles, CA, 90009; phone (213) 536-6427; Duty Officer (213) 536-6435; Duty hours 7:30-4:00 (10:30-7:00 EST)

FAA GENERAL AVIATION DISTRICT OFFICES

Unless otherwise noted, address correspondence to General Aviation District Office, Federal Aviation Administration.

Alaskan Region

Anchorage, AK—1515 East 13th Ave., 99501; phone (907) 272-1324, 265-4657, and 265-4673

Fairbanks, AK—(Flight Standards District Office), 3788 University Avenue, 99701; phone (907) 452-1276

Juneau, AK—(Flight Standards District Office), Juneau Municipal Airport, P.O. Box 2118, 99803; phone (907) 789-0231/2

Central Region

Des Moines, IA—3021 Army Post Rd., 50321; phone (515) 284-4094

Kansas City, KS—Administration Bldg., Fairfax Municipal Airport, 66115; phone (913) 281-3491

Wichita, KS—Flight Standards Bldg., Mid-Continent Airport, 67209; phone (316) 943-3244

St. Louis, MO—(Flight Standards District Office), 9275 Genaire Dr., Berkeley, MO 63134; phone (314) 425-7102

Lincoln, NE—General Aviation Bldg., Lincoln Municipal Airport, 68524; phone (402) 471-5485

Eastern Region

Washington, DC—(Flight Standards District Office), West Bldg., Room 152, National Airport, 20001; phone (202) 628-1555

Baltimore, MD—Baltimore-Washington Intl. Airport, 21240; phone (301) 761-2610

Teterboro, NJ—(Flight Standards District Office), 150 Riser Road, Teterboro Airport, 07608; phone (201) 288-1745/3597

Albany, NY—Albany County Airport, 12211; phone (518) 869-8482

Farmingdale, NY—Bldg. 53, Republic Airport, 11735; phone (516) 694-5530

Rochester, NY—(Flight Standards District Office), Rochester-Monroe County Airport, 14624; phone (716) 263-5880

Allentown, PA—Allentown-Bethlehem-Easton Airport, 18103; phone (215) 264-2888

New Cumberland, PA—Capital City Airport, Room 201, Administration Bldg., 17070, phone (717) 782-4528

Philadelphia, PA—North Philadelphia Airport, 1st Floor, Administration Bldg., 19114; phone (215) 597-9708

Pittsburgh, PA—Allegheny County Airport, West Mifflin, PA, 15122; phone (412) 461-7800 and 462-5507

Richmond, VA—Byrd Field, Sandston, VA 23150; phone (804) 222-7494

Charleston, WV—Kanawha Airport, 25311; phone (304) 343-4689

Great Lakes Region

Chicago, IL—Box H, DuPage Airport, West Chicago, IL 60185; phone (312) 584-4490

Springfield, IL—Box 3, RR #2, Capital Airport, 62707; phone (217) 525-4238

Indianapolis, IN—FAA Bldg. #1, Box 41525, Indianapolis International Airprot, 46241; phone (317) 247-2491

South Bend, IN—1843 Commerce Dr., 46628; phone (219) 232-5843

Detroit, MI—Flight Standards Bldg., Willow Run Airport, Ypsilanti, MN 48197; phone (313) 485-2250

Grand Rapids, MI—5500 44th St. S.E., Kent County Airport, 49508; phone (616) 456-2427

Minneapolis, MN—6201 34th Ave. South, 55450; phone (612) 725-3341

Cincinnati, OH—Lunken Executive Bldg., 4242 Airport Rd., 45226; phone (513) 684-2183

Cleveland, OH—Federal Office Bldg., Cleveland-Hopkins International Airport, 44135; phone (216) 267-0220

Columbus, OH—4393 E. 17th Ave., Port Columbus International Airport, 43219; phone (614) 469-7476

Milwaukee, WI—General Mitchell Field, 53207; phone (414) 747-5531

New England Region

Portland, ME—Portland International Jetport, 04102; phone (207) 774-4484

Boston, MA—Norwood Municipal Airport, Norwood, MA, 02062; phone (617) 762-2436

Westfield, MA—P.O. Box 544, 01085; phone (413) 568-3121

Northwest Region

Boise, ID—3113 Airport Way, 83705; phone (208) 384-1238

Eugene, OR—Mahlon-Sweet Airport, 90606 Greenhill Rd., 97402; phone (503) 688-9721

Portland, OR—Portland-Hillsboro Airport, 3355 N.E. Cornell Rd., Hillsboro, OR 97123; phone (503) 221-2104

Seattle, WA—(Flight Standards District Office), FAA Bldg., Boeing Field, 98108; phone (206) 767-2747/2570

Spokane, WA—5629 E. Rutter Avenue; 99206; phone (509) 456-4618

Pacific Region

Honolulu, HI—(Flight Standards District Office). P.O. Box 29728; 96820; phone 847-0615

Rocky Mountain Region

Denver, CO—Jefferson County Airport, Bldg. 1, Broomfield, CO 80020; phone (303) 466-7326

Billings, MT—Room 216, Administration Bldg., Billings Logan International Airport; 59101; phone (406) 245-6179

Helena, MT—Rm. 3, FAA Bldg., Helena Airport, 59601; phone (406) 449-5270

Fargo, ND—State University Station, P.O. Box 5496, 58102; phone (701) 232-8949

Rapid City, SD—Regional Airport, R.R. 2, Box 633B, 57701; phone (605) 343-2403

Salt Lake City, UT—116 North 2400 West; 84116; phone (801) 524-4247

Casper, WY—FAA/WB Bldg., Natrona County Int'l. Airport, 82601; phone (307) 234-8959

Southern Region

Birmingham, AL—6500 43rd Ave., North, 35206; phone (205) 254-1393

Jacksonville, FL—Craig Field, 855 St. Johns Bluff Rd., 32211; phone (904) 641-7311

Miami, FL—Bldg. 121, Opa-Locka Airport, Opa-Locka, FL, 33054; phone (305) 681-7431

St. Petersburg, FL—St. Petersburg-Clearwater Airport, 33520; phone (813) 531-1434

Atlanta, GA—FAA Bldg., Charlie Brown County Airport, 30336; phone (404) 221-6481

Louisville, KY—Bowman Field, 40205; phone (502) 582-6116

Jackson, MS—P.O. Box 6273, Pearl Branch, 39208; phone (601) 969-4633

Charlotte, NC—FAA Bldg., Municipal Airport, P.O. Box 27005, 28219; phone (704) 392-3214

Raleigh, NC—Rm. 324 Administration Bldg., Raleigh-Durham Airport, P.O. Box 486A, 27560; phone (919) 755-4240

West Columbia, SC—Box 200, Columbia Metropolitan Airport, 29169; phone (803) 765-5931

Memphis, TN—2488 Winchester, Rm. 137, 38116; phone (901) 345-0600

Nashville, TN—(Flight Standards District Office), 322 Knapp Blvd., Rm. 101, Nashville Metropolitan Airport, 37217; phone (615) 251-5661

San Juan, PR—(Flight Standards District Office), RFD 1, Box 29A, Loiza Station, 00914; phone (809) 791-5050

Southwest Region

Little Rock, AR—FAA/Weather Service Bldg., Rm. 201, Adams Field, 72202; phone (501) 372-3437

Lafayette, LA—Lafayette Airport, 70501; phone (318) 234-2321

New Orleans, LA—Rm. 227, New Orleans Lakefront Airport, 70126; phone (504) 241-2506

Shreveport, LA—Terminal Bldg., Room 137 Shreveport Downtown Airport, 71107; phone (318) 226-5379

Albuquerque, NM—P.O. Box 9045, Albuquerque Int'l Airport, 87119; phone (505) 247-0156

Oklahoma City, OK—FAA Bldg., Wiley Post Airport, Bethany, OK 73008; phone (405) 789-5220

Tulsa, OK—Room 110, Genral Aviation Terminal, Tulsa Int'l Airport, 74115; phone (918) 835-7619

Fort Worth, TX—Rm. 201, Terminal Bldg., Meacham Field, 76106; phone (817) 624-1184

Dallas, TX—8032 Air Freight La., Love Field Airport, 75235; phone (214) 357-0142

Corpus Christi, TX—Rt. 2, Box 903, 78408; phone (512) 884-9331

El Paso, TX—Room 202, FAA Bldg., 6795 Convair Rd., 79925; phone (915) 778-6389

Houston, TX—8800 Paul B. Koonce Dr., Rm. 152, 77061; phone (713) 643-6504

Lubbock, TX—Rt. 3, Box 51, 79401; phone (806) 762-0335

San Antonio, TX—1115 Paul Wilkins Rd., 78216; phone (512) 824-9535

Western Region

Phoenix, AZ—15041 North Airport Drive, Scottsdale, AZ, 85260; phone (602) 261-4763

Fresno, CA—Fresno Air Terminal, 2401 North Ashley, 93727; phone (209) 487-5306

Oakland, CA—(Flight Standards District Office), 9636 Earhart Road, P.O. Box 2397, Airport Station, 94614; phone (415) 273-7155

Riverside, CA—(Flight Standards District Office) Riverside Municipal Airport, 6961 Flight Road, 92504; phone (714) 796-1245

Sacramento, CA—Executive Airport, 95822; phone (916) 440-3169

San Diego, CA—3750 John J. Montgomery Drive, 92123; phone (714) 293-5280

San Jose, CA—1387 Airport Boulevard, 95110; phone (408) 275-7681

Santa Monica, CA—Municipal Airport, 3200 Airport Avenue, Suite 3, 90405; phone (213) 391-6701

Van Nuys, CA—7120 Hayvenhurt Avenue, Suit 316, 91406; phone (213) 997-3191

Long Beach, CA—(Flight Standards District Office), 2815 E. Spring Street, 90806; phone (213) 426-7134

Las Vegas, NV—(Flight Standards District Office), 5700-C South Haven, 89119; phone (702) 736-0666

Reno NV—Terminal Way, Room 230, Reno International Airport, 89502; phone (702) 784-5321

Federal Communications Commission

1919 M St., N.W.
Washington, DC 20554
Phone (202) 655-4000

Chairman, Charles D. Ferris

Commissioners: Robert E. Lee
Joseph R. Fogarty
Anne P. Jones
Tyrone Brown
James H. Quello
Abbott M. Washburn
Executive Director, Richard D. Lichtwardt
Chief of Aviation and Marine Licensing, Robert Mickley

FCC Field Operating Offices

Mailing addresses for Commission Field Operating Offices are listed below. Address communications to: Engineer in Charge, Federal Communications Commission.

Anchorage, AK—Federal Building & U.S. Courthouse, P.O. Box 2955, 1011 East Tudor Rd., Room 240C, Anchorage, AK, 99507; phone (907) 276-7455

Atlanta, GA—Room 440, Massell Building, 1365 Peachtree St., N.E., Atlanta, GA, 30309; phone (404) 881-3084/5

Baltimore, MD—1017 Federal Building, 31 Hopkins Plaza, Baltimore, MD, 21301; phone (301) 962-2728/9

Beaumont, TX—323 Jack Brooks Federal Building, U.S. Post Office and Courthouse, 300 Willow St., Beaumont, TX, 77701; phone (713) 838-0271

Boston, MA—1600 Customhouse, 165 State Street, Boston, MA, 02109; phone (617) 223-6609

Buffalo, NY—1307 Federal Building, 111 West Hurton St., Buffalo, NY, 14202; phone (716) 846-4511/2

Canandaigua, NY—P.O. Box 374, Canandaigua, NY, 14424; phone (716) 394-4240

Chicago, IL—230 S. Dearborn St., Room 3935, Chicago, IL, 60604; phone (312) 353-0195/6

Cincinnati, OH—8620 Winton Rd., Cincinnati, OH, 45231; phone (513) 521-1790

Dallas, TX—Earle Cabell Federal Building, U.S. Courthouse, Room 13E7, 1100 Commerce St., Dallas, TX, 75242; phone (214) 749-1719/0

Denver, CO—Suite 2925, The Executive Tower, 1405 Curtis St., Denver, CO, 80202; phone (303) 837-5137/8

Detroit, MI—1054 Federal Building, 231 W. LaFayette St., Detroit, MI, 48226; phone (313) 226-6078/9

Honolulu, HI—Prince Kuhio Federal Building, 300 Ala Moana Blvd., Room 7304, P.O. Box 50023, Honolulu, HI, 96850; phone (808) 546-5640

Houston, TX—New Federal Office Building, 515 Rusk Ave., Room 5636, Houston, TX, 77002; phone (713) 226-5624/5

Kansas City, MO—Brywood Office Tower, Room 320, 8800 East 63rd St., Kansas City, MO, 64133; phone (816) 926-5111

Long Beach, CA—Room 501, 3711 Long Beach Blvd., Long Beach, CA, 90807; phone (213) 426-4451

Miami, FL—Room 919, 51 S.W. First Ave., Miami, FL, 33130; phone (305) 350-5542

New Orleans, LA—829 F. Edward Hebert Federal Building, 600 South St., New Orleans, LA, 70130; phone (504) 589-2095/6

New York, NY—201 Varick St., New York, NY, 10014; phone (212) 620-6437/8

Norfolk, VA—Military Circle, 870 N. Military Highway, Norfolk, VA, 23502; phone (804) 441-6472.

Philadelphia, PA—11425 James A. Byrne Federal Courthouse, 601 Market St., Philadelphia, PA, 19106; phone (215) 597-4411/2

Pittsburgh, PA—3755 William Penn Highway, Monroeville, PA, 15146; phone (412) 823-3380

Portland, OR—1782 Federal Office Building, 1220 S.W. Third Ave., Portland, OR, 92704; phone (503) 221-4114

St. Paul MN—691 Federal Building & U.S. Courthouse, 316 North Robert St., St. Paul, MN, 55101; phone (612) 725-7810

San Diego, CA—7840 EL Cajon Blvd., Suite 405, La Mesa, CA, 92041; phone (714) 293-5478

San Francisco, CA—323-A Customhouse, 555 Battery St., San Francisco, CA, 94111; phone (415) 556-7701/2

San Juan, Puerto Rico—747 Federal Building, Hato Rey, Puerto Rico. 00918; phone (809) 753-4008

Savannah, GA—Room 238, Federal Building & Courthouse, P.O. Box 8004, (125 Bull St.) Savannah, GA, 31402; phone (912) 232-4321

Seattle, WA—3256 Federal Building, 915 Second Ave., Seattle, WA, 98174; phone (206) 442-7653/4

Tampa, FL—ADP Bldg., Room 601, 1211 N. Westmore Blvd., Tampa, FL, 33607; phone (813) 228-2872

Washington, DC—The Presidential Bldg., 6525 Belerest Rd., Suite 901-B, Hyattsville, MD, 20788; phone (301) 436-7590

Civil Aeronautics Board

1825 Connecticut Ave., N.W., Washington, DC, 20428
Phone (202) 673-5260

Office of Members

Marvin S. Cohen, Chairman
Elizabeth Bailey
Richard J. O'Melia
Gloria Schaffer
(Appointment to fifth seat pending)

Managing Director, Cressworth Lander
Secretary, Phyllis T. Kaylor

National Transportation Safety Board

800 Independence Ave., S.W.
Washington, DC, 20594
Phone (202) 472-6100

Board Members:

Chairman, James B. King
Elwood T. Driver, Vice Chairman
Francis H. McAdams
Patricia Goldman
Patrick Bursley (nominated)

Managing Director, Vacant
General Counsel, Fritz L. Puls
Director of Public Affairs, Edward E. Slattery, Jr.
Director of Evaluations and Safety Objectives, Roy W. Anderson
Administrative Law Judge, William E. Fowler, Jr.
Bureau of Accident Investigation, Frank T. Taylor
Bureau of Technology, Martyn V. Clarke

NTSB Field Offices

Anchorage, AK—Rm. 454, 632 Sixth Ave., 99501; phone (907) 277-0593
Los Angeles, CA—8939 South Sepulveda Blvd., Suite 426, 90045; phone (213) 536-6584
Aurora, CO—10255 East 25th Ave., 80010; phone (303) 837-4492
Washington, DC—P.O. Box 17226, Gateway Bldg. #1, Dulles Int'l. Airport, 20041; phone (703) 471-1200
Miami Springs, FL—4471 N.W. 36th St., 33166; phone (305) 526-2940
Atlanta, GA—1720 Peachtree St., N.W., 30309; phone (404) 881-7385
Des Plaines, IL—2300 E. Devon Ave., Rm. 140, 60018; phone (312) 827-8858
Kansas City, MO—Federal Bldg., Rm. 1443, 601 East 12th St., 64106; phone (816) 374-3576
Jamaica, NY—Federal Bldg., Rm. 102, John F. Kennedy Intl. Airport, 11430; phone (212) 995-3716
Fort Worth, TX—Federal Bldg., Rm. 7A07, 819 Taylor St., 76102; phone (817) 334-2616
Seattle, WA—19415 Pacific Highway South, 98188; phone (206) 764-3782
National Transportation Accident Investigation School—800 Independence Ave., S.W., Washington, DC, 20594

State Aeronautical Agencies

Alabama Dept. of Aeronautics, James ROWE, Director, State Highway Bldg., 11 S. Union St., Montgomery, AL, 36130; phone (205) 832-6290

Alaska Dept. of Transportation, James E. Moody, Special Asst. to Commissioner for Aviation, Pouch 6900, Anchorage, AK, 99502; phone (907) 266-1470

Arizona Div. of Aeronautics, Sonny Najera, Asst. Director of Transportation, 205 S. 17th Ave., Phoenix, AZ, 85007; phone (602) 261-7778

Arkansas Div. of Aeronautics, Eddie Holland, Director, Adams Field—Old Terminal Bldg., Little Rock, AR, 72202; phone (501) 376-6781

California Div. of Aeronautics, Dept. of Transportation, John West, Chief, 1120 N St., Sacramento, CA, 95814; phone (916) 322-3090

Connecticut Bureau of Aeronautics-DOT, Robert H. Carrier, Chief Exec. Officer—Aeronautics, P.O. Drawer A, Wethersfield, CT, 06109; phone (203) 566-4599

Delaware Transportation Authority, Dept. of Transportation, Rayvon Burleson, Chief of Aeronautics, P.O. Box 778, Dover, DE, 19901; phone (302) 678-4597/3

Florida Bureau of Aviation, Dept. of Transportation, Grover C. Jones, Chief, Burns Bldg., Tallahassee, FL, 32304; phone (904) 488-8444

Georgia Bureau of Aeronautics, Dept. of Transportation, William Cousins, Chief, 5025 New Peachtree Rd., N.E., Chamblee, GA, 30341; phone (404) 393-7353

Hawaii Air Transportation Facilities Div., Dept. of Transportation, Owen Miyamoto, Chief, Honolulu International Airport, Honolulu, HI, 96819; phone (808) 836-6423

Idaho Div. of Aeronautics and Public Transportation, Worthie M. Rauscher, Administrator, 3483 Rickenbacker St., Boise, ID, 83705; phone (208) 384-3183

Illinois Div. of Aeronautics, Dept. of Transportation, Robert L. Donahue, Director, Capital Airport—N. Walnut St. Rd., Springfield, IL, 62706; phone (217) 782-2880

Indiana Aeronautics Commission, Henry A. Kazimier, Director, 100 N. Senate Ave., Indianapolis IN, 46204; phone (317) 633-6545

Iowa Aeronautics Div., Dept. of Transportation, Harry A. Hoover, Director, State House, Des Moines, IA, 50319; phone (515) 281-4280

Kansas Aviation Div., Dept. of Transportation, Ray Arvin, Director, State Office Bldg., Topeka, KS, 66612; phone (913) 296-3566

Kentucky Div. of Aeronautics, Dept. of Transportation, Edward LaFontaine, Director, 419 Ann St., Frankfort, KY, 40622; phone (502) 564-4480

Louisiana Office of Aviation, Dept. of Transportation and Development, David L. Blackshear, Asst. Secretary of Transportation, P.O. Box 44245—Capitol Station, Baton Rouge, LA, 70804; phone (504) 342-7504

Maine Bureau of Aeronautics, Dept. of Transportation, Richard DiPietro, Director, State Office Bldg., Augusta, ME, 04333; phone (207) 289-3185

Maryland State Aviation Administration, Dept. of Transportation, Karl Sattler, Administrator, P.O. Box 8755, Baltimore-Washington International Airport, Baltimore, MD, 21240; phone (301) 787-7100

Massachusetts Aeronautics Commission, Crocker Snow, Consultant, Boston-Logan Airport, E. Boston, MA, 02128; phone (617) 727-5350

Michigan Aeronautics Commission, Dept. of Highways and Transportation,

Robert J. Thomas, Director, Capital City Airport, Lansing, MI, 48906; phone (517) 373-1834

Minnesota Div. of Aeronautics, Dept. of Transportation, Lawrence E. McCabe, Asst. Commissioner of Transportation, Transportation Bldg., St. Paul, MN 55155; phone (612) 296-8046

Mississippi Aeronautics Commission, Kenneth A. Barfield, Director, P.O. Box 5, 500 Robert E. Lee Bldg., Jackson, MS, 39205; phone (601) 354-7494

Missouri Dept. of Transportation, William Stephens, Director, P.O. Box 1250, Jefferson City, MO, 65102; phone (314) 751-4922

Montana Div. of Aeronautics, Dept. of Community Affairs, Michael D. Ferguson, Administrator, P.O. Box 5178, Helena, MT, 59601; phone (406) 499-2506

Nebraska Dept. of Aeronautics, Wayne C. Anderson, Director, P.O. Box 82088, Lincoln, NE, 68501; phone (402) 471-2371

New Hampshire Aeronautics Commission, John R. Sweeney, Director, Municipal Airport, Concord, NH, 03301; phone (603) 271-2551

New Jersey Div. of Aeronatutics, Dept. of Transportation, Walter G. Kies, Director, 1035 Parkway Ave., Trenton, NJ, 08625; phone (609) 292-3020

New Mexico Aviation Div., Dept. of Transportation, Bob White, Director. P.O. Box 579, Santa Fe, NM, 87503; phone (505) 827-5511

New York Airport Development Section, Dept. of Transportation, Clarence M. Cook, Supervisor, 1220 Washington Ave., Albany, NY, 12232; phone (518) 457-2820

North Carolina Div. of Aeronautics, Dept. of Transportation, Willard G. Plentl, Jr., Director, P.O. Box 25201, Raleigh, NC, 27611; phone (919) 733-2491

North Dakota Aeronautics Commission, Harold G. Vavra, Director, Box U—Bismarck Airport, Bismarck, ND, 58505; phone (701) 224-2748

Ohio Div. of Aviation, Norman Crabtree, Deputy Director of Transportation, 2829 W. Granville Rd., Worthington, OH, 43085; phone (614) 466-7120

Oklahoma Aeronautics Commission, David Jay Perry, Director, 424 United Founders Tower, Oklahoma City, OK, 73112; phone (405) 521-2377

Oregon Div. of Aeronatutics, Dept. of Transportation, Paul E. Burket, Administrator, 3040 - 25th St., S.E., Salem, OR, 97310; phone (503) 378-4880

Pennsylvania Bureau of Aviation, Dept. of Transportation, (Director vacant), Capital City Airport, New Cumberland, PA, 17070; phone (717) 787-8754

Puerto Rico Ports Authority, Wilson Loubriel, Executive Director, GPO Box 2829, San Juan, P.R. 00936; phone (809) 723-2260

Rhode Island Dept. of Transportation, Victor C. Ricci, Asst. Director of Transportation, Theodore Francis Green State Airport, Warwick, RI, 02886; phone (401) 737-4000

South Carolina Aeronautics Commission, John W. Hamilton, Director, Box 1769, Columbia Metropolitan Airport, Columbia, SC, 29202; phone (803) 758-2766

South Dakota Div. of Aeronautics, Dept. of Transportation, Monte R. Schneider, Director Transportation Bldg., Pierre, SD, 57501; phone (605)

Tennessee Bureau of Aeronautics, Dept. of Transportation, Frank P. Pledger, Director, P.O. Box 17326, Nashville Metropolitan Airport, Nashville, TN, 37217; phone (615) 741-3208

Texas Aeronautics Commission, Charles Murphy, Director, P.O. Box 12607, Capitol Station, Austin, TX, 78711; phone (512) 475-4768

Utah Div. of Aeronautical Operations, Dept. of Transportation, Phillip N. Ashbaker, Director, 135 North 2400 West, Salt Lake City, UT, 84116; phone (801) 328-2066

Vermont Agency of Transportation, Richard F. Hurd, Aeronautics Specialist, State Administration Bldg., Montpelier, VT, 05602; phone (802) 828-2828

Virginia Dept. of Aeronautics, Willard G. Plentl, Director, P.O. Box 7716, 4508 S. Laburnum Ave., Richmond, VA, 23231; phone (804) 786-3685

Washington Div. of Aeronautics, Dept. of Transportation, William H. Hamilton, Asst. Secy. for Aeronautics, 8600 Perimeter Rd., Boeing Field, Seattle, WA, 98108; phone (206) 764-4131

West Virginia Aeronautics Commission, William E. Richards, Executive Director, Kanawha Airport, Charleston, WV, 25311; phone (304) 348-2689/3790

Wisconsin Bureau of Aeronautics, Dept. of Transportation, Fritz E. Wolf, Director, P.O. Box 7914, Madison, WI, 53707; phone (608) 266-3351

Wyoming Aeronautics Commission, Casimer Krauser, Director, Cheyenne, WY, 82002; phone (307) 777-7481

Aviation Organizations

Academy of Model Aeronautics, 815 15th St., N.W., Washington, DC, 20005; phone (202) 347-2751

Aerobatic Club of America, 1401 N.E. 10th St., Pompano Beach, FL, 33060; phone (305) 943-8330

Aeronautical Radio, Inc. (ARINC), 2551 Riva Rd., Annapolis, MD, 21401; phone (301) 224-4000

Aerospace Education Foundation, c/o Dr. Herbert O. Fisher, Trustee, 628 Mountain Rd., Smoke Rise, Kinnelon, NJ, 07405; phone (201) 838-2040

Aerospace Industries Association of America, Inc., 1725 De Sales St., N.W., Washington, DC, 20036; phone (202) 347-2315

Aerospace Medical Association, c/o R. R. Hessberg, M.D., Washington National Airport, Washington, DC, 20001; phone (703) 892-2240

Airborne Law Enforcement Association, Inc., 524 Belmar Dr., Birmingham, AL, 35215; phone (205) 325-5706

Aircraft Electronics Association, P.O. Box 1981, Independence, MO, 64055; phone (816) 373-6565

Aircraft Owners and Pilots Association (AOPA), Air Rights Bldg., 7315 Wisconson Ave., Bethesda, MD, 20014; phone (301) 654-0500

Air Force Association, 1750 Pennsylvania Ave., N.W., Suite 400, Washington, DC, 20006; phone (202) 637-3300

Airline Passengers Association, P.O. Box 2758, Dallas, TX, 75221; phone (214) 438-8100

Air Line Pilots Association (ALPA), 1625 Massachusetts Ave., N.W., Washington DC, 20036; phone (202) 797-4000

Airport Operators Council International, Inc., 1700 K St., N.W., Suite 602, Washington, DC, 20006; phone (202) 296-3270

Air Traffic Control Association, 525 School St., S.W., Suite 409, Washington, DC, 20024; phone (202) 554-9135

Air Transport Association of America (ATA), 1709 New York Ave., N.W., Washington, DC, 20006; phone (202) 872-4000

Allied Pilots Association, 2621 Ave. "E" East, Suite 208, Arlington, TX, 76011; phone (817) 261-0261

American Association of Airport Executives, 2029 K St., N.W., Washington, DC, 20006; phone (202) 331-8994

American Aviation Historical Society, P.O. Box 99, Garden Grove, CA, 92642

American Bonanza Society, Reading Municipal Airport, P.O. Box 3749, Reading, PA, 19605; phone (215) 372-6967/7078

American Helicopter Society, Inc., 1325 18th St., N.W., Suite 103, Washington, DC, 20036; phone (202) 659-9524

American Navion Society. P.O. Box 1175, Municipal Airport, Banning CA, 92220; phone (714) 849-2213

American Society for Aerospace Education, Suite 432, 821 15th St., N.W., Washington, DC, 20005; phone (202) 347-5187

Animal Air Transportation Association, 6180 S.W. 56th Ct., Davie, FL, 33314; phone (305) 944-8153

Antique Airmen, Inc., Ottumwa Industrial Airport, P.O. Box 931, Ottumwa, IA, 52501; phone (515) 684-5496

Antique Airplane Association, P.O. Box H, Ottumwa, IA, 52501; phone (515) 938-2773

Association of Aviation Psychologists, c/o J. M. Koonce, Ph.D., 6920 Boysenberry Way, Colorado Spring, CO, 80918; phone (303) 598-1957

Aviation Distributors and Manufacturers Association (ADMA), 1900 Arch St., Philadelphia, PA, 19103; phone (215) 564-3484

Aviation Hall of Fame, Dayton, OH, c/o Dr. Herbert O. Fisher, National Board of Nominees, 628 Mountain Rd., Smoke Rise, Kinnelon, NJ, 07405; phone (201) 838-2040

Aviation Maintenance Foundation, P.O. Box 739, Basin, WY, 82410; phone (307) 568-2466

Aviation/Space Writers Assocation, c/o William F. Kaiser, Cliffwood Rd., Chester, NJ, 07930; phone (201) 538-0050

Balloon Federation of America, Suite 430, 821 15th St., N.W., Washington, DC, 20005; phone (202) 737-0897

Bishop Milton Wright Air Industry Awards Council, c/o Dr. Herbert O. Fisher, Director and Vice-Chairman of Awards Committee, 628 Mountain Rd., Smoke Rise, Kinnelon, NJ, 07405; phone (201) 838-2040

Cessna 120/140 Association, Box 92, Richardson, TX, 75080; phone (214) 234-2064

Cessna Skyhawk Association, c/o Paul R. Morton, Executive Director, P.O. Box 779, Delray Beach, FL, 33444; phone (305) 278-2116

Cessna Skylane Society, c/o Paul R. Morton, Executive Director, P.O. Box 779, Delray Beach, FL, 33444; phone (305) 278-2116

China Burma, India Hump Pilots Association, c/o Dr. Herbert O. Fisher, Director of Public Relations and Press, 628 Mountain Rd., Smoke Rise, Kinnelon, NJ, 07405; phone (201) 838-2040

Christian Pilots Association, Inc., (an evangelical relief agency) 802 N. Foxdale, W. Covina, CA, 91790; phone (213) 962-7591

Civil Air Patrol, Headquarters, Maxwell Air Force Base, AL, 36112; Attn: DO, phone (205) 293-5198

Civil Aviation Medical Association, 801 Green Bay Rd., Lake Bluff, IL, 60044; phone (312) 234-6330

Combat Pilots Association, c/oWilliam R. Mayo, Pres., Rt. 222, P.O. Box 8, Trexlertown, PA, 18087; phone (215) 395-0333

Commuter Airline Association of America, 1101 Conn. Ave., N.W., Suite 700, Washington, DC, 20036; phone (202) 857-1170

Confederate Air Force, Rebel Field, P.O. Box CAF, Harlingen, TX, 78550; phone (512) 425-1057

(The) Early Birds of Aviation, Inc., c/o Robert A. Warren, 60 Webster Rd., Weston, MA, 02193; phone (617) 893-2777

Ercoupe Owners Club, 3557 Roxboro Rd., P.O. Box 15058, Durham, NC, 27704; phone (919) 477-2193

Experimental Aircraft Association, Inc. (EAA), P.O. Box 229, Hales Corners, WI, 53130; phone (414) 425-4860

Flight Safety Foundation, Inc., 5510 Columbia Pike, Arlington, VA, 22204; phone (703) 820-2777

Flying Apache Assocation, c/o Marcel P. Roy, P.O. Box 461, Winona, Ontario, Canada, LOR 2LO

Flying Architects Association, Inc., c/o Harold J. Westin, First Floor, American National Bank Bldg., Fifth and Robert Streets, St. Paul, MN, 55101; phone (612) 222-3092

Flying Chiropractors Association, c/o Federic J. Miscoe, D.C., 215 Belmont St., Johnstown, PA, 15904; phone (814) 266-3314

Flying Dentists Association, 5820 Wilshire Blvd., Los Angeles, CA, 90036; phone (213) 937-5514

Flying Engineers International, P.O. Box 387, Winnebago, IL, 61088; phone (815) 335-2660 or (205) 881-5653

Flying Funeral Directors of America, c/o Phillip N. Schmidt, 10980 Reading Rd., Sharonville, OH, 45241; phone (513) 948-1113

Flying Optometrist Association of America, c/o Dr. William B. Buethe, 24953 Paseo De Valencia, Laguna Hills, CA, 92653; phone (714) 837-2200

Flying Physicians Association, 801 Green Bay Rd., Lake Bluff, IL, 60044; phone (312) 234-6330

Flying Psychologists, c/o Paul W. Clement, Ph.D., Executive Secretary, 190 N. Oakland Ave., Pasadena, CA, 91101; phone (213) 449-2182

Flying Veterinarians Association, c/o Dr. Richard Burns, 10519 Reading Rd., Cincinnati, OH, 45241; phone (513) 563-0410

General Aviation Manufacturers Association (GAMA), 1025 Connecticut Ave., N.W., Suite 517, Washington, DC, 20036; phone (202) 296-8848

Handicapped Flyers International, 1117 Rising Hill, Escondido, CA, 92025

Helicopter Association of America, 1156 15th St., N.W., Suite 610, Washington, DC, 20005; phone (202) 466-2420

International 180/185 Club, 4539 N. 49th Ave., Phoenix, AZ, 85031; phone (602) 846-6236

International Aerobatic Club, P.O. Box 229, Hales Corners, WI, 53130; phone (414) 425-4860

International Aviation Theft Bureau, 7315 Wisconsin Ave., Bethesda, MD, 20014; phone (301) 654-0500

International Cessna 170 Association, Montezuma A/P, P.O. Box 460, Camp Verde, AZ, 86322; phone (602) 567-3271

International Comanche Society, Inc., Larry T. Larkin, President, 4140 Manson Ave., Smyrna, GA, 30080; phone (404) 432-2183

International Flying Bankers Association, c/o L. B. Coward, Executive Director, P.O. Box 11187, Columbia, SC, 29211; phone (803) 252-5646

International Flying Farmers, Mid Continent Airport, P.O. Box 9124, Wichita, KS, 67277; phone (316) 943-4234

International Organization of Aviation Characters, c/o Dr. Herbert O. Fisher, Executive Vice,President, 628 Mountain Rd., Smoke Rise, Kinnelon, NJ, 07405; phone (201) 838-2040

James XD-5 Club, (BD-5 Enthusiasts) Box 151, Pasadena, CA, 91102; phone (213) 256-3542

Lawyer-Pilots Bar Association, Lloyd Ericsson, 2098 First National Bank Tower, Portland, OR, 97201; phone (503) 224-3113

(The) Lighter Than Air Society, 1800 Triplett Blvd., Akron, OH, 44306; phone (216) 325-7087, or, (216) 633-4197

Luscombe Association, c/o Bob Shelton, 339 West Pierce, Macomb, IL 61455

Mooney Aircraft Pilots Association, 314 Stardust Dr., San Antonio, TX, 78228; phone (512) 434-5959

National Aeronautic Association (NAA) 821 15th St., N.W., Suite 430, Washington, DC, 20005; phone (202) 347-2808

National Agricultural Aviation Association, Nat'l Press Bldg., Suite 459, Washington, DC, 20045; phone (202) 638-0542

National Air Transportation Association, Inc. 1010 Wisc. Ave., N.W., Suite 405, Washington, DC, 20007; phone (202) 965-8880.

National Association of Air Traffic Specialists, Wheaton Plaza North Bldg., Suite 415, Wheaton, MD, 20902; phone (301) 946-0822

National Association of Flight Instructors (NAFI), Ohio State University Airport, Box 20204, Columbus, OH, 43220; phone (614) 459-0204

National Association of Minority Aviators, c/o Tahmir T. Saladdin, Pres., 2117 Miramonte Dr., Prescott, AZ, 86301; phone (602) 778-4720

National Association of Priest Pilots, 1701 Mulberry St., Waterloo, IA, 50703; phone (319) 233-5241

National Association of State Aviation Officials (NASAO), 444 N. Capital St., N.W., Washington, DC, 20001; phone (202) 783-0588

National Business Aircraft Association, Inc. (NBAA), One Farragut Square, S., Washington, DC, 20006; phone (202) 783-9000

National Intercollegiate Flying Association (NIFA), Parks College, St. Louis University, Parks Airport, Cahokia, IL, 62206; phone (618) 337-7500

National Pilots Association (NPA), 805 15th St., N.W., Washington, DC, 20005; phone (202) 737-0773

National Police Pilots Association, Box 45, Shenorock, NY, 10587; phone (914) 682-5324

(The) National World War II Glider Pilots Association, 1516 Corinth St., Dallas, TX, 75215

National 210 Owners Association, c/o Paul E. Terry, 7726 Gloria Ave., Van Nuys, CA, 91406; phone (213) 782-4313

(The) Ninety-Nines, Inc., (international organization of women pilots), Will Rogers World Airport, Oklahoma City, OK, 73159; phone (405) 685-7969

Organized Flying Adjusters, c/o Donald E. Kehaya, President, P.O. Box 7601, Macon, GA, 31204; phone (912) 474-3332, (912) 742-6453

OX5 Aviation Pioneers, 605 Allegheny Bldg., Pittsburgh, PA, 15219; phone (412) 281-6477

P-40 Warhawk Pilots Association, c/o Dr. Herbert O. Fisher, Director of Public Relations and Press, 628 Mountain Rd., Smoke Rise, Kinnelon, NJ, 07405; phone (201) 838-2040

P-47 Thunderbolt Pilots Association, c/o Dr. Herbert O. Fisher, Director of Public Relations and Press, 628 Mountain Rd., Smoke Rise, Kinnelon, NJ, 07405; phone (201) 838-2040

Pilots International Association, Inc., 400 South County Rd. 18, Suite 500, Minneapolis, MN, 55426; phone (612) 546-4075

Professional Air Traffic Controllers Organization (PATCO), 444 N. Capitol St., Washington, DC, 20001; phone (202) 638-6500

Professional Aviation Maintenance Association, Inc., P.O. Box 12449, Greater Pittsburgh Int'l. Airport, Pittsburgh, PA, 15231; phone (412) 433-4825

Real Estate Aviation Chapter of the Farm and Land Institute, National Association of Realtors, L. R. Arie, President, 114 W. Camelback Rd., Phoenix, AZ 85013; phone (602) 279-4312

Silver Wings Fraternity, Russ Brinkley, President, Box 1228, Harrisburg, PA, 17108; phone (717) 232-9525

(The) Soaring Society of America, Inc., Box 66071, Los Angeles, CA, 90066; phone (213) 390-4447

Society of Automotive Engineers, Inc., 400 Commonwealth Dr., Warrendale, PA, 15096; phone (412) 776-4841

Society of Flight Test Engineers, Inc., P.O. Box 4047, Lancaster, CA, 93534; phone (805) 948-3067

Society of World War I Aero Historians (Aerospace), 10443 S. Memphis Ave., Whittier, CA, 90604; phone (213) 994-4003

Swift Association, McMinn County Airport, Box 644, Athens, TN, 37303; phone (615) 745-9547/3951

Taildragger Pilots Association, Hangar 5, Int'l. Airport, Box 161079, Memphis, TN, 38116; phone (901) 345-7367

United States Air Racing Association (USARA), 4895 Texas Avenue, Stead Airport, P.O. Box 60084, Reno, NV, 89512

United States Hang Gliding Association, P.O. Box 66306, Los Angeles, CA, 90066; phone (213) 390-3065

United States Parachute Association, 806 15th St., N.W., Suite 444, Washington, DC, 20005; phone (202) 347-5773

United States Seaplane Pilots Association, c/o David Quam, President, Little Ferry Seaplane Base, P.O. Box 43, Little Ferry, NJ, 07643; phone (201) 440-2175

Wheelchair Pilots Association, c/o Harold L. Treadwell, President, 11018 102nd Ave., Largo, FL, 33540; phone (813) 393-3131

(The) Whirly-Girls, Inc., (international organization of women helicopter pilots), 1725 DeSales St., N.W., Suite 700, Washington, DC, 20036; phone (202) 347-2315

Government Aviation Publications

Ordering publications from GPO: Government publications can be ordered by mail from The Superintendent of Documents, U.S. Government Printing Office, Washington, DC, 20402 or from the Public Documents Distribution Center, Pueblo Industrial Park, Pueblo, CO, 81009. Mail orders should be accompanied by a check or money order payable to The Superintendent of Documents. Unless otherwise specified, orders for mailing to foreign countries should include an additional 25% of the total price to cover postage. No C.O.D. orders are accepted. All subscription orders should go to GPO, Washington, DC. Because of increasing costs, a $1.00 minimum has been placed on all mail orders. If entire order is less than $1.00, remit additional funds to total $1.00. Prices are subject to change without notice. For this reason, Sup't Doc's recommends that customers who make frequent purchases open a prepaid deposit account. A remittance of $50 is sufficient to open such an account. Maintaining it will obviate the need to make individual remittances or to check prices before ordering.

Listed below are GPO Bookstores. They stock approximately 1500 of the most popular titles of government publications that can be purchased over-the-counter, but they do not handle mail orders, though all of them can secure the single sale publications they need from Sup't Doc's on reasonably short notice.

The bookstores vary in size from small stores displaying perhaps 1,000 titles, to larger ones which may display as many as 3,500. None of the stores carry the complete stocks of FAA publications available at Sup't Doc's.

GPO Bookstore, 9220B Parkway East, Roebuck Shopping City, Birmingham, AL, 35206.

GPO Bookstore, Federal Office Building, Room 2039, 300 North Los Angeles Street, Los Angeles, CA, 90012.

GPO Bookstore, Federal Office Building, Room 1023, 450 Golden Gate Avenue, San Francisco, CA, 94102.

GPO Bookstore, Federal Building, U.S. Courthouse, Room 117, 1961 Stout Street, Denver, CO, 80294.

GPO Bookstore, 720 North Main Street, Majestic Building, Pueblo, CO, 81003.

GPO Bookstore, Federal Building, Room 158, 400 W. Bay Street, Jacksonville, FL, 32202.

GPO Bookstore, Room 100, Federal Building, 275 Peachtree Street NE, Atlanta, GA, 30303.

GPO Bookstore, Everett McKinley Dirksen Building, Room 1463, 14th Floor, 219 South Dearborn Street, Chicago, IL, 60604.

GPO Bookstore, Room G25, John F. Kennedy Federal Building, Sudbury Street, Boston, MA, 02203.

GPO Bookstore, Patrick V. McNamara Federal Building, 477 Michigan Avenue, Suite 160, Detroit, MI, 48226

GPO Bookstore, Federal Office Building, Room 144, 601 East 12th Street, Kansas City, MO, 64106.

GPO Bookstore, Room 110, 26 Federal Plaza, New York, NY, 10007.

GPO Bookstore, Federal Office Building, Room 207, 200 N. High Street, Columbus, OH, 43215.

GPO Bookstore, Federal Building, Room 171, 1240 East Ninth Street, Cleveland, OH, 44114.

GPO Bookstore, Federal Office Building, Room 1214, 600 Arch Street, Philadelphia, PA, 19106.

GPO Bookstore, Room 1C50, Federal Building, U.S. Courthouse, 1100 Commerce Street, Dallas, TX, 75242.

GPO Bookstore, 45 College Center, 9319 Gulf Freeway, Houston, TX, 77017.

GPO Bookstore, Federal Building, Room 194, 915 Second Avenue, Seattle, WA, 98104.

GPO Bookstore, Federal Building, Room 190, 517 E. Wisconsin Avenue, Milwaukee, WI, 53202.

GPO Main Bookstore, 710 North Capitol Street, NW, Washington, DC, 20402.

GPO Sales Agencies:
  Anchorage—Rm. 412, Hill Bldg., 632 Sixth Avenue, Anchorage, AK, 99501.
  Honolulu—286 Alexander Young Bldg., 1015 Bishop Street, Honolulu, HI, 96813.
  San Juan, Puerto Rico—Rm 659, Federal Bldg., Hato Rey, PR.

Listing more than 5000 publications, the "Guide to Federal Aviation Administration Publications" (June 1979; FAA-APA-PG-2) has been updated to make it easier for the public to acquire FAA documents as well as civil aviation-related publications issued by other Federal agencies. Prices for each publication are included in the guide along with instructions on how to order material. The guide is free and may be obtained by writing the Department of Transportation Publications Section, M-443.1, Washington, DC 20590 or FAA Public Inquiry Center, APA-430, 800 Independence Ave., S.W., Washington, DC 20591.

FAA also publishes a considerable amount of good material in the form of Advisory Circulars, some 400 of which are available free from FAA. Over 60 Advisory Circulars are also sold through GPO. An Advisory Circular Checklist (AC 00-2), published three times a year, can be obtained from the Department of Transportation, Publications Section, M-443.1, Washington, DC 20590.

The following are some government aviation publications of particular interest, with an indication of where to order them.

Flight Information

Airman's Information Manual (AIM):

Basic Flight Information and ATC Procedures (formerly AIM Part 1) (issued semi-annually—Jan., July). Annual subscription $5.00 domestic; $6.25 foreign—GPO.

Airport/Facility Directory (replaces AIM Parts 2 and 3) is issued every 56 days. Regional editions $2.00 apiece (Northeast, Southeast, East Central, South Central, North Central, Northwest, Southwest). Book subscription $12.50, each additional region $5.00 per book. 7 book subscription (complete U.S.) $37.50—AOPA Chart Department forwards orders to NOS.

Notices to Airmen (formerly AIM Part 3A) is issued every 14 days. Annual subscription $26.00 domestic; $32.50 foreign—GPO.

Graphic Notices and Supplemental Data (formerly AIM Part 4) is issued quarterly—Jan., April, July, Oct. Annual subscription $14.40 domestic; $18.00 foreign—GPO.

Alaska Supplement (issued every 56 days). Annual subscription $15.00 first class; $2.25 single copy. National Ocean Survey, Distribution Division (C-44), Riverdale, MD 20840. (Make check or money order payable to NOS, Dept. of Commerce, C-44.)

Alaska Terminal (Procedures) Publication (issued every 56 days, with amendment on 28th day as required). Annual subscription $13.25, single copy $2.10—NOS.

Pacific Chart Supplement (published every 56 days with amendment notice between issues). Annual subscription $15.00 first class. $3.75 single copy.—NOS.

Visual Aeronautical Chart Symbols. $1.50—NOS.

International Flight Information Manual (published annually in April, quarterly supplement in July, Oct., Jan.) is available by subscription. $9.00 domestic; $11.25 foreign.—GPO.

International Notices to Airmen (issued bi-weekly). Annual subscription $31.00 domestic; $38.75 foreign—GPO.

NOS orders to foreign countries (excluding Canada and Mexico), add 10%

to total cost of order for foreign surface shipment. For faster foreign delivery, write NOS for a transportation cost quotation.

Miscellaneous FAA Publications

Acceptable Methods, Techniques, and Practices—Aircraft Alterations (AC 43.13-2A). 1977. Subscription with changes $2.75—GPO.

Acceptable Methods, Techniques, and Practices—Aircraft Inspection and Repair (AC 43.13-1A). 1973, $3.70 plus .65 for Change 1 and .35 for Change 2—GPO.

Aviation Weather (AC 00-6A). Published 1975. $4.55—GPO.

Aviation Weather Services (AC-0045A). Published 1977. $3.00—GPO.

Census of U.S. Civil Aircraft (issued annually; calendar year 1977). $12.00—National Technical Information Service, 5285 Port Royal Rd., Springfield, Va. 22151.

Contractions Handbook (word and phrase contractions used by FAA). (7340.1G) 1980. Issued biennially with 3 annual changes. Subscription, $12.00 domestic; $15.00 foreign—GPO.

Denalt Performance Computer (specify whether for fixed-pitch or variable-pitch propeller aircraft). 1966. 70¢—GPO.

FAA Air Traffic Activity (fiscal year 1978). $11.00—NTIS.

FAA General Aviation News (bi-monthly magazine). Annual subscription $6.20 domestic; $7.75 foreign. Single copy 55¢; foreign single copy 70¢—GPO.

FAA Statistical Handbook of Aviation (issued annually, calendar year 1977). $9.00—NTIS.

Flight Training Handbook (AC 61-21). Published 1966; reprinted 1969. $2.15—GPO.

Instrument Flying Handbook (AC 61-27A). 1971. $3.25—GPO.

Pilot's Handbook of Aeronautical Knowledge (AC 61-23A). Published 1971. $5.30—GPO.

Summary of Airworthiness Directives (ADs are summarized in two volumes available separately: Vol. 1, for small aircraft and Vol. 2, for large aircraft.) Subscription consists of the volume ordered plus bi-weekly updates for a 2 year period. Vol. 1, $12.50 domestic; $15.65 foreign. Vol. 2, $10.75 domestic; $13.45 foreign—both U.S. Dept. of Transportation, FAA, P.O. Box 25461, Attn: AAC-23, Okla. City, OK, 73125 (Make check or money order payable to Federal Aviation Administration.)

U.S. Civil Aircraft Register (AC 20-6EE, July '78; AC 20-6FF, Jan. '79). $21.00 for 3-vol. set. (Temporarily suspended publication before Jan. 1979 edition.)

Films

All films available from the FAA are in 16mm sound. They are loaned free of charge for a maximum period of one week, unless special permission is obtained for longer use. It is important to send your request as far in advance as possible. Requests should be mailed in time to reach the FAA Film Service at least a month prior to desired show date. No admission charge may be made for viewing these films.

Order requests should be sent to FAA Film Service, c/o Modern Talking Picture Service, Inc., 5000 Park Street N., St. Petersburg, FL, 33709, and should include the following information: title and film number, complete address where the film is to be sent, and first and alternate show dates.

Airports Mean Business (11111), 28 minutes. Illustrates how airports attract new industry, provide new jobs, generate additional revenue and a strengthened tax base, offer increased recreational opportunities, and enable a community to enjoy services that depend on air access.

All It Takes Is Once (11112), 25 min. Dramatic presentation of the effect five psychological problems frequently encountered by general aviation pilots can have on flight performance.

Aloft (11113), 11 minutes. Offers an upbeat view of FAA's safety mission and the highly trained men and women who carry it out.

Area Navigation (11114), 25 min. Gives better understanding of the area navigation concept and its advantages in expediting air traffic control.

Basic Radio Procedures for Pilots (11116), 30 minutes. Designed to familiarize private pilots, and particularly novices, with proper radio procedures while communicating with FAA flight service stations and airport traffic control towers.

Brother (11117), 13½ min. Stresses the FAA's need to recruit bright young men and women of minority groups into professional careers in agency technical areas—particularly air traffic control and electronic maintenance.

Caution: Wake Turbulence (11118), 16 min. Information on wake turbulence, particularly with respect to hazards for general aviation aircraft operating in a mixed-traffic environment.

Charlie (11119), 22 min. Illustrates how alcohol can affect judgment of a pilot in flight.

Density Altitude (11121), 29 min. Dramatizes effects of high altitude and high temperature on light-aircraft performance

Discrete Address Beacon System (11122), 12½ min. Describes the principles, applications and add-on features, such as data-link, of DABS.

Disorientation (11123), 19 min. Alerts pilots to the way this physiological phenomenon can dangerously distort flying judgments.

Dusk To Dawn (11124), 28½ min. Demonstrates that night flying is physiologically and operationally different from day flying.

Eagle Eyed Pilot (11125), 24½ min. Shows that pilot safety and "eagle vision" go hand in hand. Points out limitations of the eye in flight and other factors that can impair vision.

Flight 52 (11127), 14½ min. Provides a behind-the-scenes look at air traffic control, with emphasis on computer technology as applied to the U.S. aviation system.

Flying Clubs (11128), 20 minutes. States the advantages belonging to a flying club and emphasizes the safety factors associated with its operations.

Flying Floats (11129), 19 min. Gives a few pointers for safe float plane operations.

General Aviation Fact or Fiction (11130), 14½ min. Shows the role of general aviation—its importance and its contributions to the Nation's economy.

How Airplanes Fly (11131), 18 min. Basic aerodynamics for general aviation pilots and high school students.

How to Succeed Without Really Flying (11132), 28 minutes. Describes what air traffic control offers as a profession and how it provides rapid career advancement, professional status, high pay, and a sense of personal achievement.

Hypoxia (11133), 16 min. Illustrates the danger of insufficient oxygen and shows the subtle and insidious symptoms of hypoxia, and how they can be prevented.

In Celebration of Flight (11134), 28½ min. A dramatic tribute to the individuals and institutions that have helped make American aviation what it is today.

It Pays To Stay Open (11135), 23 min. Documents how low-cost lighting for utility airports can be of economic benefit to the community.

Kites To Capsules (11136), 5 min. A fast-moving, humorous film that contrasts early flying attempts with modern, successful commercial and general aviation.

Looking Up To Your Aviation Career (10314), 14 min. This film is a lively exploration of young people in aviation. Illustrates how careers in aviation present a wide-ranging opportunity for achievement, challenge, responsibility, and fun.

Low-Level Wind Shear (11137), 16 min. A fairly technical film describing current research on wind shear detection techniques being sponsored by the Federal Government.

Medical Facts For Pilots (11138), 25 min. Fundamental physical, physiological, and psychological limitations in flight.

Meteorology—Ice Formation On Aircraft (11155), 20 min. Discusses structural, carburetor, pitot-tube, and turbojet-engine icing problems.

Meteorology—Fog And Low Ceiling Clouds: Advection Fog And Ground Fog (11156), 25 min. Characteristics of, and conditions conductive to, fog formation.

Meteorology—Fog And Low Ceiling Clouds: Upslope Fog And Frontal Fog (11157), 10 min. Illustrates how upslope fog, frontal fog, and low stratus clouds are generated.

Meteorology—The Cold Front (11158), 15 min. Explains flight hazards of cold fronts, and how to avoid them.

Meteorology—The Warm Front (11159), 20 min. Flight hazards of warm fronts, and how to avoid them.

Microwave Landing Systems (11139), 15 minutes. Explains how the new Microwave Landing System (MLS) functions and highlights its advantages over the conventional Instrument Landing Systems (ILS).

Mountain Flying (11140), 23 minutes. It's a film that has valuable tips for anyone considering a trip that involves mountain flying.

Overwater Flying (11141), 25 min. Aimed at pilots planning to fly overwater in light aircraft. Covers such topics as emergency survival gear, optical illusions over water, minimal navigational and radio equipment, proper ditching procedures, water survival techniques.

Path To Safety (11142), 20 min. Actor Cliff Robertson in this presentation of some common mistakes made by general aviation pilots.

Profile Descent and Metering (11143), 20 minutes. Describes new operational procedures that are expected to be in effect at all terminals served by high performance aircraft by 1979.

Put Wings On Your Career (11144), 15 min. Illustrates the diversity of aviation-related jobs, both in government and private industry. Outlines basic technical requirements and gives contact addresses for those desiring more information.

Red Alert (10316), 16 min. Describes current FAA regulations relating to crash fire rescue; illustrates basic principles and techniques; demonstrates new forms of agents and agent applicators, protective suits and equipment; and underscores the critical importance of having a well-trained crash fire rescue force available.

Rx For Flight (11145), 20 min. Discussion of some basic aeromedical concerns: alcohol, drugs, hypoxia, disorientation, smoking, safety equipment.

Safety By The Numbers (11146), 31 minutes. Shows the use of a twin-engine aircraft for a rescue operation. Illustrates the proper in-flight procedures to follow in the event of engine failure.

The Silver Eagle: Master of the Skies (10318), 16 min. Through the eyes of "Silver Eagle", a pilot who envisions himself with extraordinary judgement and flying prowess, other pilots can see the adverse effects of alcohol, medicines, stress, and fatigue on flying ability. (A black and white film.)

Some Thoughts on Winter Flying (11147), 21 min. Experienced Alaskan bush pilots share their expertise on hazards and safety precautions involved with winter flying.

A Sound Approach (11148), 14 min. Outlines the technological, operational, and regulatory procedures leading to significant aircraft noise reduction. Aimed at the role of the community in helping to make airports better neighbors.

Stable and Safe (11149), 20 minutes. Reveals what frequently happens when VFR pilots inadvertently fly into marginal or IFR weather and lose their visual reference, becoming dangerously disoriented.

Stalling for Safety (11150), 18 min. Shows how stalls and spins occur, demonstrates warning signs of approaching stalls, and reviews recovery actions.

Start-Up (11151), 17 minutes. Reminds pilots of what to look for, check out, and do before they start up in the spring.

Takeoffs and Landings (11152), 12 min. Three short films on one reel which highlight short field, soft field, and crosswind techniques.

These Special People (10315), 14 min. Explores the work and career opportunities of electronics technicians who work for the FAA. Describes their technical skills and craftsmanship, and provides a look at how they install, operate, and maintain the airway facilities network.

Other sources of aviation films are the Armed Forces film libraries. To obtain information, write:

Commander, AAVS, Attn. USAF Film Library, Hq AAVS, Norton AFB, CA. 92409.

Commanding General, (nearest) Army Headquarters, Attn: Central Audio-Visual Support Center.

Commander, (local) Naval District, Attn: Assistant for Information.

Some state aeronautics commissions and airframe and equipment manufacturers also have films to loan.

INTERNATIONAL OPERATIONS

INTERNATIONAL COUNCIL OF AIRCRAFT OWNER AND PILOT ASSOCIATIONS (IAOPA)

Officers:

President, J. B. Hartranft, Jr., Washington, DC

Vice President, Africa-Indian Ocean Region, Guillaume H. Marais, Pretoria, Republic of South AFRICA.

Vice President, Pacific Region, R. C. Adams, Sydney, Australia.

Vice President, European-Mediterranean Region, R. A. S. Ames, London, England.

Vice President, North Atlantic Region, Russell Beach, Smith Falls, Ontario, Canada

Vice President, South American-South Atlantic Region, Jorge A. Römer, Caracas, Venezuela.

Vice President, Southeast Asia Region, Oscar D. Ramos, Manilla, Philippines

Secretary, Victor J. Kayne, Washingtpn, DC

Treasurer, William S. Brassel, Washington, DC

Headquarters address:

7315 Wisconsin Ave., Washington, DC 20014; phone: (202) 654-0500; Telex 89—8468.

Cable address:

IAOPA

European Secretariat:

IAOPA European Branch Office, P.O. Box 55, 2110 AB Aerdenhout, Netherlands. Hubert M. Koemans, Secretary; Phone Haarlem (023)

24 42 84, Cable address: GENERAVIA AERDENHOUT NETHER-
LANDS.

IAOPA Member Organizations

Australia

AOPA of Australia, Box 2912, G.P.O., Sydney, 2001, Australia; R. C. Adams,
President; phone 29-6168; Cables: same as mailing address.

Austria

AOPA of Austria, Postfach 114, Vienna A-1171, Austria; J. Meinl, President;
phone (0222) 46 80/217. Telex: 74914.

Belgium

AOPA of Belgium, 24 Blvd. de L'Empereur, B-1000 Brussels, Belgium; Rene
Thierry, President.

Brazil

Associaçao de Pilotos e Proprietarios de Aeronaves, Rua Maestro Elias Lobo
121, Sao Paulo, 01433 Brazil; Mario Amaral, President.

Canada

Canadian Owners and Pilots Association, P.O. Box 734, Station B, Ottawa,
Ontario, KIP 5S4 Canada; Russell Beach, President; William Peppler,
Manager; phone (613) 236-4901; Cables: same as mailing address.

Denmark

AOPA of Denmark, Box 52, DK 4930 Maribo, Denmark; Holger Nicolaisen,
President; Bent Stig Møller, Vice President; phone (03) 88 19 89.

France

Association des Pilotes Privés, Bureau No. 10, Batiment Paul-Bert, 93350
Aeroport Le Bourget, France; Hubert Avran, President; phone 837-36-70;
Cables: same as mailing address.

Germany, Federal Republic of

AOPA of Germany, Haus Nr. 1, 6073 Egelsbach/Flugplatz, Germany;
Wolfgang Trinkaus, President; phone (06103) 4 91 92, Telex 4150 23.

Ireland, Republic of

AOPA of Ireland, P.O. Box 927, Nassau St., Dublin 2, Ireland; Anthony
Leonard, President; Maurice Cronin, Hon. Secretary.

Italy

AOPA of Italy, Via Bandello 4/2, 20123 Milan, Italy; Dr. Enrico Massimo
Carle, President; phone (020) 34.07.36.

Luxembourg

Union des Pilotes d'Aviation du Grande-Duche de Luxembourg, B.P. 300,
Esch/Alzette, Luxembourg; Jean Claude Weber, President; Cables: same as
mailing address.

Netherlands

AOPA Netherlands, Dorpshuisstraat 10, Nieuwe Pekela, Netherlands; J van der Veen, President; E. Kuijl, Secretary; phone (05978) 6013; Cables: same as mailing address.

Norway

AOPA Norway, P.O. Box 1604, Vika Oslo 1, Norway; Per Holter-Sorensen, President; phone 41 41 17.

Philippines

AOPA-Philippines, P.O. Box 7070, Manila International Airport 3120, Philippines; Judge Onofre Villaluz, President; phone 83-15-46; Cables: same as mailing address.

South Africa, Republic of

AOPA of South Africa, P.O. Box 1789, Pretoria 0001, Republic of South Africa; W. J. Seymore, President; phone 31651. Telex: 3-0524 SA.

Sweden

AOPA Sweden, Fack, 161 10 Bromma, Sweden; Claes Borg, President; phone 08/29-29-20; Cables: same as mailing address. Telex: 10725 FFA S.

Switzerland

AOPA of Switzerland, P.O. Box 113, 8302 Kloten, Switzerland; Christian P. Tschudi, President; phone 01-813-01-85; Cables: AOPASWISS ZURICH.

United Kingdom

AOPA of the U.K., 50 Cambridge Street, London, SW1V 4QQ, England; Ronald D. Campbell, Chairman; phone 01-834-5631; Cables: AVIACENTRE LONDON; Telex: 262284, Ref. 2290.

United States of America

Aircraft Owners and Pilots Association, 7315 Wisconsin Avenue, Washington, DC 20014, U.S.A.; John L. Baker, President; phone (301) 654-0500; Cables: AOPA Washington; Telex: 89-8468.

Venezuela

Federación Venezolona de Aeroclubes, Aeropuerto La Carlota, Caracas, 107 Venezuela; Pedro Luis Angarita, President; phone 91 78 06; Cables: same as mailing address; Telex: 25 336-LAFAR.

FAA INTERNATIONAL OFFICES

Europe, Africa, Middle East Region

FAA Brussels, Belgium—Assistant Administrator. APO Address: c/o American Embassy, APO New York, NY 09667. Location/International Mail Address: FAA, c/o American Embassy, 1 Place Madou 1030, Brussels, Belgium. Phone: (Switchboard, all hours) 513,38.30.

FAA Europe, Africa, Middle East Offices

Berlin, Germany—U.S. Administrator for Aeronautics. APO Address: U.S. Mission, Berlin, APO New York, NY, 09742. Location/International Mail Address: Tempelhof Airport, 1 Berlin, Germany. Phone: Berlin Civil 819-5351 or 6909-220; Berlin-Military 018-5635.

Bonn, Germany—FAA Representative. APO Address: c/o American Embassy, APO NY 09080. International Mail Address: Box 365, Deichmannsaue, 5300 Bonn, Germany. Phone: 02221-8955.

Frankfort, Germany—FAA Representative, c/o American Consultant, APO, NY 09757; or, Siesmeyer Str 21, D 6000, Frankfort/Mame.

Paris, France—FAA Representative. APO Address: c/o American Embassy, APO New York, NY 09777. Location/International Mail Address: FAA, c/o American Embassy, 2 Avenue Gabriel 75382, Paris, Cedex 08, France. Phone: 296-1202 or 261-8075, Ext. 2901/37.

London, England—FAA Representative. APO Address: c/o American Embassy, Box 40, FPO NY 09510. International Mail Address: FAA, c/o American Embassy, Grosvenor Square, London, W1A 1AE. Location: American Embassy. Phone: 499-9000, Ext. 494.

Rome, Italy—FAA Representative. APO Address c/o American Embassy, APO NY 09794. Location/International Mail Address: FAA, VIA V. Veneto 119, Rome, Italy. Phone: 39 64674.

Monrovia, Liberia—FAA Representative, c/o American Embassy, APO NY 09155. Location/International Mail Address: 56½ Broad St., 1st Floor, Monrovia, Liberia. Phone: 222335 or Embassy phone 222991.

Pacific-Asia Region

FAA Honolulu, Hawaii—Director. Address: P.O. Box 50109, Honolulu, HI, 96850. Location: Prince Jonah Kuhio Kalanianaole Federal Bldg., 300 Ala Moana Blvd., Honolulu, Hawaii 96850. Phone (808) 547-9741/7544.

FAA Pacific-Asia Region Offices

Tokyo, Japan—FAA Representative. APO Address: East Asian International Field Office, c/o American Embassy, APO San Francisco, California 96503. Phone: 583-7141 Ext. 7625/7833/7346, 583-0157 (direct line).

Guam, Mariana Islands—Resident Director. Address: Route 008, Guam M.I. 96912. Phone: 355-5820. For Chief, International Field Officer, use Zip Code 96910. Phone: 355-5715/5719/5980.

American Samoa—Resident Director. Address: P.O. Box 8, Pago Pago, American Samao, 96799. Phone: Samoa 688-9485.

Southern Region

(Responsible for South America, Canal Zone, Caribbean Sea and Central America excluding Mexico.)

FAA Southern Region—Director. APO Address: P.O. Box 20636, Atlanta, GA, USA, 30320. Location: 3400 Whipple St., East Point, Atlanta, Ga. Phone: (404) 763-7222.

FAA Southern Region Offices

Rio de Janeiro, Brazil—FAA Representative. APO Address: APO Miami, FL, 34030. Location/International Mail Address: 147 Avenida Presidente Wilson, Rio de Janeiro, Brazil. Phone (305) 252-8055, ext. 240.

Lima, Peru—FAA Representative, APO Address: APO Miami, FL, 34031. Location/International Mail Address: Corner Avenidas Inca Garcilaso de la Vega & Espana, P.O. Box 1995, Lima, Peru. Phone: 28600, ext. 211.

Balboa, Canal Zone—Area Manager. Address: FAA, Balboa Area Office, Drawer H, Balboa Heights, U.S. Canal Zone. Location: Room 206, FAA Bldg., Albrook AFB, C.Z. Phone: Panama Canal Co. Exchange 52-6104; Military Exchange 85-4501.

San Juan, Puerto Rico—Area Manager. Address: RFD 1, Box 29A, Loiza Street Station, San Juna, Puerto Rico 00914. Location: Isla Verde Caroling Rd., San Juan, P.R. Phone (809) 791-2310.

Buenos Aires, Argentina—FAA Representative. APO Address: APO Miami, FL, 34034. Location/International Mail Address: Saramiento 1425, Colcmbia 4300 Esquina, Buenos Aires, Argentina.

Southwest Region

(Responsible for Mexico.)

FAA Southwest Region—Director. APO Address: P.O. Box 1689, Fort Worth, TX, 76101. Location: 4400 Blue Mound Road, Fort Worth, Texas. Phone: (817) 624-4911.

International Travel

For detailed information and passport agency addresses, see Section 1.

International Aircraft Markings

A–2–	Botswana	D–	Germany (Fed. Rep.)
A6–	United Arab Emirates	D2–	Angola
A7–	Qatar	DQ–	Fiji
A40–	Oman	DZ–	Angola
AN–	Nicaragua	EC–	Spain
AP–	Pakistan	EI–,EJ–	Ireland
B–	China	EL–	Liberia
C–2–	Nauru	EP–	Iran
C5–	Gambia	ET–	Ethiopia
CC–	Chile	F–	France
CCCP–	U.S.S.R.	G–	United Kingdom
C–,CF–	Canada	HA–	Hungary
CN–	Morocco	HB–*	Switzerland
CP–	Bolivia	HB–*	Liechtenstein
CR–,CS–	Portugal	HC–	Ecuador
CU–	Cuba	HH–	Haiti
CX–	Uruguay	HI–	Dominican Republic

HK–	Colombia	TY–	Benin
HL–	Korea (Rep. of)	TZ–	Mali
HP–	Panama	VH–	Australia
HR–	Honduras	VP–,VQ–,	U.K. Colonies &
HS–	Thailand	VR–	Protectorates
HZ–	Saudi Arabia	VT–	India
I–	Italy	XA–,XB–,	Mexico
JA–	Japan	XC–	
JY–	Jordan	XT–	Upper Volta
LN–	Norway	XU–	Democratic Kampucha
LV–,LQ–	Argentina	XV–	Vietnam
LX–	Luxembourg	XY–,XZ–	Burma
LZ–	Bulgaria	YA–	Afghanistan
N–	U.S.A.	YI–	Iraq
OB–	Peru	YK–	Syrian Arab Rep.
OD–	Lebanon	YR–	Romania
OE–	Austria	YS–	El Salvador
OH–	Finland	YU–	Yugloslavia
OK–	Czechoslovakia	YV–	Venezuela
OO–	Belgium	ZK–,ZL–,Z	New Zealand
OY–	Denmark	M–	
P–	North Korea	ZP–	Paraguay
P2–	Papua New Guinea	ZS–,ZT–,Z	South Africa
PDRL–	Laos	U–	
PH–	Netherlands	3A–	Monaco
PJ–	Netherlands Antilles	3B–	Mauritius
PK–	Indonesia	3C–	Equatorial Guinea
PK–	West Irian	3D–	Swaziland
PP–,PT–	Brazil	3X–	Guinea
PZ–	Surinam	4R–	Sri Lanka
RP–	Philippines	4W–	Yemen
S–2–	Bangladesh	4X–	Israel
SE–	Sweden	5A–	Libya
SP–	Poland	5B–	Cyprus
ST–	Sudan	5H–	Tanzania
SU–	Egypt	5N–	Nigeria
SX–	Greece	5R–	Madagascar
TC–	Turkey	5T–	Mauritania
TF–	Iceland	5U–	Niger
TG–	Guatemala	5V–	Togo
TI–	Costa Rica	5W–	Western Samoa
TJ–	Cameroon	5X–	Uganda
TL–	Central African Rep.	5Y–	Kenya
TN–	Congo	6O–	Somalia
TR–	Gabon	6V–,6W–	Senegal
TS–	Tunisia	6Y–	Jamaica
TT–	Chad	7O–	Democratic Yemen
TU–	Ivory Coast	7P–	Lesotho

7QY–	Malawi	9L–	Sierra Leone
7T–	Algeria	9M–	Malaysia
8P–	Barbados	9N–	Nepal
8Q–	Maldives	9Q–	Zaire
8R–	Guyana	9U–	Burundi
9G–	Ghana	9V–	Singapore
9H–	Malta	9XR–	Rwanda
9J–	Zambia	9Y–	Trinidad and Tobago
9K–	Kuwait	*Plus national emblem	

SECTION 6

FEDERAL AVIATION REGULATIONS

(Compiled and edited by John S. Yodice, AOPA's Washington Counsel)

NOTE: *This section contains all of the regulations of Parts 1, 61, 67, 91, 93, and 830 to which the general aviation pilot needs ready reference. Those regulations not generally applicable have been deleted and are indicated by an asterisk (*). Changes from the 1979 edition are shown in boldface brackets. The regulations are current as of Oct. 1, 1979. Regulatory changes subsequent to that date will be noted in The AOPA PILOT.*

Part 1

Definitions and Abbreviations

CONTENTS

1.1 General Definitions
1.2 Abbreviations and Symbols
1.3 Rules of Construction

1.1 GENERAL DEFINITIONS

As used in Subchapters A through K of this chapter, unless the context requires otherwise:

Administrator means the Federal Aviation Administrator or any person to whom he has delegated his authority in the matter concerned.

[Aerodynamic coefficients means nondimensional coefficients for aerodynamic forces and moments.]

Air carrier means a person who undertakes directly by lease, or other arrangement, to engage in air transportation.

Air commerce means interstate, overseas, or foreign air commerce or the transportation of mail by aircraft, or any operation or navigation of aircraft within the limits of any Federal airway, or any operation or navigation of aircraft which directly affects, or which may endanger safety in, interstate, overseas, or foreign air commerce.

Aircraft means a device that is used or intended to be used for flight in the air.

Aircraft engine means an engine that is used or intended to be used for propelling aircraft. It includes turbosuperchargers, appurtenances, and accessories necessary for its functioning, but does not include propellers.

Airframe means the fuselage, booms, nacelles, cowlings, fairings, airfoil surfaces (including rotors but excluding propellers and rotating airfoils of engines), and landing gear of an aircraft and their accessories and controls.

Airplane means an engine-driven fixed-wing aircraft heavier than air, that is supported in flight by the dynamic reaction of the air against its wings.

Airport means an area of land or water that is used or intended to be used for the landing and takeoff of aircraft, and includes its buildings and facilities, if any.

Airport traffic area means, unless otherwise specifically designated in Part 93, that airspace within a horizontal radius of 5 statute miles from the geographical center of any airport at which a control tower is operating, extending from the surface up to, but not including, an altitude of 3,000 feet above the elevation of the airport.

Airship means an engine-driven lighter-than-air aircraft that can be steered.

Air traffic means aircraft operating in the air or on an airport surface, exclusive of loading ramps and parking areas.

Air traffic clearance means an authorization by air traffic control, for the purpose of preventing collision between known aircraft, for an aircraft to proceed under specified traffic conditions within controlled airspace.

Air traffic control means a service operated by appropriate authority to promote the safe, orderly, and expeditious flow of air traffic.

Air transportation means interstate, overseas, or foreign air transportation or the transportation of mail by aircraft.

Alternate airport means an airport at which an aircraft may land if a landing at the intended airport becomes inadvisable.

[**Altitude engine** means a reciprocating aircraft engine having a rated takeoff power that is producible from sea level to an established higher altitude.]

Appliance means any instrument, mechanism, equipment, part, apparatus, appurtenance, or accessory, including communications equipment, that is used or intended to be used in operating or controlling an aircraft in flight, is installed in or attached to the aircraft, and is not part of an airframe, engine, or propeller.

Approved, unless used with reference to another person, means approved by the Administrator.

Area navigation (RNAV) means a method of navigation that permits aircraft operations on any desired course within the coverage of station-referenced navigation signals or within the limits of self-contained system capability.

Area navigation high route means an area navigation route within the airspace extending upward from, and including, 18,000 feet MSL to flight level 450.

Area navigation low route means an area navigation route within the airspace extending upward from 1,200 feet above the surface of the earth to, but not including, 18,000 feet MSL.

Armed Forces means the Army, Navy, Air Force, Marine Corps, and Coast Guard, including their regular and reserve components and members serving without component status.

Autorotation means a rotorcraft flight condition in which the lifting rotor is driven entirely by action of the air when the rotorcraft is in motion.

Auxiliary rotor means a rotor that serves either to counteract the effect of the main rotor torque on a rotorcraft or to maneuver the rotorcraft about one or more of its three principal axes.

Balloon means a lighter-than-air aircraft that is not engine driven.

Brake horsepower means the power delivered at the propeller shaft (main drive or main output) of an aircraft engine.

Calibrated airspeed means indicated airspeed of an aircraft, corrected for position and instrument error. Calibrated airspeed is equal to true airspeed in standard atmosphere at sea level.

Category—

(1) As used with respect to the certification, ratings, privileges, and limitations of airmen, means a broad classification of aircraft. Examples include: airplane; rotorcraft; glider; and lighter-than-air; and

(2) As used with respect to the certification of aircraft, means a grouping of aircraft based upon intended use or operating limitations. Examples include: transport; normal; utility; acrobatic; limited; restricted; and provisional.

Category II operations, with respect to the operation of aircraft, means a straight-in ILS approach to the runway of an airport under a Category II ILS instrument approach procedure issued by the Administrator or other appropriate authority.

Ceiling means the height above the earth's surface of the lowest layer of clouds or obscuring phenomena that is reported as "broken", "overcast", or "obscuration", and not classified as "thin" or "partial."

Civil aircraft means aircraft other than public aircraft.

Class—

(1) As used with respect to the certification, ratings, privileges, and limitations of airmen, means a classification of aircraft within a category having similar operating characteristics. Examples include: single engine; multiengine; land; water; gyroplane; helicopter; airship; and free balloon; and

(2) As used with respect to the certification of aircraft, means a broad grouping of aircraft having similar characteristics of propulsion, flight, or landing. Examples include: airplane; rotorcraft; glider; balloon; landplane; and seaplane.

[Clearway means:

(1) For turbine engine powered airplanes certificated after August 29, 1959, an area beyond the runway, not less than 500 feet wide, centrally located about the extended centerline of the runway, and under the control of the airport authorities. The clearway is expressed in terms of a clearway plane, extending from the end of the runway with an upward slope not exceeding 1.25 percent, above which no object nor any terrain protrudes. However, threshold lights may protrude above the plane if their height above the end of the runway is 26 inches or less and if they are located to each side of the runway.

(2) For turbine engine powered airplanes certificated after September

261

30, 1958 but before August 30, 1959, an area beyond the takeoff runway extending no less than 300 feet on either side of the extended centerline of the runway, at an elevation no higher than the elevation of the end of the runway, clear of all fixed obstacles, and under the control of the airport authorities.]

Commercial operator means a person who, for compensation or hire, engages in the carriage by aircraft in air commerce of persons or property, other than as an air carrier or foreign air carrier or under the authority of Part 375 of this Title. Where it is doubtful that an operation is for "compensation or hire," the test applied is whether the carriage by air is merely incidental to the person's other business or is, in itself, a major enterprise for profit.

Controlled airspace means airspace designated as a continental control area, control area, control zone, terminal control area, or transition area, within which some or all aircraft may be subject to air traffic control.

Crewmember means a person assigned to perform duty in an aircraft during flight time.

Critical altitude means the maximum altitude at which, in standard atmosphere, it is possible to maintain, at a specified rotational speed, a specific power or a specified manifold pressure. Unless otherwise stated, the critical altitude is the maximum altitude at which it is possible to maintain, at the maximum continuous rotational speed, one of the following:

(1) The maximum continuous power, in the case of engines for which this power rating is the same at sea level and at the rated altitude.

(2) The maximum continuous rated manifold pressure, in the case of engines, the maximum continuous power of which is governed by a constant manifold pressure.

Critical engine means the engine whose failure would most adversely affect the performance or handling qualities of an aircraft.

Decision height, with respect to the operation of aircraft, means the height at which a decision must be made, during an ILS or PAR instrument approach, to either continue the approach or to execute a missed approach.

Equivalent airspeed means the calibrated airspeed of an aircraft corrected for adiabatic compressible flow for the particular altitude. Equivalent airspeed is equal to calibrated airspeed in standard atmosphere at sea level.

Extended over-water operation means—

(1) With respect to aircraft other than helicopters, an operation over water at a horizontal distance of more than 50 nautical miles from the nearest shoreline; and

(2) With respect to helicopters, an operation over water at a horizontal distance of more than 50 nautical miles from the nearest shoreline and more than 50 nautical miles from an offshore heliport structure.

External load means a load that is carried, or extends, outside of the aircraft fuselage.

External-load attaching means means the structural components used to attach an external load to an aircraft, including external-load containers, the backup structure at the attachment points, and any quick-release device used to jettison the external load.

[**Fireproof**—

(1) With respect to materials and parts used to confine fire in a designated fire zone, means the capacity to withstand at least as well as steel in dimensions appropriate for the purpose for which they are used, the heat produced when there is a severe fire of extended duration in that zone; and

(2) With respect to other materials and parts, means the capacity to withstand the heat associated with fire at least as well as steel in dimensions appropriate for the purpose for which they are used.]

[**Fire resistant**—

(1) With respect to sheet or structural members means the capacity to withstand the heat associated with fire at least as well as aluminum alloy in dimensions appropriate for the purpose for which they are used; and

(2) With respect to fluid-carrying lines, fluid system parts, wiring, air ducts, fittings, and powerplant controls, means the capacity to perform the intended functions under the heat and other conditions likely to occur when there is a fire at the place concerned.]

[**Flame resistant** means not susceptible to combustion to the point of propagating a flame, beyond safe limits, after the ignition source is removed.]

[**Flammable,** with respect to a fluid or gas, means susceptible to igniting readily or to exploding.]

Flap extended speed means the highest speed permissible with wing flaps in a prescribed extended position.

[**Flash resistant** means not susceptible to burning violently when ignited.]

Flight crewmember means a pilot, flight engineer, or flight navigator assigned to duty in an aircraft during flight time.

Flight level means a level of constant atmospheric pressure related to a reference datum of 29.92 inches of mercury. Each is stated in three digits that represent hundreds of feet. For example, flight level 250 represents a barometric altimeter indication of 25,000 feet; flight level 255, an indication of 25,500 feet.

Flight plan means specified information, relating to the intended flight of an aircraft, that is filed orally or in writing with air traffic control.

Flight time means the time from the moment the aircraft first moves under its own power for the purpose of flight until the moment it comes to rest at the next point of landing. ("Block-to-block" time).

Flight visibility means the average forward horizontal distance, from the cockpit of an aircraft in flight, at which prominent unlighted objects may be seen and identified by day and prominent lighted objects may be seen and identified by night.

[**Foreign air carrier** means any person other than a citizen of the United States, who undertakes directly, by lease or other arrangement, to engage in air transportation.]

[**Foreign air commerce** means the carriage by aircraft of persons or property for compensation or hire, or the carriage of mail by aircraft, or the operation or navigation of aircraft in the conduct or furtherance of a business or vocation, in commerce between a place in the United States and any place outside thereof; whether such commerce moves wholly by aircraft or partly by aircraft and partly by other forms of transportation.]

[Foreign air transportation means the carriage by aircraft of persons or property as a common carrier for compensation or hire, or the carriage of mail by aircraft, in commerce between a place in the United States and any place outside of the United States, whether that commerce moves wholly by aircraft or partly by aircraft and partly by other forms of transportation.]

Glider means a heavier-than-air aircraft that is supported in flight by the dynamic reaction of the air against its lifting surfaces and whose free flight does not depend principally on an engine.

Ground visibility means prevailing horizonal visibility near the earth's surface as reported by the National Weather Service or an accredited observer.

Gyrodyne means a rotorcraft whose rotors are normally engine-driven for takeoff, hovering, and landing, and for forward flight through part of its speed range, and whose means of propulsion, consisting usually of conventional propellers, is independent of the rotor system.

Gyroplane means a rotorcraft whose rotors are not engine-driven except for initial starting, but are made to rotate by action of the air when the rotorcraft is moving; and whose means of propulsion, consisting usually of conventional propellers, is independent of the rotor system.

Helicopter means a rotorcraft that, for its horizontal motion, depends principally on its engine-driven rotors.

Heliport means an area of land, water, or structure used or intended to be used for the landing and takeoff of helicopters.

Idle thrust means the jet thrust obtained with the engine power control lever set at the stop for the least thrust position at which it can be placed.

IFR conditions means weather conditions below the minimum for flight under visual flight rules.

IFR over-the-top, with respect to the operation of aircraft, means the operation of an aircraft over-the-top on an IFR flight plan when cleared by air traffic control to maintain "VFR conditions" or "VFR conditions on top".

Indicated airspeed means the speed of an aircraft as shown on its pitot static airspeed indicator calibrated to reflect standard atmosphere adiabatic compressible flow at sea level, uncorrected for airspeed system errors.

Instrument means a device using an internal mechanism to show visually or aurally the attitude, altitude, or operation of an aircraft or aircraft part. It includes electronic devices for automatically controlling an aircraft in flight.

Interstate air commerce means the carriage by aircraft of persons or property for compensation or hire, or the carriage of mail by aircraft, or the operation or navigation of aircraft in the conduct or furtherance of a business or vocation, in commerce between a place in any State of the United States, or the District of Columbia, and a place in any other State of the United States, or the District of Columbia; or between places in the same State of the United States through the airspace over any place outside thereof; or between places in the same territory or possession of the United States, or the District of Columbia.

Interstate air transportation means the carriage by aircraft of persons or property as a common carrier for compensation or hire, or the carriage of mail by aircraft, in commerce—

(1) Between a place in a State or the District of Columbia and another place in another State or the District of Columbia;

(2) Between places in the same State through the airspace of any place outside that State; or

(3) Between places in the same possession of the United States; whether that commerce moves wholly by aircraft or partly by aircraft and partly by other forms of transportation.

[**Intrastate air transportation** means the carriage of persons or property as a common carrier for compensation or hire, by turbojet-powered aircraft capable of carrying thirty or more persons, wholly within the same State of the United States.]

[**Kite** means a framework, covered with paper, cloth, metal, or other material, intended to be flown at the end of a rope or cable, and having as its only support the force of the wind moving past its surfaces.]

Landing gear extended speed means the maximum speed at which an aircraft can be safely flown with the landing gear extended.

Landing gear operating speed means the maximum speed at which the landing gear can be safely extended or retracted.

Large aircraft means aircraft of more than 12,500 pounds, maximum certificated takeoff weight.

Lighter-than-air aircraft means aircraft that can rise and remain suspended by using contained gas weighing less than the air that is displaced by the gas.

Load factor means the ratio of a specified load to the total weight of the aircraft. The specified load is expressed in terms of any of the following: aerodynamic forces, inertia forces, or ground or water reactions.

Mach number means the ratio of true airspeed to the speed of sound.

Main rotor means the rotor that supplies the principal lift to a rotorcraft.

Maintenance means inspection, overhaul, repair, preservation, and the replacement of parts, but excludes preventive maintenance.

Major alteration means an alteration not listed in the aircraft, aircraft engine, or propeller specifications—

(1) That might appreciably affect weight, balance, structural strength, performance, powerplant operation, flight characteristics, or other qualities affecting airworthiness; or

(2) That is not done according to accepted practices or cannot be done by elementary operations.

Major repair means a repair—

(1) That, if improperly done, might appreciably affect weight, balance, structural strength, performance, powerplant operation, flight characteristics, or other qualities affecting airworthiness; or

(2) That is not done according to accepted practices or cannot be done by elementary operations.

Manifold pressure means absolute pressure as measured at the appropriate point in the induction system and usually expressed in inches of mercury.

Medical certificate means acceptable evidence of physical fitness on a form prescribed by the Administrator.

Minimum descent altitude means the lowest altitude, expressed in feet above mean sea level, to which descent is authorized on final approach or during circle-to-land maneuvering in execution of a standard instrument approach procedure, where no electronic guide slope is provided.

Minor alteration means an alteration other than a major alteration.

Minor repair means a repair other than a major repair.

Navigable airspace means airspace at and above the minimum flight altitudes prescribed by or under this chapter, including airspace needed for safe takeoff and landing.

Night means the time between the end of evening civil twilight and the beginning of morning civil twilight, as published in The Air Almanac, converted to local time.

Nonprecision approach procedure means a standard instrument approach procedure in which no electronic guide slope is provided.

Operate, with respect to aircraft, means use, cause to use or authorize to use aircraft, for the purpose (except as provided in 91.10 of this chapter) of air navigation including the piloting of aircraft, with or without the right of legal control (as owner, leasee, or otherwise).

Operational control, with respect to a flight, means the exercise of authority over initiating, conducting, or terminating a flight.

Overseas air commerce means the carriage by aircraft of persons or property for compensation or hire, or the carriage of mail by aircraft, or the operation or navigation of aircraft in the conduct or furtherance of a business or vocation, in commerce between a place in any State of the United States, or the District of Columbia, and any place in a territory or possession of the United States; or between a place in a territory or possession of the United States, and a place in any other territory or possession of the United States.

Overseas air transportation means the carriage by aircraft of persons or property as a common carrier for compensation or hire, or the carriage of mail by aircraft, in commerce—

(1) Between a place in a State or the District of Columbia and a place in a possession of the United States; or

(2) Between a place in a possession of the United States and a place in another possession of the United States; whether that commerce moves wholly by aircraft or partly by aircraft and partly by other forms of transportation.

Over-the-top means above the layer of clouds or other obscuring phenomena forming the ceiling.

Parachute means a device used or intended to be used to retard the fall of a body or object through the air.

Person means an individual, firm, partnership, corporation, company, association, joint-stock association, or governmental entity. It includes a trustee, receiver, assignee, or similar representative of any of them.

Pilotage means navigation by visual reference to landmarks.

Pilot in command means the pilot responsible for the operation and safety of an aircraft during flight time.

266

Pitch setting means the propeller blade setting as determined by the blade angle measured in a manner, and at a radius, specified by the instruction manual for the propeller.

Positive control means control of all air traffic, within designated airspace, by air traffic control.

Precision approach procedure means a standard instrument approach procedure in which an electronic glide slope is provided, such as ILS and PAR.

Preventive maintenance means simple or minor preservation operations and the replacement of small standard parts not involving complex assembly operations.

Prohibited area means designated airspace within which the flight of aircraft is prohibited.

Propeller means a device for propelling an aircraft that has blades on an engine-driven shaft and that, when rotated, produces by its action on the air, a thrust approximately perpendicular to its plane of rotation. It includes control components normally supplied by its manufacturer, but does not include main and auxiliary rotors or rotating airfoils of engines.

Public aircraft means aircraft used only in the service of a government, or a political subdivision. It does not include any government-owned aircraft engaged in carrying persons or property for commercial purposes.

[**Rated maximum continuous augmented thrust,** with respect to turbojet engine type certification, means the approved jet thrust that is developed statically or in flight, in standard atmosphere at a specified altitude, with fluid injection or with the burning of fuel in a separate combustion chamber, within the engine operating limitations established under Part 33 of this chapter, and approved for unrestricted periods of use.]

Rated maximum continuous power, with respect to reciprocating, turbopropeller, and turboshaft engines, means the approved brake horsepower that is developed statically or in flight, in standard atmosphere at a specified altitude, within the engine operating limitations established under Part 33, and approved for unrestricted periods of use.

Rated maximum continuous thrust, with respect to turbojet engine type certification, means the approved jet thrust that is developed statically or in flight, in standard atmosphere at a specified altitude, without fluid injection and without the burning of fuel in a separate combustion chamber, within the engine operating limitations established under Part 33 of this chapter, and approved for unrestricted periods of use.

[**Rated takeoff augmented thrust,** with respect to turbojet engine type certification, means the approved jet thrust that is developed statically under standard sea level conditions, with fluid injection or with the burning of fuel in a separate combustion chamber, within the engine operating limitations established under Part 33 of this chapter, and limited in use to periods of not over 5 minutes for takeoff operation.]

Rated takeoff power, with respect to reciprocating, turbopropeller, and turboshaft engine type certification, means the approved brake horsepower that is developed statically under standard sea level conditions, within the engine operating limitations established under Part 33, and limited in use to periods of not over 5 minutes for takeoff operation.

Rated takeoff thrust, with respect to turbojet engine type certification, means the approved jet thrust that is developed statically under standard sea level conditions, without fluid injection and without the burning of fuel in a separate combustion chamber, within the engine operating limitations established under Part 33 of this chapter, and limited in use to periods of not over 5 minutes for takeoff operation.

Rated 30-minute power, with respect to helicopter turbine engines, means the maximum brake horsepower, developed under static conditions at specified altitudes and atmospheric temperatures, under the maximum conditions or rotor shaft rotational speed and gas temperature, and limited in use to periods of not over 30 minutes as shown on the engine data sheet.

Rated 2½-minute power, with respect to helicopter turbine engines, means the brake horsepower, developed statically in standard atmosphere at sea level, or at a specified altitude, for one-engine-out operation of multi-engine helicopters for 2½ minutes at rotor shaft rotation speed and gas temperature established for this rating.

Rating means a statement that, as a part of a certificate, sets forth special conditions, privileges, or limitations.

Reporting point means a geographical location in relation to which the position of an aircraft is reported.

Restricted area means airspace designated under Part 73 of this chapter within which the flight of aircraft, while not wholly prohibited, is subject to restriction.

RNAV way point (W/P) means a predetermined geographical position used for route or instrument approach definition or progress reporting purposes that is defined relative to a VORTAC station position.

Rocket means an aircraft propelled by ejected expanding gases generated in the engine from self-contained propellants and not dependent on the intake of outside substances. It includes any part which becomes separated during the operation.

Rotorcraft means a heavier-than-air aircraft that depends principally for its support in flight on the lift generated by one or more rotors.

Rotorcraft-load combination means the combination of a rotorcraft and an external load, including the external load attaching means. Rotorcraft-load combinations are designated as Class A, Class B, and Class C, as follows:

(1) "Class A rotorcraft-load combination" means one in which the external load cannot move freely, cannot be jettisoned, and does not extend below the landing gear.

(2) "Class B rotorcraft-load combination" means one in which the external load is jettisonable and is lifted free of land or water during the rotorcraft operation.

(3) "Class C rotorcraft-load combination" means one in which the external load is jettisonable and remains in contact with land or water during the rotorcraft operation.

Route segment means a part of a route. Each end of that part is identified by—

(1) a continental or insular geographical location; or

(2) a point at which a definite radio fix can be established.

[**Sea level engine** means a reciprocating aircraft engine having a rated takeoff power that is producible only at sea level.]

Second in command means a pilot who is designated to be second in command of an aircraft during flight time.

Show, unless the context otherwise requires, means to show to the satisfaction of the Administrator.

Small aircraft means aircraft of 12,500 pounds or less, maximum certificated takeoff weight.

Standard atmosphere means the atmosphere defined in U.S. Standard Atmosphere, 1962 (Geopotential altitude tables).

Stopway means an area beyond the takeoff runway, no less wide than the runway and centered upon the extended centerline of the runway, able to support the airplane during an aborted takeoff, without causing structural damage to the airplane, and designated by the airport authorities for use in decelerating the airplane during an aborted takeoff.

Takeoff power—

(1) With respect to reciprocating engines, means the brake horsepower that is developed under standard sea level conditions, and under the maximum conditions of crankshaft rotational speed and engine manifold pressure approved for the normal takeoff, and limited in continuous use to the period of time shown in the approved engine specification; and

(2) With respect to turbine engines, means the brake horsepower that is developed under static conditions at a specified altitude and atmospheric temperature, and under the maximum conditions of rotorshaft rotational speed and gas temperature approved for the normal takeoff, and limited in continuous use to the period of time shown in the approved engine specification.

Takeoff thrust, with respect to turbine engines, means the jet thrust that is developed under static conditions at a specific altitude and atmospheric temperature under the maximum conditions of rotorshaft rotational speed and gas temperature approved for the normal takeoff, and limited in continuous use to the period of time shown in the approved engine specification.

Time in service, with respect to maintenance time records, means the time from the moment an aircraft leaves the surface of the earth until it touches it at the next point of landing.

Traffic pattern means the traffic flow that is prescribed for aircraft landing at, taxiing on, or taking off from, an airport.

True airspeed means the airspeed of an aircraft relative to undisturbed air. True airspeed is equal to equivalent airspeed multiplied by $(po/p)^{1/2}$.

Type—

(1) As used with respect to the certification, ratings, privileges, and limitations of airmen, means a specific make and basic model of aircraft, including modifications thereto that do not change its handling or flight characteristics. Examples include: DC-7, 1049, and F-27; and

(2) As used with respect to the certification of aircraft, means those aircraft which are similar in design. Examples include: DC-7 and DC-7C;

1049G and 1049H; and F-27 and F-27F.

(3) As used with respect to the certification of aircraft engines, means those engines which are similar in design. For example, JT8D and JT8D-7 are engines of the same type, and JT9D-3A and JT9D-7 are engines of the same type.

United States, in a geographical sense, means (1) the States, the District of Columbia, Puerto Rico, and the possessions, including the territorial waters, and (2) the airspace of those areas.

[**United States air carrier** means a citizen of the United States who undertakes directly by lease, or other arrangement, to engage in air transportation.]

VFR over-the-top, with respect to the operation of aircraft, means the operation of an aircraft over-the-top under VFR when it is not being operated on an IFR flight plan.

1.2 ABBREVIATIONS AND SYMBOLS

In Subchapters A through K of this chapter:

"AGL"—above ground level.

"ALS"—approach light system.

"ASR"—airport surveillance radar.

"ATC"—air traffic control.

"CAS"—calibrated airspeed.

"CAT II"—Category II.

"CONSOL or CONSOLAN"—a kind of low or medium frequency long range navigational aid.

"DH"—decision height.

"DME"—distance measuring equipment compatible with TACAN.

"EAS"—equivalent airspeed.

"FAA"—Federal Aviation Administration.

"FM"—fan marker.

"GS"—glide slope.

"HIRL"—high-intensity runway light system.

"IAS"—indicated airspeed.

"ICAO"—International Civil Aviation Organization.

"IFR"—instrument flight rules.

"ILS"—instrument landing system.

"IM"—ILS inner marker.

"INT"—intersection.

"LDA"—localizer-type directional aid.

"LFR"—low-frequency radio range.

"LMM"—compass locator at middle marker.

"LOC"—ILS localizer.

"LOM"—compass locator at outer marker.

"*M*"—mach number.

"MAA"—maximum authorized IFR altitude.

"MALS"—medium intensity approach light system.

"MALSR"—medium intensity approach light system with runway alignment indicator lights.

"MCA"—minimum crossing altitude.

"MDA"—minimum descent altitude.

"MEA"—minimum en route IFR altitude.

"MM"—ILS middle marker.

"MOCA"—minimum obstruction clearance altitude.

"MRA"—minimum reception altitude.

"MSL"—mean sea level.

"NDB(ADF)"—nondirectional beacon (automatic direction finder).

"NOPT"—no procedure turn required.

"OM"—ILS outer marker.

"PAR"—precision approach radar.

"RAIL"—runway alignment indicator light system.

"RBN"—radio beacon.

"RCLM"—runway centerline marking.

"RCLS"—runway centerline light system.

"REIL"—runway end identification lights.

"RR"—low or medium frequency radio range station.

"RVR"—runway visual range as measured in the touchdown zone area.

"SALS"—short approach light system.

"SSALS"—simplified short approach light system.

"SSALSR"—simplified short approach light system with runway alignment indicator lights.

"TACAN"—ultra-high frequency tactical air navigational aid.

"TAS"—true airspeed.

"TDZL"—touchdown zone lights.

"TVOR"—very high frequency terminal omnirange station.

"VFR"—visual flight rules.

"VHF"—very high frequency.

"VOR"—very high frequency omnirange station.

"VORTAC"—collocated VOR and TACAN.

"Va"—design maneuvering speed.

"Vb"—design speed for maximum gust intensity.

"Vc"—design cruising speed.

"Vd"—design diving speed.

"Vd/Mdf"—demonstrated flight diving speed.

"Vf"—design flap speed.

"Vfc/Mfc"—maximum speed for stability characteristics.

"Vfe"—maximum flap extended speed.

"Vh"—maximum speed in level flight with maximum continuous power.

"Vle"—maximum landing gear extended speed.

"Vlo"—maximum landing gear operating speed.

"Vlof"—lift-off-speed.

"Vmc"—minimum control speed with the critical engine inoperative.

"Vmo/Mmo"—maximum operating limit speed.

"Vmu"—minimum upstick speed.

"Vne"—never-exceed speed.

"Vno"—maximum structural cruising speed.

"Vr"—rotation speed.

"Vs"—the stalling speed or the minimum steady flight speed at which the airplane is controllable.

"Vso"—the stalling speed or the minimum steady flight speed in the landing configuration.

"Vs^1"—the stalling speed or the minimum steady flight speed obtained in a specified configuration.

"Vx"—speed for best angle of climb.

"Vy"—speed for best rate of climb.

"V^1"—takeoff decision speed (formerly denoted as critical engine failure speed).

"V^2"—takeoff safety speed.

"V^2 min"—minimum takeoff safety speed.

1.3 RULES OF CONSTRUCTION

(a) In Subchapters A through K of this chapter, unless the context requires otherwise:

(1) Words importing the singular include the plural;

(2) Words importing the plural include the singular; and

(3) Words importing the masculine gender include the feminine.

(b) In Subchapters A through K of this chapter, the word:

(1) "Shall" is used in an imperative sense;

(2) "May" is used in a permissive sense to state authority or permission to do the act prescribed, and the words "no person may . . ." or "a person may not . . ." means that no person is required, authorized, or permitted to do the act prescribed; and

(3) "Includes" means "includes but is not limited to".

Part 61
Certification: Pilots and Flight Instructors
CONTENTS

SUBPART A—GENERAL

Subpart A — General

61.1 APPLICABILITY.

(a) This Part prescribes the requirements for issuing pilot and flight instructor certificates and ratings, the conditions under which those certificates and ratings are necessary, and the privileges and limitations of those certificates and ratings.

(b) Except as provided in 61.71 of this part, an applicant for a certificate or rating may, until November 1, 1974, meet either the requirements of this Part, or the requirements in effect immediately before November 1, 1973. However, the applicant for a private pilot certificate with a free balloon class rating must meet the requirements of this Part.

61.3 REQUIREMENT FOR CERTIFICATES, RATINGS, AND AUTHORIZATIONS.

(a) **Pilot certificate.** No person may act as pilot in command or in any other capacity as a required pilot flight crewmember of a civil aircraft of United States registry unless he has in his personal possession a current pilot certificate issued to him under this part. However, when the aircraft is operated within a foreign country a current pilot license issued by the country in which the aircraft is operated may be used.

(b) **Pilot certificate: foreign aircraft.** No person may, within the United States, act as pilot in command or in any other capacity as a required pilot flight crewmember of a civil aircraft of foreign registry unless he has in his personal possession a current pilot certificate issued to him under this Part, or a pilot license issued to him or validated for him by the country in which the aircraft is registered.

(c) **Medical certificate.** Except for free balloon pilots piloting balloons and glider pilots piloting gliders, no person may act as pilot in command or in any other capacity as a required pilot flight crewmember of an aircraft under a certificate issued to him under this part, unless he has in his personal possession an appropriate current medical certicate issued under Part 67 of this chapter. However, when the aircraft is operated within a foreign country with a current pilot license issued by that country, evidence of current medical qualification for that license, issued by that country, may be used. In the case of a pilot certificate issued on the basis of a foreign pilot license under 61.75, evidence of current medical qualification accepted for the issue of that license is used in place of a medical certificate.

(d) **Flight instructor certificate.** Except for lighter-than-air flight instruction in lighter-than-air aircraft, and for instruction in air transportation service given by the holder of an Airline Transport Pilot Certificate under 61.169, no person other than the holder of a flight instructor certificate issued by the Administrator with an appropriate rating on that certificate may—

(1) Give any of the flight instruction required to qualify for a solo flight, solo cross-country flight, or for the issue of a pilot or flight instructor certificate or rating;

(2) Endorse a pilot logbook to show that he has given any flight instruction; or

(3) Endorse a student pilot certificate or log book for solo operating privileges.

(e) **Instrument rating.** No person may act as pilot in command of a civil aircraft under instrument flight rules, or in weather conditions less than the minimums prescribed for VFR flight unless—

(1) In the case of an airplane, he holds an instrument rating or an airline transport pilot certificate with an airplane category rating on it;

(2) In the case of a helicopter, he holds a helicopter instrument rating or an airline transport pilot certificate with a rotorcraft category and helicopter class rating not limited to VFR;

(3) In the case of a glider, he holds an instrument rating (airplane) or an airline transport pilot certificate with an airplane category rating; or

(4) In the case of an airship, he holds a commercial pilot certificate with lighter-than-air category and airship class ratings.

(f) **Category II pilot authorization.** (1) No person may act as pilot in command of a civil aircraft in a Category II operation unless he holds a current Category II pilot authorization for that type aircraft or, in the case of a civil aircraft of foreign registry, he is authorized by the country of registry to act as pilot in command of that aircraft in Category II operations.

(2) No person may act as second in command of a civil aircraft in a Category II operation unless he holds a current appropriate instrument rating or an airline transport pilot certificate (airplane) or, in the case of a civil aircraft of foreign registry, he is authorized by the country of registry to act as second in command of that aircraft in Category II operations.

This paragraph does not apply to operations conducted by the holder of a certificate issued under Part 121 of this chapter.

(g) **Category A aircraft pilot authorization.** The Administrator may issue a certificate of authorization to the pilot of a small airplane identified as a Category A aircraft in 97.3(b)(1) of this chapter to use that airplane in a Category II operation, if he finds that the proposed operation can be safely conducted under the terms of the certificate. Such authorization does not permit operation of the aircraft carrying persons or property for compensation or hire.

(h) **Inspection of certificate.** Each person who holds a pilot certificate, flight instructor certificate, medical certificate, authorization, or license required by this Part shall present it for inspection upon the request of the Administrator, an authorized representative of the National Transportation Safety Board, or any Federal, State, or local law enforcement officer.

61.5 CERTIFICATES AND RATINGS ISSUED UNDER THIS PART.

(a) The following certificates are issued under this Part:

(1) Pilot certificates:
  (i) Student pilot.
  (ii) Private pilot.
  (iii) Commercial pilot.
  (iv) Airline transport pilot.
(2) Flight instructor certificates.

(b) The following ratings are placed on pilot certificates (other than student pilot) where applicable:

 (1) Aircraft category ratings:

  (i) Airplane.

  (ii) Rotorcraft.

  (iii) Glider.

  (iv) Lighter-than-air.

 (2) Airplane class ratings:

  (i) Single-engine land.

  (ii) Multiengine land.

  (iii) Single-engine sea.

  (iv) Multiengine sea.

 (3) Rotorcraft class ratings:

  (i) Helicopter.

  (ii) Gyroplane.

 (4) Lighter-than-air class ratings:

  (i) Airship.

  (ii) Free balloon.

 (5) Aircraft type ratings are listed in Advisory Circular 61-1 entitled "Aircraft Type Ratings." This list includes ratings for the following:

  (i) Large aircraft, other than lighter-than-air.

  (ii) Small turbojet-powered airplanes.

  (iii) Small helicopters for operations requiring an airline transport pilot certificate.

  (iv) Other aircraft type ratings specified by the Administrator through aircraft type certificate procedures.

 (6) Instrument ratings (on private and commercial pilot certificates only):

  (i) Instrument—airplanes.

  (ii) Instrument—helicopter.

 (c) The following ratings are placed on flight instructor certificates where applicable:

 (1) Aircraft category ratings:

  (i) Airplane.

  (ii) Rotorcraft.

  (iii) Glider.

 (2) Airplane class ratings:

  (i) Single-engine

  (ii) Multiengine

 (3) Rotorcraft class ratings:

  (i) Helicopter.

  (ii) Gyroplane.

 (4) Instrument ratings:

  (i) Instrument—airplane.

  (ii) Instrument—helicopter.

61.7 OBSOLETE CERTIFICATES AND RATINGS.

(a) The holder of a free balloon pilot certificate issued before November 1, 1973, may not exercise the privileges of that certificate.

(b) The holder of a pilot certificate that bears any of the following category ratings without an associated class rating, may not exercise the privileges of that category rating:

(1) Rotorcraft.

(2) Lighter-than-air.

(3) Helicopter.

(4) Autogiro.

61.9 EXCHANGE OF OBSOLETE CERTIFICATES AND RATINGS FOR CURRENT CERTIFICATES AND RATINGS.

(a) The holder of an unexpired free ballon pilot certificate, or an unexpired pilot certificate with an obsolete category rating listed in 61.7(b) may exchange that certificate for a certificate with the following applicable category and class ratings, without a further showing of competency, until October 31, 1975. After that date, a free balloon pilot certificate or certificate with an obsolete rating expires.

(b) **Private or commercial pilot certificate with rotorcraft category rating.** The holder of a private or commercial pilot certificate with a rotorcraft category rating is issued that certificate with a rotorcraft category rating, and a helicopter or gyroplane class rating, depending upon whether a helicopter or a gyroplane is used to qualify for the rotorcraft category rating.

(c) **Private or commercial pilot certificate with helicopter or autogiro category rating.** The holder of a private or commercial pilot certificate with a helicopter or autogiro category rating is issued that certificate with a rotorcraft category rating and a helicopter class rating (in the case of a helicopter category rating), or a gyroplane class rating (in the case of an autogiro rating).

(d) **Airline transport pilot certificate with helicopter or autogiro category rating.** The holder of an airline transport pilot certificate with a helicopter or autogiro category rating is issued that certificate with a rotorcraft category rating (limited to VFR) and a helicopter class and type rating (in the case of a helicopter category rating), or a gyroplane class rating (in the case of an autogiro category rating).

(e) **Airline transport pilot certificate with a rotorcraft category rating (without a class rating).** The holder of an airline transport pilot certificate with a rotorcraft category rating (without a class rating) is issued that certificate with a rotorcraft category rating limited to VFR, and a helicopter and type rating or a gyroplane class rating, depending upon whether a helicopter or gyroplane is used to qualify for the rotorcraft category rating.

(f) **Free balloon pilot certificate.** The holder of a free balloon pilot certificate is issued a commercial pilot certificate with a lighter-than-air category rating and a free balloon class rating. However, a free balloon class rating may be issued with the limitations provided in 61.141.

(g) **Lighter-than-air pilot certificate or pilot certificate with lighter-than-air category (without a class rating).** (1) In the case of an application made before November 1, 1975, the holder of a lighter-than-air pilot certificate or a pilot certificate with a lighter-than-air category rating (without a class rating) is issued a private or commercial pilot certificate, as appropriate, with a lighter-than-air category rating and airship and free balloon class ratings.

(2) In the case of an application made after October 31, 1975, the holder of a lighter-than-air pilot certificate with an airship rating issued prior to November 1, 1973, may be issued a free balloon class rating upon passing the appropriate flight test in a free balloon.

61.11 EXPIRED PILOT CERTIFICATES AND REISSUANCE.

(a) No person who holds an expired pilot certificate or rating may exercise the privileges of that pilot certificate, or rating.

(b) Except as provided, the following certificates and ratings have expired and are not reissued:

(1) An airline transport pilot certificate issued before May 1, 1949, or containing a horsepower rating. However, an airline transport pilot certificate bearing an expiration date and issued after April 30, 1949, may be reissued without an expiration date if it does not contain a horsepower rating.

(2) A private or commercial pilot certificate, or a lighter-than-air or free balloon pilot certificate, issued before July 1, 1945. However, each of those certificates issued after June 30, 1945, and bearing an expiration date, may be reissued without an expiration date.

(c) A private or commercial pilot certificate or a special purpose pilot certificate, issued on the basis of a foreign pilot license, expires on the expiration date stated thereon. A certificate without an expiration date is issued to the holder of the expired certificate only if he meets the requirements of 61.75 for the issue of a pilot certificate based on a foreign pilot license.

61.13 APPLICATION AND QUALIFICATION.

(a) Application for a certificate and rating, or for an additional rating under this Part is made on a form and in a manner prescribed by the Administrator.

(b) An applicant who meets the requirements of this Part is entitled to an appropriate pilot certificate with aircraft ratings. Additional aircraft category, class, type and other ratings, for which the applicant is qualified, are added to his certificate. However, the Administrator may refuse to issue certificates to persons who are not citizens of the United States and who do not reside in the United States.

(c) An applicant who cannot comply with all of the flight proficiency requirements prescribed by this Part because the aircraft used by him for his flight training or flight test is characteristically incapable of performing a required pilot operation, but who meets all other requirements for the certificate or rating sought, is issued the certificate or rating with appropriate limitations.

(d) An applicant for a pilot's certificate who holds a medical certificate under 67.19 of this chapter with special limitations on it, but who meets all other requirements for that pilot certificate, is issued a pilot certificate containing such operating limitations as the Administrator determines are necessary because of the applicant's medical deficiency.

(e) A Category II pilot authorization is issued as a part of the applicant's instrument rating or airline transport pilot certificate. Upon original issue the authorization contains a limitation for Category II operations of 1,600 feet RVR and a 150 foot decision height. This limitation is removed when the holder shows that since the beginning of the sixth preceding month he has made three Category II ILS approaches to a landing under actual or simulated instrument conditions with a 150 foot decision height.

(f) Unless authorized by the Administrator—

(1) A person whose pilot certificate is suspended may not apply for any pilot or flight instructor certificate or rating during the period of suspension; and

(2) A person whose flight instructor certificate only is suspended may not apply for any rating to be added to that certificate during the period of suspension.

(g) Unless the order of revocation provides otherwise—

(1) A person whose pilot certificate is revoked may not apply for any pilot or flight instructor certificate or rating for 1 year after the date of revocation; and

(2) A person whose flight instructor certificate only is revoked may not apply for any flight instructor certificate for 1 year after the date of revocation.

61.15 OFFENSES INVOLVING NARCOTIC DRUGS, MARIJUANA, AND DEPRESSANT OR STIMULANT DRUGS OR SUBSTANCES.

(a) No person who is convicted of violating any Federal or State statute relating to the growing, processing, manufacture, sale, disposition, possession, transportation, or importation of narcotic drugs, marijuana, and depressant or stimulant drugs or substances, is eligible for any certificate or rating issued under this Part for a period of 1 year after the date of final conviction.

(b) No person who commits an act prohibited by 91.12(a) of this chapter is eligible for any certificate or rating issued under this Part for a period of 1 year after the date of that act.

(c) Any conviction specified in paragraph (a) of this section or the commission of the act referenced in paragraph (b) of this section, is grounds for suspending or revoking any certificate or rating issued under this Part.

61.17 TEMPORARY CERTIFICATE.

(a) A temporary pilot or flight instructor certificate, or a rating, effective for a period of not more than 120 days, is issued to a qualified applicant pending a review of his qualifications and the issuance of a permanent certificate by the Administrator. The permanent certificate or rating is issued to an applicant found qualified and a denial thereof is issued to an applicant found not qualified.

(b) A temporary certificate issued under paragraph (a) of this section expires—

(1) At the end of the expiration date stated thereon; or

(2) Upon receipt by the applicant, of—

    (i) The certificate or rating sought; or

    (ii) Notice that the certificate or rating sought is denied.

61.19 DURATION OF PILOT AND FLIGHT INSTRUCTOR CERTIFICATES.

(a) **General.** The holder of a certificate with an expiration date may not, after that date, exercise the privileges of that certificate.

(b) **Student pilot certificate.** A student pilot certificate expires at the end of the 24th month after the month in which it is issued.

(c) **Other pilot certificates.** Any pilot certificate (other than a student pilot certificate) issued under this Part is issued without a specific expiration date. However, the holder of a pilot certificate issued on the basis of a foreign pilot license may exercise the privileges of that certificate only while the foreign pilot license on which that certificate is based is effective.

(d) **Flight instructor certificate.** A flight instructor certificate—

(1) Is effective only while the holder has a current pilot certificate and a medical certificate appropriate to the pilot privileges being exercised; and

(2) Expires at the end of the 24th month after the month in which it was last issued or renewed.

(e) **Surrender, suspension, or revocation.** Any pilot certificate or flight instructor certificate issued under this Part ceases to be effective if it is surrendered, suspended, or revoked.

(f) **Return of certificate.** The holder of any certificate issued under this Part that is suspended or revoked shall, upon the Administrator's request, return it to the Administrator.

61.21 DURATION OF CATEGORY II PILOT AUTHORIZATION.

A Category II pilot authorization expires at the end of the sixth month after it was last issued or renewed. Upon passing a practical test it is renewed for each type airplane for which an authorization is held. However, an authorization for any particular type airplane for which an authorization is held will not be renewed to extend beyond the end of the 12th month after the practical test was passed in that type airplane. If the holder of the authorization passes the practical test for a renewal in the month before the authorization expires, he is considered to have passed it during the month the authorization expired.

61.23 DURATION OF MEDICAL CERTIFICATES.

(a) A first-class medical certificate expires at the end of the last day of—

(1) The sixth month after the month of the date of examination shown on the certificate, for operations requiring an airline transport pilot certificate;

(2) The 12th month after the month of the date of examination shown on the certificate, for operations requiring only a commercial pilot certificate; and

(3) The 24th month after the month of the date of examination shown on the certificate, for operations requiring only a private or student pilot certificate.

(b) A second-class medical certificate expires at the end of the last day of—

(1) The 12th month after the month of the date of examination shown

on the certificate, for operations requiring a commercial pilot certificate; and

(2) The 24th month after the month of the date of examination shown on the certificate, for operations requiring only a private or student pilot certificate.

(c) A third-class medical certificate expires at the end of the last day of the 24th month after the month of the date of examination shown on the certificate, for operations requiring a private or student pilot certificate.

61.25 CHANGE OF NAME.

An application for the change of a name on a certificate issued under this Part must be accompanied by the applicant's current certificate and a copy of the marriage license, court order, or other document verifying the change. The documents are returned to the applicant after inspection.

61.27 VOLUNTARY SURRENDER OR EXCHANGE OF CERTIFICATE.

The holder of a certificate issued under this Part may voluntarily surrender it for cancellation, or for the issue of a certificate of lower grade, or another certificate with specific ratings deleted. If he so requests, he must include the following signed statement or its equivalent:

This request is made for my own reasons, with full knowledge that my (insert name of certificate or rating, as appropriate) may not be reissued to me unless I again pass the tests prescribed for its issue.

61.29 REPLACEMENT OF LOST OR DESTROYED CERTIFICATE.

(a) An application for the replacement of a lost or destroyed airman certificate issued under this Part is made by letter to the Department of Transportation, Federal Aviation Administration, Airman Certification Branch, Post Office Box 25082, Oklahoma City, OK 73125. The letter must—

(1) State the name of the person to whom the certificate was issued, the permanent mailing address (including zip code), social security number (if any), date and place of birth of the certificate holder, and any available information regarding the grade, number, and date of issue of the certificate, and the ratings on it; and

(2) Be accompanied by a check or money order for $2, payable to the Federal Aviation Administration.

(b) An application for the replacement of a lost or destroyed medical certificate is made by letter to the Department of Transportation, Federal Aviation Adminstration, Aeromedical Certification Branch, Post Office Box 25082, Oklahoma City, OK 73125, accompanied by a check or money order for $2.

(c) A person who has lost a certificate issued under this Part, or a medical certificate issued under Part 67 of this chapter, or both, may obtain a telegram from the FAA confirming that it was issued. The telegram may be carried as a certificate for a period not to exceed 60 days pending his request of a duplicate certificate under paragraph (a) or (b) of this section, unless he has been notified that the certificate has been suspended or revoked. The request for such a telegram may be made by letter or prepaid telegram, including the date upon which a duplicate certificate was previously requested, if a request had been made, and a money order for the cost of the duplicate certificate. The request for a telegraphic certificate is sent to the office listed in paragraph (a) or (b) of this section, as appropriate. However, a request for both airman and medical certificates at the same time must be sent to the office prescribed in paragraph (a) of this section.

61.31 GENERAL LIMITATIONS.

(a) **Type ratings required.** A person may not act as pilot in command of any of the following aircraft unless he holds a type rating for that aircraft:

(1) A large aircraft (except lighter-than-air).

(2) A helicopter, for operations requiring an airline transport pilot certificate.

(3) A turbojet powered airplane.

(4) Other aircraft specified by the Administrator through aircraft type certificate procedures.

(b) **Authorization in lieu of a type rating.** (1) In lieu of a type rating required under paragraphs (a) (1), (3), and (4) of this section, an aircraft may be operated under an authorization issued by the Administrator, for a flight or series of flights within the United States, if—

(i) The particular operation for which the authorization is requested involves a ferry flight, a practice or training flight, a flight test for a pilot type rating, or a test flight of an aircraft, for a period that does not exceed 60 days;

(ii) The applicant shows that compliance with paragraph (a) of this section is impracticable for the particular operation; and

(iii) The Administrator finds that an equivalent level of safety may be achieved through operating limitations on the authorization.

(2) Aircraft operated under an authorization issued under this paragraph—

(i) May not be operated for compensation or hire; and

(ii) May carry only flight crewmembers necessary for the flight.

(3) An authorization issued under this paragraph may be reissued for an additional 60-day period for the same operation if the applicant shows that he was prevented from carrying out the purpose of the particular operation before his authorization expired. The prohibition of paragraph (b)(2)(i) of this section does not prohibit compensation for the use of an aircraft by a pilot solely to prepare for or take a flight test for a type rating.

(c) **Category and class rating: Carrying another person or operating for compensation or hire.** Unless he holds a category and class rating for that aircraft, a person may not act as pilot in command of an aircraft that is carrying another person or is operated for compensation or hire. In addition, he may not act as pilot in command of that aircraft for compensation or hire.

(d) **Category and class rating: Other operations.** No person may act as pilot in command of an aircraft in solo flight in operations not subject to paragraph (c) of this section, unless he meets at least one of the following:

(1) He holds a category and class rating appropriate to that aircraft.

(2) He has received flight instruction in the pilot operations required

by this part, appropriate to the category and class of aircraft for first solo, given to him by a certified flight instructor who found him competent to solo that category and class of aircraft and has so endorsed his pilot logbook.

(3) He has soloed and logged pilot-in-command time in that category and class of aircraft before November 1, 1973.

(e) **High performance airplanes.** A person holding a private or commercial pilot certificate may not act as pilot in command of an airplane that has more than 200 horsepower, or that has a retractable landing gear, flaps, and a controllable propeller, unless he has received flight instruction from an authorized flight instructor who certified in his logbook that he is competent to pilot an airplane that has more than 200 horse-power, or that has a retractable landing gear, flaps, and a controllable propeller, as the case may be. However, this instruction is not required if he has logged flight time as pilot in command in high performance airplanes before November 1, 1973.

(f) **Exception.** This section does not require a class rating for gliders, or category and class ratings for aircraft that are not type certified as airplanes, rotorcraft, or lighter-than-air aircraft. In addition, the rating limitations of this section do not apply to—

(1) The holder of a student pilot certificate;

(2) The holder of a pilot certificate when operating an aircraft under the authority of an experimental or provisional type certificate;

(3) An applicant when taking a flight test given by the Administrator; or

(4) The holder of a pilot certificate with a lighter-than-air category rating when operating a hot air balloon without an airborne heater.

61.33 TESTS: GENERAL PROCEDURE.

Tests prescribed by or under this Part are given at times and places, and by persons, designated by the Administrator.

61.35 WRITTEN TEST: PREREQUISITES AND PASSING GRADES.

(a) An applicant for a written test must—

(1) Show that he has satisfactorily completed the ground instruction or home study course required by this Part for the certificate or rating sought;

(2) Present as personal identification an airman certificate, driver's license, or other official document; and

(3) Present a birth certificate or other official document showing that he meets the age requirement prescribed in this Part for the certificate sought not later than 2 years from the date of application for the test.

(b) The minimum passing grade is specified by the Administrator on each written test sheet or booklet furnished to the applicant.

This section does not apply to the written test for an airline transport pilot certificate or a rating associated with that certificate.

61.37 WRITTEN TESTS: CHEATING OR OTHER UNAUTHORIZED CONDUCT.

(a) Except as authorized by the Administrator, no person may—

(1) Copy, or intentionally remove, a written test under this Part;

(2) Give to another, or receive from another, any part or copy of that test;

(3) Give help on that test to, or receive help on that test from, any person during the period that test is being given;

(4) Take any part of that test in behalf of another person;

(5) Use any material or aid during the period that test is being given; or

(6) Intentionally cause, assist, or participate in any act prohibited by this paragraph.

(b) No person whom the Administrator finds to have committed an act prohibited by paragraph (a) of this section is eligible for any airman or ground instructor certificate or rating, or to take any test therefor, under this chapter for a period of 1 year after the date of that act. In addition, the commission of that act is a basis for suspending or revoking any airman or ground instructor certificate or rating held by that person.

61.39 PREREQUISITES FOR FLIGHT TESTS.

(a) To be eligible for a flight test for a certificate, or an aircraft or instrument rating issued under this Part, the applicant must—

(1) Have passed any required written test since the beginning of the 24th month before the month in which he takes the flight test;

(2) Have the applicable instruction and aeronautical experience prescribed in this part;

(3) Hold a current medical certificate appropriate to the certificate he seeks or, in the case of a rating to be added to his pilot certificate, at least a third-class medical certificate issued since the beginning of the 24th month before the month in which he takes the flight test;

(4) Except for a flight test for an airline transport pilot certificate, meet the age requirement for the issuance of the certificate or rating he seeks; and

(5) Have a written statement from an appropriately certificated flight instructor certifying that he has given the applicant flight instruction in preparation for the flight test within 60 days preceding the date of application, and finds him competent to pass the test and to have satisfactory knowledge of the subject areas in which he is shown to be deficient by his FAA airman written test report. However, an applicant need not have this written statement if he—

(i) Holds a foreign pilot license issued by a contracting State to the Convention on International Civil Aviation that authorizes at least the pilot privileges of the airman certificate sought by him;

(ii) Is applying for a type rating only, or a class rating with an associated type rating; or

(iii) Is applying for an airline transport pilot certificate or an additional aircraft rating on that certificate.

(b) Notwithstanding paragraph (a)(1) of this section, an applicant for an airline transport pilot certificate or an additional aircraft rating on that certificate who has been, since passing the written examination, continuously employed as a pilot, or as a pilot assigned to flight engineer duties by, and is participating in an approved pilot training program of a U.S. air carrier or commercial operator, or who is rated as a pilot by, and is participating in a pilot training program of a U.S. scheduled military air transportation service, may take the flight test for that certificate or rating.

61.41 FLIGHT INSTRUCTION RECEIVED FROM FLIGHT INSTRUCTORS NOT CERTIFICATED BY FAA.

Flight instruction may be credited toward the requirements for a pilot certificate or rating issued under this Part if it is received from—

(a) An Armed Force of either the United States or a foreign contracting State to the Convention on International Civil Aviation in an program for training military pilots; or

(b) A flight instructor who is authorized to give that flight instruction by the licensing authority of a foreign contracting State to the Convention on International Civil Aviation and the flight instruction is given outside the United States.

61.43 FLIGHT TESTS: GENERAL PROCEDURES.

(a) The ability of an applicant for a private or commercial pilot certificate, or for an aircraft or instrument rating on that certificate, to perform the required pilot operations is based on the following:

(1) Executing procedures and maneuvers within the aircraft's performance capabilities and limitations, including use of the aircraft's systems.

(2) Executing emergency procedures and maneuvers appropriate to the aircraft.

(3) Piloting the aircraft with smoothness and accuracy.

(4) Exercising judgment.

(5) Applying his aeronautical knowledge.

(6) Showing that he is the master of the aircraft, with the successful outcome of a procedure or maneuver never seriously in doubt.

(b) If the applicant fails any of the required pilot operations in accordance with the applicable provisions of paragraph (a) of this section, the applicant fails the flight test. The applicant is not eligible for the certificate or rating sought until he passes any pilot operations he has failed.

(c) The examiner or the applicant may discontinue the test at any time when the failure of a required pilot operation makes the applicant ineligible for the certificate or rating sought. If the test is discontinued the applicant is entitled to credit for only those entire pilot operations that he has successfully performed.

61.45 FLIGHT TESTS: REQUIRED AIRCRAFT AND EQUIPMENT.

(a) **General.** An applicant for a certificate or rating under this part must furnish, for each flight test that he is required to take, an appropriate aircraft of United States registry that has a current standard or limited airworthiness certificate. However, the applicant may, at the discretion of the inspector or examiner conducting the test, furnish an aircraft of U.S. registry that has a current airworthiness certificate other than standard or limited, an aircraft of foreign registry that is properly certificated by the country of registry, or a military aircraft in an operational status if its use is allowed by an appropriate military authority.

(b) **Required equipment (other than controls).** Aircraft furnished for a flight test must have—

(1) The equipment for each pilot operation required for the flight test;

(2) No prescribed operating limitations that prohibit its use in any pilot operation required on the test;

(3) Pilot seats with adequate visibility for each pilot to operate the aircraft safely, except as provided in paragraph (d) of this section; and

(4) Cockpit and outside visibility adequate to evaluate the performance of the applicant, where an additional jump seat is provided for the examiner.

(c) **Required controls.** An aircraft (other than lighter-than-air) furnished under paragraph (a) of this section for any pilot flight test must have engine power controls and flight controls that are easily reached and operable in a normal manner by both pilots, unless after considering all the factors, the examiner determines that the flight test can be conducted safely without them. However, an aircraft having other controls such as nose-wheel steering, brakes, switches, fuel selectors, and engine air flow controls that are not easily reached and operable in a normal manner by both pilots may be used, if more than one pilot is required under its airworthiness certificate, or if the examiner determines that the flight can be conducted safely.

(d) **Simulated instrument flight equipment.** An applicant for any flight test involving flight maneuvers solely by reference to instruments must furnish equipment satisfactory to the examiner that excludes the visual reference of the applicant outside of the aircraft.

(e) **Aircraft with single controls.** At the discretion of the examiner, an aircraft furnished under paragraph (a) of this section for a flight test may, in the cases listed herein, have a single set of controls. In such case, the examiner determines the competence of the applicant by observation from the ground or from another aircraft.

(1) A flight test for addition of a class or type rating, not involving demonstration of instrument skills, to a private or commercial pilot certificate.

(2) A flight test in a single-place gyroplane for—

(i) A private pilot certificate with a rotorcraft category rating and gyroplane class rating, in which case the certificate bears the limitation "rotorcraft single-place gyroplane only"; or

(ii) Addition of a rotorcraft category rating and gyroplane class rating to a pilot certificate, in which case a certificate higher than a private pilot certificate bears the limitation "rotorcraft single-place gyroplane, private pilot privileges, only."

The limitations prescribed by this subparagraph may be removed if the holder of the certificate passes the appropriate flight test in a gyroplane with two pilot stations or otherwise passes the appropriate flight test for a rotorcraft category rating.

61.47 FLIGHT TESTS: STATUS OF FAA INSPECTORS AND OTHER AUTHORIZED FLIGHT EXAMINERS.

An FAA inspector or other authorized flight examiner conducts the flight test of an applicant for a pilot certificate or rating for the purpose of observing the applicant's ability to perform satisfactorily the procedures and maneuvers on the flight test. The inspector or other examiner is not pilot in command of the aircraft during the flight test unless he acts in that capacity for the flight, or portion of the flight, by prior arrangement with the applicant or other person who would otherwise act as pilot in command of the flight, or portion of the flight. Notwithstanding the type of aircraft used during a flight test, the applicant and the inspector or other examiner are not, with respect to each other (or other occupants authorized by the inspector or other examiner), subject to the requirements or limitations for the carriage of passengers specified in this chapter.

61.49   RETESTING AFTER FAILURE.

An applicant for a written or flight test who fails that test may not apply for retesting until 30 days after the date he failed the test. However, in the case of his first failure he may apply for retesting before the 30 days have expired upon presenting a written statement from an authorized instructor certifying that he has given flight or ground instruction as appropriate to the applicant and finds him competent to pass the test.

61.51   PILOT LOGBOOKS.

   (a) The aeronautical training and experience used to meet the requirements for a certificate or rating, or the recent flight experience requirements of this Part must be shown by a reliable record. The logging of other flight time is not required.

   (b) **Logbook entries.** Each pilot shall enter the following information for each flight or lesson logged:

   (1) **General**
      (i)   Date.
      (ii) Total time of flight.
      (iii) Place, or points of departure and arrival.
      (iv) Type and identification of aircraft.

   (2) **Type of pilot experience or training.**
      (i)   Pilot in command or solo.
      (ii) Second in command.
      (iii) Flight instruction received from an authorized flight instructor.
      (iv) Instrument flight instruction from an authorized flight instructor.
      (v)   Pilot ground trainer instruction.
      (vi) Participating crew (lighter-than-air).
      (vii) Other pilot time.

   (3) **Conditions of flight.**
      (i)   Day or night.
      (ii) Actual instrument.
      (iii) Simulated instrument conditions.

   (c) **Logging of pilot time—(1) Solo flight time.** A pilot may log as solo flight time only that flight time when he is the sole occupant of the aircraft. However, a student pilot may also log as solo flight time that time during which he acts as the pilot in command of an airship requiring more than one flight crewmember.

(2) **Pilot-in-command flight time.**

(i) A private or commercial pilot may log as pilot-in-command-time only that flight time during which he is the sole manipulator of the controls of an aircraft for which he is rated, or when he is the sole occupant of the aircraft, or when he acts as pilot in command of an aircraft on which more than one pilot is required under the type certification of the aircraft, or the regulations under which the flight is conducted.

(ii) An airline transport pilot may log as pilot-in-command-time all of the flight time during which he acts as pilot-in-command.

(iii) A certificated flight instructor may log as pilot-in-command-time all flight time during which he acts as a flight instructor.

(3) **Second-in-command flight time.** A pilot may log as second-in-command-time all flight time during which he acts as second in command of an aircraft on which more than one pilot is required under the type certification of the aircraft, or the regulations under which the flight is conducted.

(4) **Instrument flight time.** A pilot may log as instrument flight time only that time during which he operates the aircraft solely by reference to instruments, under actual or simulated instrument flight conditions. Each entry must include the place and type of each instrument approach completed, and the name of the safety pilot for each simulated instrument flight. An instrument flight instructor may log as instrument time that time during which he acts as instrument flight instructor in actual instrument weather conditions.

(5) **Instruction time.** All time logged as flight instruction, instrument flight instruction, pilot ground trainer instruction, or ground instruction time must be certified by the appropriately rated and certificated instructor from whom it was received.

(d) **Presentation of logbook.**

(1) A pilot must present his logbook (or other record required by this section) for inspection upon reasonable request by the Administrator, an authorized representative of the National Transportation Safety Board, or any State or local law enforcement officer.

(2) A student pilot must carry his logbook (or other record required by this section) with him on all solo cross-country flights, as evidence of the required instructor clearances and endorsements.

61.53 OPERATIONS DURING MEDICAL DEFICIENCY.

No person may act as pilot in command, or in any other capacity as a required pilot flight crewmember while he has a known medical deficiency, or increase of a known medical deficiency, that would make him unable to meet the requirements for his current medical certificate.

61.55 SECOND IN COMMAND QUALIFICATIONS: OPERATION OF LARGE AIRPLANES OR TURBOJET-POWERED MULTIENGINE AIRPLANES.

(a) Except as provided in paragraph (d) of this section, no person may serve as second in command of a large airplane, or a turbojet-powered multiengine airplane type certificated for more than one required pilot flight crewmember unless he holds—

(1) At least a current private pilot certificate with appropriate category and class ratings; and

(2) An appropriate instrument rating in the case of flight under IFR.

(b) Except as provided in paragraph (d) of this section, no person may serve as second in command of a large airplane, or a turbojet-powered multiengine airplane type certificated for more than one required pilot flight crewmember, unless since the beginning of the 12th calendar month before the month in which he serves, he has, with respect to that type airplane:

(1) Familiarized himself with all information concerning the airplane's powerplant, major components and systems, major appliances, performance and limitations, standard and emergency operating procedures and the contents of the approved airplane flight manual, if one is required.

(2) Except as provided in paragraph (e) of this section, performed and logged—

(i) Three takeoffs and three landings to a full stop as the sole manipulator of the flight controls; and

(ii) Engine-out procedures and maneuvering with an engine out while executing the duties of a pilot in command. This requirement may be satisfied in an airplane simulator acceptable to the Administrator.

For the purpose of meeting the requirements of subparagraph (2) of this paragraph, a person may act as second in command of a flight under day VFR or day IFR, if no persons or property, other than as necessary for the operations, are carried.

(c) If a pilot complies with the requirements in paragraph (b) of this section in the calender month before, or the calendar month after, the month in which compliance with those requirements is due, he is considered to have complied with them in the month they are due.

(d) This section does not apply to a pilot who—

(1) Meets the pilot in command proficiency check requirements of Part 121, 123, or 135 of this chapter;

(2) Is designated as the second in command of an airplane operated under the provisions of Part 121, 123, or 135 of this chapter; or

(3) Is designated as the second in command of an airplane for the purpose of receiving flight training required by this section and no passengers or cargo are carried on that airplane.

(e) The holder of a commercial or airline transport pilot certificate with appropriate category and class ratings need not meet the requirements of paragraph (b) (2) of this section for the conduct of ferry flights, aircraft flight tests, or airborne equipment evaluation, if no persons or property other than as necessary for the operation are carried.

61.57 RECENT FLIGHT EXPERIENCE: PILOT IN COMMAND.

(a) **Flight review.** After November 1, 1974, no person may act as pilot in command of an aircraft unless, within the preceding 24 months, he has—

(1) Accomplished a flight review given to him, in an aircraft for which he is rated, by an appropriately certificated instructor or other person

designed by the Administrator; and

(2) Had his log book endorsed by the person who gave him the review certifying that he has satisfactorily accomplished the flight review.

However, a person who has, within the preceding 24 months, satisfactorily completed a pilot proficiency check conducted by the FAA, an approved pilot check airman, or a U.S. Armed Force for a pilot certificate, rating or operating privilege, need not accomplish the flight review required by this section.

(b) **Meaning of flight review.** As used in this section, a flight review consists of—

(1) A review of the current general operating and flight rules of Part 91 of this chapter; and

(2) A review of those maneuvers and procedures which in the discretion of the person giving the review are necessary for the pilot to demonstrate that he can safely exercise the privileges of his pilot certificate.

(c) **Gerenal experience.** No person may act as pilot in command of an aircraft carrying passengers, nor of an aircraft certificated for more than one required pilot flight crewmember, unless within the preceding 90 days, he has made three takeoffs and three landings as the sole manipulator of the flight controls in an aircraft of the same category and class and, if a type rating is required, of the same type. If the aircraft is a tailwheel airplane, the landings must have been made to a full stop in a tailwheel airplane. For the purpose of meeting the requirements of the paragraph a person may act as pilot-in-command of a flight under day VFR or day IFR if no persons or property other than as necessary for his compliance thereunder, are carried. This paragraph does not apply to operations requiring an airline transport pilot certificate, or to operations conducted under Part 135 of this chapter.

(d) **Night experience.** No person may act as pilot in command of an aircraft carrying passengers during the period beginning 1 hour after sunset and ending 1 hour before sunrise (as published in the Air Almanac) unless, within the preceding 90 days, he has made at least three takeoffs and three landings to a full stop during that period in the category and class of aircraft to be used. This paragraph does not apply to operations requiring an airline transport pilot certificate.

(e) **Instrument—**(1) **Recent IFR experience.** No pilot may act as pilot in command under IFR, nor in weather conditions less than the minimums prescribed for VFR, unless he has, within the past 6 months—

(i) In the case of an aircraft other than a glider, logged at least 6 hours of instrument time under actual or simulated IFR conditions, at least 3 of which were in flight in the category of aircraft involved, including at least six instrument approaches, or passed an instrument competency check in the category of aircraft involved.

(ii) In the case of a glider, logged at least 3 hours of instrument time, at least half of which were in a glider or an airplane. If a passenger is carried in the glider, at least 3 hours of instrument flight time must have been in gliders.

(2) **Instrument competency check.** A pilot who does not meet the recent instrument experience requirements of paragraph (e)(1) of this section

during the prescribed time or 6 months thereafter may not serve as pilot in command under IFR, nor in weather conditions less than the minimum presecribed for VFR, until he passes an instrument competency check in the category of aircraft involved, given by an FAA inspector, a member of an armed force of the United States authorized to conduct flight tests, an FAA-approved check pilot, or a certificated instrument flight instructor. The Administrator may authorize the conduct of part or all of this check in a pilot ground trainer equipped for instruments or an aircraft simulator.

61.58 PILOT-IN-COMMAND PROFICIENCY CHECK: OPERATION OF AIRCRAFT REQUIRING MORE THAN ONE REQUIRED PILOT.

(a) Except as provided in paragraph (e) of this section, after November 1, 1974, no person may act as pilot in command of an aircraft that is type certificated for more than one required pilot crewmember unless he has satisfactorily completed the proficiency checks or flight checks prescribed in paragraphs (b) and (c) of this section.

(b) Since the beginning of the 12th calendar month before the month in which a person acts as pilot in command of an aircraft that is type certificated for more than one required pilot crewmember he must have completed one of the following:

(1) For an airplane—a proficiency or flight check in either an airplane that is type certificated for more than one required pilot crewmember, or in an approved simulator or other training device, given to him by an FAA inspector or designated pilot examiner and consisting of those maneuvers and procedures set forth in Appendix F of Part 121 of this chapter whch may be performed in a simulator or training device.

(2) For other aircraft—a proficiency or flight check in an aircraft that is type certificated for more than one required pilot crewmember given to him by an FAA inspector or designated pilot examiner which includes those maneuvers and procedures required for the original issuance of a type rating for the aircraft used in the check.

(3) A pilot in command proficiency check given to him in accordance with the provisions for that check under Parts 121, 123, or 135 of this chapter. However, in the case of a person acting as pilot in command of a helicopter he may complete a proficiency check given to him in accordance with Part 127 of this chapter.

(4) A flight test required for an aircraft type rating.

(5) An initial or periodic check for the purpose of the issuance of a pilot examiner or check airman designation.

(6) A military proficiency check required for pilot in command and instrument privileges in an aircraft which the military requires to be operated by more than one pilot.

(c) Except as provided in paragraph (d) of this section, since the beginning of the 24th calendar month before the month in which a person acts as pilot in command of an aircraft that is type certificated for more than one required pilot crewmember he must have completed one of the following proficiency or flight checks in the particular type aircraft in which he is to serve as pilot in command:

(1) A proficiency check or flight check given to him by an FAA inspector or a designated pilot examiner which includes the maneuvers, procedures, and standards required for the original issuance of a type rating for the aircraft used in the check.

(2) A pilot in command proficiency check given to him in accordance with the provisions for that check under Parts 121, 123, or 135 of this chapter. However, in the case of a person acting as pilot in command of a helicopter he may complete a proficiency check given to him in accordance with Part 127 of this chapter.

(3) A flight test required for an aircraft type rating.

(4) An initial or periodic flight check for the purpose of the issuance of a pilot examiner or check airman designation.

(5) A military proficiency check required for pilot in command and instrument privileges in an aircraft which the military requires to be operated by more than one pilot.

(d) For airplanes, the maneuvers and procedures required for the checks and test prescribed in paragraphs (c) (1), (2), (4), and (5) of this section, and paragraph (c)(3) of this section in the case of type ratings obtained in conjunction with a Part 121 of this chapter training program may be performed in a simulator or training device if—

(1) The maneuver or procedure can be performed in a simulator or training device as set forth in Appendix F to Part 121 of this chapter; and

(2) The simulator or training device is one that is approved for the particular maneuver or procedure.

(e) This section does not apply to persons conducting operations subject to Parts 121, 123, 127, 133, and 135, and 137 of this chapter.

(f) For the purpose of meeting the proficiency check requirements of paragraphs (b) and (c) of this section, a person may act as pilot in command of a flight under day VFR or day IFR if no persons or property, other than as necessary for his compliance thereunder, are carried.

(g) If a pilot takes the proficiency check required by paragraph (a) of this section in the calender month before, or the calendar month after, the month in which it is due, he is considered to have taken it in the month it is due.

61.59 FALSIFICATION, REPRODUCTION, OR ALTERATION OF APPLICATIONS, CERTIFICATES, LOGBOOKS, REPORTS, OR RECORDS.

(a) No person may make or cause to be made—

(1) Any fraudulent or intentionally false statement on any application for a certificate, rating, or duplicate thereof, issued under this Part;

(2) Any fraudulent or intentionally false entry in any logbook, record, or report that is required to be kept, made, or used, to show compliance with any requirement for the issuance, or exercise of the privileges, of any certificate or rating under this Part;

(3) Any reproduction, for fraudulent purpose, of any certificate or rating under this Part,

(4) Any alteration of any certificate or rating under this Part.

(b) The commission by any person of an act prohibited under paragraph

(a) of this section is a basis for suspending or revoking any airman or ground instructor certificate or rating held by that person.

61.60   CHANGE OF ADDRESS.
The holder of a pilot or flight instructor certificate who has made a change in his permanent mailing address may not after 30 days from the date he moved, exercise the privileges of his certificate unless he has notified in writing the Department of Transportation, Federal Aviation Administration, Airman Certification Branch, Box 25082, Oklahoma City, OK 73125, of his new address.

Subpart B — Aircraft Ratings and Special Certificates

61.61   APPLICABILITY.
This subpart prescribes the requirements for the issuance of additional aircraft ratings after a pilot or instructor certificate is issued, and the requirements and limitations for special pilot certificates and ratings issued by the Administrator.

61.63   ADDITIONAL AIRCRAFT RATINGS (OTHER THAN AIRLINE TRANSPORT PILOT).
(a) **General.** To be eligible for an aircraft rating after his certificate is issued to him an applicant must meet the requirements of paragraphs (b) through (d) of this section, as appropriate to the rating sought.

(b) **Category rating.** An applicant for a category rating to be added on his pilot certificate must meet the requirements of this Part for the issue of the pilot certificate appropriate to the privileges for which the category rating is sought. However, the holder of a category rating for powered aircraft is not required to take a written test for the addition of a category rating on his pilot certificate.

(c) **Class rating.** An applicant for an aircraft class rating to be added on his pilot certificate must—

(1) Present a logbook record certified by an authorized flight instructor showing that the applicant has received flight instruction in the class of aircraft for which a rating is sought and has been found competent in the pilot operations appropriate to the pilot certificate to which his category rating applies; and

(2) Pass a flight test appropriate to his pilot certificate and applicable to the aircraft category and class rating sought.

A person who holds a lighter-than-air category rating with a free balloon class rating, who seeks an airship class rating, must meet the requirements of paragraph (b) of this section as though seeking a lighter-than-air category rating.

(d) **Type rating.** An applicant for a type rating to be added on his pilot certificate must meet the following requirements:

(1) He must hold, or concurrently obtain, an instrument rating appropriate to the aircraft for which a type rating is sought.

(2) He must pass a flight test showing competence in pilot operations appropriate to the pilot certificate he holds and to the type rating sought.

(3) He must pass a flight test showing competence in pilot operations under instrument flight rules in an aircraft of the type for which the type rating is sought or, in the case of a single pilot station airplane, meet the requirements of paragraph (d)(3) (i) or (ii) of this section, whichever is applicable.

(i) The applicant must have met the requirements of this subparagraph in a multiengine airplane for which the type rating is required.

(ii) If he does not meet the requirements of paragraph (d)(3)(i) of this section and he seeks a type rating for a single-engine airplane, he must meet the requirements of this subparagraph in either a single or multiengine airplane, and have the recent instrument experience set forth in 61.57(e), when he applies for the flight test under paragraph (d)(2) of this section.

(4) An applicant who does not meet the requirements of paragraphs (d) (1) and (3) of this section may obtain a type rating limited to "VFR only." Upon meeting these instrument requirments or the requirements of 61.73(e)(2), the "VFR only" limitation may be removed for the particular type of aircraft in which competence is shown.

(5) When an instrument rating is issued to the holder of one or more type ratings, the type ratings on the amended certificate bear the limitation described in paragraph (d)(4) of this section for each airplane type rating for which he has not shown his instrument competency under this paragraph.

61.65 INSTRUMENT RATING REQUIREMENTS.

(a) **General.** To be eligible for an instrument rating (airplane) or an instrument rating (helicopter), an applicant must—

(1) Hold a current private or commercial pilot certificate with an aircraft rating appropriate to the instrument rating sought;

(2) Be able to read, speak, and understand the English language; and

(3) Comply with the applicable requirements of this section.

(b) **Ground instruction.** An applicant for the written test for an instrument rating must have received ground instruction, or have logged home study in at least the following areas of aeronautical knowledge appropriate to the rating sought.

(1) The regulations of this chapter that apply to flight under IFR conditions, the Airman's Information Manual, and the IFR air traffic system and procedures;

(2) Dead reckoning appropriate to IFR navigation, IFR navigation by radio aids using the VOR, ADF, and ILS systems, and the use of IFR charts and instrument approach plates;

(3) The procurement and use of aviation weather reports and forecasts, and the elements of forecasting weather trends on the basis of that information and personal observation of weather conditions; and

(4) The safe and efficient operation of airplanes or helicopters, as appropriate, under instrument weather conditons.

(c) **Flight instruction and skill—airplanes.** An applicant for the flight test for an instrument rating (airplane) must present a logbook record certified by an authorized flight instructor showing that he has received instrument flight instruction in an airplane in the following pilot operations, and has been found competent in each of them:

(1) Control and accurate maneuvering of an airplane solely by reference to instruments.

(2) IFR navigation by the use of the VOR and ADF systems, including compliance with air traffic control instructions and procedures.

(3) Instrument approaches to published minimums using the VOR, ADF, and ILS systems (instruction in the use of the ADF and ILS may be received in an instrument ground trainer and instruction in the use of the ILS glide slope may be received in an airborne ILS simulator).

(4) Cross-country flying in simulated or actual IFR conditions, on Federal airways or as routed by ATC, including one such trip of at least 250 nautical miles, including VOR, ADF, and ILS approaches at different airports.

(5) Simulated emergencies, including the recovery from unusual attitudes, equipment or instrument malfunctions, loss of communications, and engine-out emergencies if a multiengine airplane is used, and missed approach procedures.

(d) **Instrument instruction and skill—(helicopter).** An applicant for the flight test for an instrument rating (helicopter) must present a logbook record certified to by an authorized flight instructor showing that he has received instrument flight instruction in a helicopter in the following pilot operations, and has been found competent in each of them:

(1) The control and accurate maneuvering of a helicopter solely by reference to instruments.

(2) IFR navigation by the use of the VOR and ADF systems, including compliance with air traffic instructions and procedures.

(3) Instrument approaches to published minimums using the VOR, ADF, and ILS systems (instruction in the use of the ADF and ILS may be received in an instrument ground trainer, and instruction in the use of the ILS glide slope may be received in an airborne ILS simulator).

(4) Cross-country flying under simulated or actual IFR conditions, on Federal airways or as routed by ATC, including one flight or at least 100 nautical miles, including VOR, ADF, and ILS approaches at different airports.

(5) Simulated IFR emergencies, including equipment malfunctions, missed approach procedures, and deviations to unplanned alternates.

(e) **Flight experience.** An applicant for an instrument rating must have at least the following flight time as a pilot:

(1) A total of 200 hours of pilot flight time, including 100 hours as pilot in command, of which 50 hours are cross-country in the category of aircraft for which an instrument rating is sought.

(2) 40 hours of simulated or actual instrument time, of which not more than 20 hours may be instrument instruction by an authorized instructor in an instrument ground trainer acceptable to the Administrator.

(3) 15 hours of instrument flight instruction by an authorized flight instructor, including at least 5 hours in an airplane or a helicopter, as appropriate.

(f) **Written test.** An applicant for an instrument rating must pass a written test appropriate to the instrument rating sought on the subjects in which ground instruction is required by paragraph (b) of this section.

(g) **Practical test.** An applicant for an instrument rating must pass a flight test in an airplane or a helicopter, as appropriate. The test must include instrument flight procedures selected by the inspector or examiner conducting the test to determine the applicant's ability to perform competently the IFR operations on which instruction is required by paragraph (c) or (d) of this section.

61.67 CATEGORY II PILOT AUTHORIZATION REQUIREMENTS.

(a) **General.** An applicant for a Category II pilot authorization must hold—

(1) A pilot certificate with an instrument rating or an airline transport pilot certificate; and

(2) A type rating for the airplane type if the authorization is requested for a large airplane or a small turbojet airplane.

(b) **Experience requirements.** Except for the holder of an airline transport pilot certificate, an applicant for a Category II authorization must have at least—

(1) 50 hours of night flight time under VFR conditions as pilot in command;

(2) 75 hours of instrument time under actual or simulated conditions that may include 25 hours in a synthetic trainer; and

(3) 250 hours of cross-country flight time as pilot in command. Night flight and instrument flight time used to meet the requirements of paragraphs (b) (1) and (2) of this section may also be used to meet the requirements of paragraph (b)(3) of this section.

(c) **Practical test required.** (1) The practical test must be passed by—

(i) An applicant for issue or renewal of an authorization; and

(ii) An applicant for the addition of another type airplane to his authorization.

(2) To be eligible for the practical test an applicant must meet the requirements of paragraph (a) of this section and, if he has not passed a practical test since the beginning of the twelfth month before the test, he must meet the following recent experience requirements:

(i) The requirements of 61.57(e).

(ii) At least six ILS approaches since the beginning of the sixth month before the test. These approaches must be under actual or simulated instrument flight conditions down to the minimum landing altitude for the ILS approach in the type airplane in which the flight test is to be conducted. However, the approaches need not be conducted down to the decision heights authorized for Category II operations. At least three of these approaches must have been conducted manually, without the use of an approach coupler.

The flight time acquired in meeting the requirements of paragraph (c)(2)(ii) of this section may be used to meet the requirements of paragraph (c)(2)(i) of this section.

(d) **Practice test procedures.** The practical test consists of two phases:

(1) **Phase I—oral operational test.** The applicant must demonstrate his knowledge of the following:

(i) Required landing distance.

(ii) Recognition of the decision height.

(iii) Missed approach procedures and techniques utilizing computed or fixed attitude guidance displays.

(iv) RVR, its use and limitations.

(v) Use of visual clues, their availability or limitations, and altitudes at which they are normally discernible at reduced RVR readings.

(vi) Procedures and techniques related to transition from nonvisual to visual flights during a final approach under reduced RVR.

(vii) Effects of vertical and horizontal wind shear.

(viii) Characteristics and limitations of the ILS and runway lighting system.

(ix) Characteristics and limitations of the flight director system, auto approach coupler (including split axis type if equipped), auto throttle system (if equipped), and other required Category II equipment.

(x) Assigned duties of the second in command during Category II approaches.

(xi) Instrument and equipment failure warning systems.

(2) **Phase II—flight test.** The flight test must be taken in an airplane that meets the requirements of Part 91 of this chapter for Category II operations. The test consists of at least two ILS approaches to 100 feet including at least one landing and missed approach. All approaches must be made with the approved flight control guidance system. However, if an approved automatic approach coupler is installed, at least one approach must be made manually. In the case of a multiengine airplane that has performance capability to execute a missed approach with an engine out, the missed approach must be executed with one engine set in idle or zero thrust position before reaching the middle marker. The required flight maneuvers must be performed solely by reference to instruments and in coordination with a second in command who holds a class rating and, in the case of a large airplane or a small turbojet airplane, a type rating for that airplane.

61.69 GLIDER TOWING: EXPERIENCE AND INSTRUCTION REQUIREMENTS.

No person may act as pilot in command of an aircraft towing a glider unless he meets the following requirements:

(a) He holds a current pilot certificate (other than a student pilot certificate) issued under this Part.

(b) He has an endorsement in his pilot log book from a person authorized to give flight instruction in gliders, certifying that he has received ground and flight instruction in gliders and is familiar with the techniques and procedures essential to the safe towing of gliders, including airspeed limitations, emergency procedures, signals used, and maximum angles of bank.

(c) He has made and entered in his pilot logbook—

(1) At least three flights as sole manipulator of the controls of an

aircraft towing a glider (while accompanied by a pilot who has met the requirements of this section), and made and logged at least 10 flights as pilot in command of an aircraft towing a glider; or

(2) At least three flights as sole manipulator of the controls of an aircraft simulating glider towing flight procedures (while accompanied by a pilot who meets the requirements of this section) and at least three flights as pilot or observer in a glider being towed by an aircraft.

However, any person who, before May 17, 1967, made, and entered in his pilot logbook, 10 or more flights as pilot in command of an aircraft towing a glider in accordance with a certificate of waiver need not comply with paragraphs (c)(1) and (2) of this section.

(d) If he holds only a private pilot certificate he must have had, and entered in his pilot logbook at least—

(1) 100 hours of pilot flight time in powered aircraft; or

(2) 200 total hours of pilot flight time in powered or other aircraft.

(e) Within the preceding 12 months he has—

(1) Made at least three actual or simulated glider tows while accompanied by a qualified pilot who meets the requirements of this section; or

(2) Made at least three flights as pilot in command of a glider towed by an aircraft.

61.71 GRADUATES OF CERTIFICATED FLYING SCHOOLS: SPECIAL RULES.

(a) A graduate of a flying school that is certified under Part 141 of this chapter is considered to meet the applicable aeronautical experience requirements of this part if he presents an appropriate graduation certificate within 60 days after the date he is graduated. However, if he applies for a flight test for an instrument rating he must hold a commercial pilot certificate, or hold a private pilot certificate and meet the requirements of 61.65(e)(1) and 61.123 (except paragraphs (d) and (e) thereof). In addition, if he applies for a flight instructor certificate he must hold a commercial pilot certificate.

(b) An applicant for a certificate or rating under this Part is considered to meet the aeronautical knowledge or skill requirements, or both, applicable to that certificate or rating, if he applies within 90 days after graduation from an appropriate course given by a flying school that is certificated under Part 141 of this chapter and is authorized to test applicants on aeronautical knowledge or skill, or both. However, until January 1, 1977, a graduate of a flying school certificated and operated under the provisions of 141.29 of this chapter, is considered to meet the requirements of this Part, and may be tested under the requirements of Part 61 that were in effect prior to November 1, 1973.

61.73 MILITARY PILOTS OR FORMER MILITARY PILOTS: SPECIAL RULES.

(a) **General.** A rated military pilot or former rated military pilot who applies for a private or commercial pilot certificate, or an aircraft or instrument rating, is entitled to that certificate with appropriate ratings or to the addition of a rating on the pilot certificate he holds, if he meets the applicable requirements of this section. This section does not apply to a military pilot or former military pilot who has been removed from flying status for lack of proficiency or because of disciplinary action involving aircraft operations.

(b) **Military pilots on active flying status within 12 months.** A rated military pilot or former rated military pilot who has been on active flying status within the 12 months before he applies must pass a written test on the parts of this chapter relating to pilot privileges and limitations, air traffic and general operating rules, and accident reporting rules. In addition, he must present documents showing that he meets the requirements of paragraph (d) of this section for at least one aircraft rating, and that he is, or was at any time since the beginning of the twelfth month before the month in which he applies—

(1) A rated military pilot on active flying status in an armed force of the United States; or

(2) A rated military pilot of an armed force of a foreign contracting State to the Convention on International Civil Aviation, assigned to pilot duties (other than flight training) with an armed force of the United States who holds, at the time he applies, a current civil pilot license issued by that foreign State authorizing at last the privileges of the pilot certificate he seeks.

(c) **Military pilots not on active flying status within previous 12 months.** A rated military pilot or former military pilot who has not been on active flying status within the 12 months before he applies must pass the appropriate written and flight tests prescribed in this Part for the certificate or rating he seeks. In addition, he must show that he holds an FAA medical certificate appropriate to the pilot certificate he seeks and present documents showing that he was, before the beginning of the twelfth month before the month in which he applies, a rated military pilot as prescribed by either paragraph (b) (1) or (2) of this section.

(d) **Aircraft ratings: Other than airplane category and type.** An applicant for a category, class, or type rating (other than airplane category and type rating) to be added on the pilot certificate he holds, or for which he has applied, is issued that rating if he presents documentary evidence showing one of the following:

(1) That he has passed an official United States military checkout as pilot in command of aircraft of the category, class, or type for which he seeks a rating since the beginning of the twelfth month before the month in which he applies.

(2) That he has had at least 10 hours of flight time serving as pilot in command of aircraft of the category, class, or type for which he seeks a rating since the beginning of the twelfth month before the month in which he applies and previously has had an official United States military checkout as pilot in command of that aircraft.

(3) That he has met the requirements of paragraph (b) (1) or (2) of this section, has had an official United States military checkout in the category of aircraft for which he seeks a rating, and that he passes an FAA flight test appropriate to that category and the class or type rating he seeks. To be eligible for that flight test, he must have a written statement from an authorized flight instructor, made not more than 60 days before he applies

for the flight test, certifying that he is competent to pass the test.

A type rating is issued only for aircraft types that the Administraor has certificated for civil operations. Any rating placed on an airline transport pilot certificate is limited to commercial pilot privileges.

(e) **Airplane category and type ratings.** (1) An applicant for a commercial pilot certificate with an airplane category rating, or an applicant for the addition of an airplane category rating on his commercial pilot certificate, must hold an airplane instrument rating, or his certificate is endorsed with the following limitation: "not valid for the carriage of passengers or property for hire in airplanes on cross-country flights of more than 50 nautical miles, or at night."

(2) An applicant for a private or commercial pilot certificate with an airplane type rating, or for the addition of an airplane type rating on his private or commercial pilot certificate who holds an instrument rating (airplane), must present documentary evidence showing that he has demonstrated instrument competency in the type of airplane for which the type rating is sought, or his certificate is endorsed with the following limitation: "VFR only."

(f) **Instrument rating.** An applicant for an airplane instrument rating or a helicopter instrument rating to be added on the pilot certificate he holds, or for which he has applied, is entitled to that rating if he has, within the 12 months preceding the month in which he applies, satisfactorily accomplished an instrument flight check of a U.S. Armed Force in an aircraft of the category for which he seeks the instrument rating and is authorized to conduct IFR flights on Federal airways. A helicopter instrument rating added on an airline transport pilot certificate is limited to commercial pilot privileges.

(g) **Evidentiary documents.** The following documents are satisfactory evidence for the purposes indicated:

(1) To show that the applicant is a member of the armed forces, an official identification card issued to the applicant by an Armed Force may be used.

(2) To show the applicant's discharge or release from an Armed Force, or his former membership therein, an original or a copy of a certificate of discharge or release may be used.

(3) To show current or previous status as a rated military pilot on flying status with a U.S. Armed Force, one of the following may be used:

(i) An official U.S. Armed Force order to flight duty as a military pilot.

(ii) An official U.S. Armed Force form or logbook showing military pilot status.

(iii) An official order showing that the applicant graduated from a U.S. military pilot school and is rated as a military pilot.

(4) To show flight time in military aircraft as a member of a U.S. Armed Force, an appropriate U.S. Armed Force form or summary of it, or a certified United States military logbook may be used.

(5) To show pilot-in-command status, an official U.S. Armed Force record of a military checkout as pilot in command, may be used.

(6) To show instrument pilot qualification, a current instrument card issued by a U.S. Armed Force, or an official record of the satisfactory completion of an instrument flight check within the 12 months preceding the month of the application may be used. However, a Tactical (Pink) instrument card issued by the U.S. Army is not acceptable.

61.75 PILOT CERTIFICATE ISSUED ON BASIS OF A FOREIGN PILOT LICENSE.

(a) **Purpose.** The holder of a current private, commercial, senior commercial, or airline transport pilot license issued by a foreign contracting State to the Convention on International Civil Aviation may apply for a pilot certificate under this section authorizing him to act as a pilot of a civil aircraft of U.S. registry.

(b) **Certificate issued.** A pilot certificate is issued to an applicant under this section, specifying the number and State of issuance of the foreign pilot license on which it is based. An applicant who holds a foreign private pilot license is issued a private pilot certificate, and an applicant who holds a foreign commercial, senior commercial, or airline transport pilot license is issued a commercial pilot certificate, if—

(1) He meets the requirements of this section;

(2) His foreign pilot license does not contain an endorsement that he has not met all of the standards of ICAO for that license; and

(3) He does not hold a U.S. pilot certificate of private pilot grade or higher.

(c) **Limitation on licenses used as basis for U.S. certificate.** Only one foreign pilot license may be used as a basis for issuing a pilot certificate under this section.

(d) **Aircraft ratings issued.** Aircraft ratings listed on the applicant's foreign pilot license, in addition to any issued after testing under the provisions of this Part, are placed on the applicant's pilot certificate.

(e) **Instrument rating issued.** An instrument rating is issued to an applicant if—

(1) His foreign pilot license authorizes instrument privileges; and

(2) Within 24 months preceding the month in which he makes application for a certificate, he passed a test on the instrument flight rules in Subpart B of Part 91 of this chapter, including the related procedures for the operation of the aircraft under instrument flight rules.

(f) **Medical standards and certification.** An applicant must submit evidence that he currently meets the medical standards for the foreign pilot license on which the application for a certificate under this section is based. A current medical certificate issued under Part 67 of this chapter is accepted as evidence that the applicant meets those standards. However, a medical certificate issued under Part 67 of this chapter is not evidence that the applicant meets those standards outside the United States, unless the State that issued the applicant's foreign pilot license also accepts that medical certificate as evidence of meeting the medical standards for his foreign pilot license.

(g) **Limitations placed on pilot certificate.** (1) If the applicant cannot read, speak, and understand the English language, the Administrator places any limitation on the certificate that he considers necessary for safety.

(2) A certificate issued under this section is not valid for agricultural aircraft operations, or the operation of an aircraft in which persons or property are carried for compensation or hire. This limitation is also placed on the certificate.

(h) **Operating privileges and limitations.** The holder of a pilot certificate issued under this section may act as a pilot of a civil aircraft of U.S. registry in accordance with the pilot privileges authorized by the foreign pilot license on which that certificate is based, subject to the limitations of this Part and any additional limitations placed on his certificate by the Administrator. He is subject to these limitations while he is acting as a pilot of the aircraft within or outside the United States. However, he may not act as pilot in command, or in any other capacity as a required pilot flight crewmember, of a civil aircraft of U.S. registry that is carrying persons or property for compensation or hire.

(i) **Flight instructor certificate.** A pilot certificate issued under this section does not satisfy any of the requirements of this Part for the issuance of a flight instructor certificate.

Subpart C—Student Pilots

61.81 APPLICABILITY.

This subpart prescribes the requirements for the issuance of student pilot certificates, the conditions under which those certificates are necessary and the general operating rules for the holders of those certificates.

61.83 ELIGIBILITY REQUIREMENTS: GENERAL.

To be eligible for a student pilot certificate, a person must—

(a) Be at least 16 years of age, or at least 14 years of age for a student pilot certificate limited to the operation of a glider or free balloon;

(b) Be able to read, speak, and understand the English language, or have such operating limitations placed on his pilot certificate as are necessary for the safe operation of aircraft, to be removed when he shows that he can read, speak, and understand the English language; and

(c) Hold at least a current third-class medical certificate issued under Part 67 of this chapter, or, in the case of glider or free balloon operations, certify that he has no known medical defect that makes him unable to pilot a glider or a free balloon.

61.85 APPLICATION.

An application for a student pilot certificate is made on a form and in a manner provided by the Administrator and is submitted to—

(a) A designated aviation medical examiner when applying for an FAA medical certificate; or

(b) An FAA operations inspector or designated pilot examiner, accompanied by a current FAA medical certificate, or in the case of an application for a glider or free balloon pilot certificate it may be accompanied by a certification by the applicant that he has no known medical defect that makes him unable to pilot a glider or free balloon.

61.87 REQUIREMENTS FOR SOLO FLIGHT.

(a) **General.** A student pilot may not operate an aircraft in solo flight until he has complied with the requirements of this section. As used in this subpart the term solo flight means that flight time during which a student pilot is the sole occupant of the aircraft, or that flight time during which he acts as pilot in command of an airship requiring more than one flight crewmember.

(b) **Aeronautical knowledge.** He must have demonstrated to an authorized instructor that he is familiar with the flight rules of Part 91 of this chapter which are pertinent to student solo flights.

(c) **Flight proficiency training.** He must have received ground and flight instruction in at least the following procedures and operations:

(1) **In airplanes.** (i) Flight preparation procedures, including preflight inspection and powerplant operation;

(ii) Ground maneuvering and runups;

(iii) Straight and level flight, climbs, turns, and descents;

(iv) Flight at minimum controllable airspeeds, and stall recognition and recovery;

(v) Normal takeoffs and landings;

(vi) Airport traffic patterns, including collision avoidance precautions and wake turbulence; and

(vii) Emergencies, including elementary emergency landings. Instruction must be given by a flight instructor who is authorized to give instruction in airplanes.

(2) **In rotorcraft.** (i) Flight preparation procedures, including preflight inspections and powerplant operation;

(ii) Ground handling and runups;

(iii) Hovering turns and air taxi (helicopter only);

(iv)) Straight and level flight, turns, climbs, and descents;

(v) Maneuvering by ground references, airport traffic patterns including collision avoidance precautions;

(vi) Normal takeoffs and landings; and

(vii) Emergencies, including autorotational descents.

Instruction must be given by a flight instructor who is authorized to give instruction in helicopters or gyroplanes, as appropriate.

(3) **In single-place gyroplanes.** (i) Flight preparation procedures, including preflight inspection and powerplant operation;

(ii) Ground handling and runups; and

(iii) At least three successful flights in a gyroplane towed from the ground under the observation of the instructor involved.

Instruction must be given by a flight instructor who is authorized to give instruction in airplanes or rotorcraft.

(4) **In gliders.** (i) Flight preparation procedures, including preflight inspections, towline rigging, signals, and release procedures;

(ii) Aero tows or ground tows;

(iii) Straight glides, turns, and spirals;

(iv) Flight at minimum controllable airspeeds, and stall recognition and recoveries;

(v) Traffic patterns, including collision avoidance precautions; and

(vi) Normal landings.

Instruction must be given by a flight instructor who is authorized to give instruction in gliders.

(5) **In airships.** (i) Flight preparation procedures, including preflight inspection and powerplant operation;

(ii) Rigging, ballasting, controlling pressure in the ballonets, and superheating;

(iii) Takeoffs and ascents;

(iv) Straight and level flights, climbs, turns, and descents; and

(v) Landings with positive and with negative static balance.

Instruction must be given by an authorized flight instructor or the holder of a commercial pilot certificate with a lighter-than-air category and airship class rating.

(6) **In free balloons.** (i) Flight preparation procedures, including preflight operations;

(ii) Operations of hot air or gas source, ballast, valves, and rip panels, as appropriate;

(iii) Liftoffs and climbs; and

(iv) Descents, landings, and emergency use of rip panel (may be simulated).

Instruction may be given by an authorized flight instructor or the holder of a commercial pilot certificate with a lighter-than-air category and free balloon class rating.

(d) **Flight instructor endorsements.** A student pilot may not operate an aircraft in solo flight unless his student pilot certificate is endorsed, and unless within the preceding 90 days his pilot logbook has been endorsed, by an authorized flight instructor who—

(1) Has given him instruction in the make and model of aircraft in which the solo flight is made;

(2) Finds that he has met the requirements of this section; and

(3) Finds that he is competent to make a safe solo flight in that aircraft.

61.89 GENERAL LIMITATIONS.

(a) A student pilot may not act as pilot in command of an aircraft—

(1) That is carrying a passenger;

(2) That is carrying property for compensation or hire;

(3) For compensation or hire;

(4) In furtherance of a business; or

(5) On an international flight, except that a student pilot may make solo training flights from Haines, Gustavus, or Juneau, Alaska, to White Horse, Yukon, Canada, and return, over the province of British Columbia.

(b) A student may not act as a required pilot flight crewmember on any aircraft for which more than one pilot is required, except when receiving flight instruction from an authorized flight instructor on board an airship and no person other than a required flight crewmember is carried on the aircraft.

61.91 AIRCRAFT LIMITATIONS: PILOT IN COMMAND.

A student pilot may not serve as pilot in command of any airship requiring more than one flight crewmember unless he has met the pertinent requirements prescribed in 61.87.

61.93 CROSS-COUNTRY FLIGHT REQUIREMENTS.

(a) **General.** A student pilot may not operate an aircraft in a solo cross-country flight, nor may he, except in an emergency, make a solo flight landing at any point other than the airport of takeoff, until he meets the requirements prescribed in this section. However, an authorized flight instructor may allow a student pilot to practice solo landings and takeoffs at another airport within 25 nautical miles from the airport at which the student pilot receives instruction if he finds that the student pilot is competent to make those landings and takeoffs. As used in this section the term cross-country flight means a flight beyond a radius of 25 nautical miles from the point of takeoff.

(b) **Flight training.** A student pilot must receive instruction from an authorized instructor in at least the following flight operations pertinent to the aircraft to be operated in a solo cross-country flight:

(1) For solo cross-country in airplanes—

(i) The use of aeronautical charts, pilotage, and elementary dead reckoning using the magnetic compass;

(ii) The use of radio for VFR navigation, and for two-way communication;

(iii) Control of an airplane by reference to flight instruments; takeoffs and landings;

(iv) Short field and soft field procedures, and crosswind takeoffs and landings;

(v) Recognition of critical weather situations, estimating visibility while in flight, and the procurement and use of aeronautical weather reports and forecasts; and

(vi) Cross-country emergency procedures.

(2) For solo cross-country in rotorcraft—

(i) The use of aeronautical charts and the magnetic compass for pilotage and for elementary dead reckoning;

(ii) The recognition of critical weather situations, estimating visibility while in flight, and the procurement and use of aeronautical weather reports and forecasts; and

(iii) Radio communications; and

(iv) Cross-country emergenices.

(3) For solo cross-country in gliders—

(i) The recognition of critical weather situations and conditions favorable for soaring flight, and the procurement and use of aeronautical weather reports and forecasts;

(ii) The use of aeronautical charts and the magnetic compass for pilotage; and

(iii) Cross-country emergency procedures.

(4) For student cross-country in airships—

(i) The use of aeronautical charts and the magnetic compass for pilotage and dead reckoning, and the use of radio for navigation and two-way communications;

(ii) The control of an airship solely by reference to flight instruments;

(iii) The control of gas pressures, with regard to superheating and altitude changes;

(iv) The recognition of critical weather situations, and the procurement and use of aeronautical weather reports and forecasts; and

(v) Cross-country emergency procedures.

(5) For solo cross-country in free balloons—

(i) The use of aeronautical charts and the magnetic compass for pilotage;

(ii) The recognition of critical weather situations, and the procurement and use of aeronautical weather reports and forecasts; and

(iii) Cross-country emergency procedures.

(c) **Flight instructor endorsements.** A student pilot must have the following endorsements from an authorized flight instructor:

(1) An endorsement on his student pilot certificate stating that he has received instruction in solo cross-country flying and the applicable training requirements of this section, and is competent to make cross-country solo flights in the category of aircraft involved.

(2) An endorsement in his pilot logbook that the instructor has reviewed the preflight planning and preparation for each solo cross-country flight, and he is prepared to make the flight safely under the known circumstances and the conditions listed by the instructor in the logbook. The instructor may also endorse the logbook for repeated solo cross-country flights under stipulated conditions over a course not more than 50 nautical miles from the point of departure if he has given the student flight instruction in both directions over the route, including takeoffs and landings at the airports to be used.

Subpart D—Private Pilots

61.101 APPLICABILITY.

This subpart prescribes the requirements for the issuance of private pilot certificates and ratings, the conditions under which those certificates and ratings are necessary, and the general operating rules for the holders of those certificates and ratings.

61.103 ELIGIBILITY REQUIREMENTS: GENERAL

To be eligible for a private pilot certificate, a person must—

(a) Be at least 17 years of age, except that a private pilot certificate with a free balloon or a glider rating only may be issued to a qualified applicant who is at least 16 years of age;

(b) Be able to read, speak, and understand the English language, or have such operating limitations placed on his pilot certificate as are necessary for the safe operation of aircraft, to be removed when he shows that he can read, speak, and understand the English language;

(c) Hold at least a current third-class medical certificate issued under Part

67 of this chapter, or, in the case of a glider or free balloon rating, certify that he has no known medical defect that makes him unable to pilot a glider or free balloon, as appropriate;

(d) Pass a written test on the subject areas on which instruction or home study is required by 61.105;

(e) Pass an oral and flight test on procedures and maneuvers selected by an FAA inspector or examiner to determine the applicant's competency in the flight operations on which instruction is required by the flight proficiency provisions of 61.107; and

(f) Comply with the sections of this Part that apply to the rating he seeks.

61.105 AERONAUTICAL KNOWLEDGE.

An applicant for a private pilot certificate must have logged ground instruction from an authorized instructor, or must present evidence showing that he has satisfactorily completed a course of instruction or home study in at least the following areas of aeronautical knowledge appropriate to the category of aircraft for which a rating is sought.

(a) **Airplanes.** (1) The Federal Aviation Regulations applicable to private pilot privileges, limitations, and flight operations, accident reporting requirements of the National Transporatation Safety Board, and the use of the "Airman's Information Manual" and the FAA Advisory Circulars;

(2) VFR navigation, using pilotage, dead reckoning, and radio aids;

(3) The recognition of critical weather situations from the ground and in flight and the procurement and use of aeronautical weather reports and forecasts; and

(4) The safe and efficient operation of airplanes, including high density airport operations, collision avoidance precautions, and radio communication procedures.

(b) **Rotorcraft.** (1) The accident reporting requirements of the National Transportation Safety Board and the Federal Aviation Regulations applicable to private pilot privileges, limitations, and helicopter or gyroplane operations, as appropriate;

(2) The use of aeronautical charts and the magnetic compass for pilotage, and elementary dead reckoning, and the use of radio aids;

(3) Recognition of critical weather situations from the ground and in flight, and the procurement and use of aeronautical weather reports and forecasts; and

(4) The safe and efficient operation of helicopters or gyroplanes, as appropriate, including high density airport operations.

(c) **Gliders.** (1) The accident reporting requirements of the National Transportation Safety Board and the Federal Aviation Regulations applicable to glider pilot privileges, limitations, and flight operations;

(2) Glider navigation, including the use of aeronautical charts and the magnetic compass;

(3) Recognition of weather situations of concern to the glider pilot, and the procurement and use of aeronautical weather reports and forecasts; and

(4) The safe and efficient operation of gliders, including ground and aero tow procedures, signals, and safety precautions.

(d) **Airships.** (1) The Federal Aviation Regulations applicable to private lighter-than-air pilot privileges, limitations, and airship flight operations;

(2) Airship navigation, including pilotage, dead reckoning, and the use of radio aids;

(3) The recognition of weather conditions of concern to the airship pilot, and the procurement and use of aeronautical weather reports and forecasts; and

(4) Airship operations, including free ballooning, the effects of super-heating, and positive and negative lift.

(e) **Free balloons.** (1) The Federal Aviation Regulations applicable to private free balloon pilot privileges, limitations, and flight operations;

(2) The use of aeronautical charts and the magnetic compass for free balloon navigation;

(3) The recognition of weather conditions of concern to the free balloon pilot, and the procurement and use of aeronautical weather reports and forecasts appropriate to free balloon operations; and

(4) Operating principles and procedures of free balloons, including gas and hot air inflation systems.

61.107 FLIGHT PROFICIENCY.

The applicant for a private pilot certificate must have logged instruction from an authorized flight instructor in at least the following pilot operations. In addition, his logbook must contain an endorsement by an authorized flight instructor who has found him competent to perform each of those operations safely as a private pilot.

(a) **In airplanes.** (1) Preflight operations, including weight and balance determination, line inspection, and airplane servicing;

(2) Airport and traffic pattern operations, including operations at controlled airports, radio communications, and collision avoidance precautions;

(3) Flight maneuvering by reference to ground objects;

(4) Flight at critically slow airspeeds, and the recognition of and recovery from imminent and full stalls entered from straight flight and from turns;

(5) Normal and crosswind takeoffs and landings;

(6) Control and maneuvering an airplane solely by reference to instruments, including descents and climbs using radio aids or radar directives;

(7) Cross-country flying, using pilotage, dead reckoning, and radio aids, including one 2-hour flight;

(8) Maximum performance takeoffs and landings;

(9) Night flying, including takeoffs, landings, and VFR navigation; and

(10) Emergency operations, including simulated aircraft and equipment malfunctions.

(b) **In helicopters.** (1) Preflight operations, including the line inspection and servicing of helicopters;

(2) Hovering, air taxiing, and maneuvering by ground references;

(3) Airport and traffic pattern operations, including collision avoidance precautions;

(4) Cross-country flight operations;

(5) High altitude takeoffs and roll-on landings, and rapid decelerations; and

(6) Emergency operations, including autorotative descents.

(c) **In gyroplanes.** (1) Preflight operations, including the line inspection and servicing of gyroplanes;

(2) Flight maneuvering by ground references;

(3) Maneuvering at critically slow airspeeds, and the recognition of and recovery from high rates of descent at low airspeeds;

(4) Airport and traffic pattern operations, including collision avoidance precautions and radio communication procedures;

(5) Cross-country flying by pilotage, dead reckoning, and the use of radio aids; and

(6) Emergency procedures, including maximum performance takeoffs and landings.

(d) **In gliders.** (1) Preflight operations, including line inspection;

(2) Ground (auto or winch) tow or aero tow (the applicant's certificate is limited to the kind of tow selected);

(3) Precision maneuvering, including steep turns and spirals in both directions;

(4) The correct use of critical sailplane performance speeds;

(5) Flight at critically slow airspeeds, and the recognition of and recovery from imminent and full stalls entered from straight and from turning flight; and

(6) Accuracy approaches and landings with the nose of the glider stopping short of and within 200 feet of a line or mark.

(e) **In airships.** (1) Ground handling, mooring, rigging, and preflight operations;

(2) Takeoffs and landings with static lift, and with negative and positive lift, and the use of two-way radio;

(3) Straight and level flight, climbs, turns, and descents;

(4) Precision flight maneuvering;

(5) Navigation, using pilotage, dead reckoning, and radio aids; and

(6) Simulated emergencies, including equipment malfunction, the valving of gas, and the loss of power on one engine.

(f) **In free balloons.** (1) Rigging and mooring;

(2) Operation of burner, if airborne heater used;

(3) Ascents and descents;

(4) Landing; and

(5) Emergencies, including the use of the ripcord (may be simulated).

61.109 AIRPLANE RATING: AERONAUTICAL EXPERIENCE.

An applicant for a private pilot certificate with an airplane rating must have had at least a total of 40 hours of flight instruction and solo flight time which must include the following:

(a) Twenty hours of flight instruction from an authorized flight instructor, including at least—

(1) Three hours of cross country:

(2) Three hours at night, including 10 takeoffs and landings for applicants seeking night flying privileges; and

(3) Three hours in airplanes in preparation for the private pilot flight test within 60 days prior to that test.

An applicant who does not meet the night flying requirements in paragraph (a)(2) of this section is issued a private pilot certificate bearing the limitation "Night flying prohibited." This limitation may be removed if the holder of the certificate shows that he has met the requirements of paragraph (a)(2) of this section.

(b) Twenty hours of solo flight time, including at least—

(1) Ten hours in airplanes;

(2) Ten hours of cross-country flights, each flight with a landing more than 50 nautical miles from the point of departure, and one with landings at three points, each of which is more than 100 nautical miles from each of the other two points; and

(3) Three solo takeoffs and landings to a full stop at an airport with an operating control tower.

61.111 CROSS-COUNTRY FLIGHTS: PILOTS BASED ON SMALL ISLANDS.

(a) An applicant who shows that he is located on an island from which the required flights cannot be accomplished without flying over water more than 10 nautical miles from the nearest shoreline need not comply with paragraph (b)(2) of 61.109. However, if other airports that permit civil operations are available to which a flight may be made without flying over water more than 10 nautical miles from the nearest shoreline, he must show that he has completed two round trip solo flights between those two airports that are farthest apart, including a landing at each airport on both flights.

(b) The pilot certificate issued to a person under paragraph (a) of this section contains an endorsement with the following limitation which may be subsequently amended to include another island if the applicant complies with paragraph (a) of this section with respect to that island:

Passenger carrying prohibited on flights more than 10 nautical miles from (appropriate island).

(c) If an applicant for a private pilot certificate under paragraph (a) of this section does not have at least 3 hours of solo cross-country flight time, including a round trip flight to an airport at least 50 nautical miles from the place of departure with at least two full stop landings at different points along the route, his pilot certificate is also endorsed, as follows:

Holder does not meet the cross-country flight requirements of ICAO.

(d) The holder of a private pilot certificate with an endorsement described in paragraph (b) or (c) of this section, is entitled to a removal of the endorsement, if he presents satisfactory evidence to an FAA inspector or designated pilot examiner that he has complied with the applicable solo cross-country flight requirements and has passed a practical test on cross-country flying.

61.113 ROTORCRAFT RATING: AERONAUTICAL EXPERIENCE.

An applicant for a private pilot certificate with a rotorcraft category rating must have at least the following aeronautical experience:

(a) For a helicopter rating an applicant must have at least a total of 40 hours of flight instruction and solo flight time in aircraft with at least 15 hours of solo flight time in helicopters, which must include—

(1) A takeoff and landing at an airport which serves both airplanes and helicopters;

(2) A flight with a landing at a point other than an airport; and

(3) Three hours of cross-country flying, including one flight with landings at three or more points, each of which must be more than 25 nautical miles from each of the other two points.

(b) For a gyroplane rating an applicant must have at least a total of 40 hours of flight instruction and solo flight time in aircraft with at least 10 hours of solo flight time in a gyroplane, which must include—

(1) Flights with takeoffs and landings at paved and unpaved airports; and

(2) Three hours of cross-country flying, including a flight with landings at three or more points, each of which must be more than 25 nautical miles from each of the other two points.

61.115 GLIDER RATING: AERONAUTICAL EXPERIENCE.

An applicant for a private pilot certificate with a glider rating must have logged at least one of the following:

(a) Seventy solo glider flights, including 20 flights during which 360° turns were made.

(b) Seven hours of solo flight in gliders, including 35 glider flights launched by ground tows, or 20 glider flights launched by aero tows.

(c) Forty hours of flight time in gliders and single-engine airplanes, including 10 solo glider flights during which 360° turns were made.

61.117 LIGHTER-THAN-AIR RATING: AERONAUTICAL EXPERIENCE.

An applicant for a private pilot certificate with a lighter-than-air category rating must have at least the aeronautical experience prescribed in paragraph (a) and (b) of this section, appropriate to the rating sought.

(a) **Airships.** A total of 50 hours of flight time as pilot with at least 25 hours in airships, which must include 5 hours of solo flight time in airships, or time performing the functions of pilot in command of an airship for which more than one pilot is required.

(b) **Free balloons.** (1) If a gas balloon or a hot air balloon with an airborne heater is used, a total of 10 hours in free balloons with at least six flights under the supervision of a person holding a commercial pilot certificate with a free balloon rating. These flights must include—

(i) Two flights, each of at least 1 hour's duration, if a gas balloon is used, or of 30 minutes' duration, if a hot air balloon with an airborne heater is used;

(ii) One ascent under control to 5,000 feet above the point of takeoff, if a gas balloon is used, or 3,000 feet above the point of takeoff, if a hot air balloon with an airborne heater is used; and

(iii) One solo flight in a free balloon.

(2) If a hot air balloon without an airborne heater is used, six flights in a free balloon under the supervision of a commercial balloon pilot, including at least one solo flight.

61.118 PRIVATE PILOT PRIVILEGES AND LIMITATIONS: PILOT IN COMMAND.

Except as provided in paragraphs (a) through (d) of this section, a private pilot may not act as pilot in command of an aircraft that is carrying passengers or property for compensation or hire; nor may he, for compensation or hire, act as pilot in command of an aircraft.

(a) A private pilot may, for compensation or hire, act as pilot in command of an aircraft in connection with any business or employment if the flight is only incidental to that business or employment and the aircraft does not carry passengers or property for compensation or hire.

(b) A private pilot may share the operating expenses of a flight with his passengers.

(c) A private pilot who is an aircraft salesman and who has at least 200 hours of logged flight time may demonstrate an aircraft in flight to a prospective buyer.

(d) A private pilot may act as pilot in command of an aircraft used in a passenger-carrying airlift sponsored by a charitable organization, and for which the passengers make a donation to the organization, if—

(1) The sponsor of the airlift notifies the FAA General Aviation District Office having jurisdiction over the area concerned, at least 7 days before the flight, and furnishes any essential information that the office requests;

(2) The flight is conducted from a public airport adequate for the aircraft used, or from another airport that has been approved for the operation by an FAA inspector;

(3) He has logged at least 200 hours of flight time;

(4) No aerobatic or formation flights are conducted;

(5) Each aircraft used is certified in the standard category and complies with the 100-hour inspection requirement of 91.169 of this chapter; and

(6) The flight is made under VFR during the day.

For the purpose of paragraph (d) of this section, a "charitable organization" means an organization listed in Publication No. 78 of the Department of the Treasury called the "Cumulative List of Organizations described in section 170(c) of the Internal Revenue Code of 1954," as amended from time to time by published supplemental lists.

61.119 FREE BALLOON RATINGS: LIMITATIONS.

(a) If the applicant for a free balloon rating takes his flight test in a hot air balloon with an airborne heater, his pilot certificate contains an endorsement restricting the exercise of the privilege of that rating to hot air balloons with airborne heaters. The restriction may be deleted when the holder of the certificate obtains the pilot experience required for a rating on a gas balloon.

(b) If the applicant for a free balloon rating takes his flight test in a hot air balloon without an airborne heater, his pilot certificate contains an endorsement restricting the exercise of the privileges of that rating to hot air balloons without airborne heaters. The restriction may be deleted when the holder of the certificate obtains the pilot experience and passes the tests required for a rating on a free balloon with an airborne heater or a gas balloon.

61.120 PRIVATE PILOT PRIVILEGES AND LIMITATIONS: SECOND IN COMMAND OF AIRCRAFT REQUIRING MORE THAN ONE REQUIRED PILOT.

Except as provided in paragraphs (a) through (d) of 61.118 a private pilot may not, for compensation or hire, act as second in command of an aircraft that is type certificated for more than one required pilot, nor may he act as second in command of such an aircraft that is carrying passengers or property for compensation or hire.

Subpart E – Commercial Pilots

61.121 APPLICABILITY.

This subpart prescribes the requirements for the issuance of commercial pilot certificates and ratings, the conditions under which those certificates and ratings are necessary, and the limitations upon those certificates and ratings.

61.123 ELIGIBILITY REQUIREMENTS: GENERAL.

To be eligible for a commercial pilot certificate, a person must—
  (a) Be at least 18 years of age;
  (b) Be able to read, speak, and understand the English language, or have such operating limitations placed on his pilot certificate as are necessary for safety, to be removed when he shows that he can read, speak and understand the English language;
  (c) Hold at least a valid second-class medical certificate issued under Part 67 of this chapter, or, in the case of a glider or free balloon rating, certify that he has no known medical deficiency that makes him unable to pilot a glider or a free balloon, as appropriate;
  (d) Pass a written examination appropriate to the aircraft rating sought on the subjects in which ground instruction is required by 61.125;
  (e) Pass an oral and flight test, appropriate to the rating he seeks, covering items selected by the inspector or examiner from those on which training is required by 61.127; and
  (f) Comply with the provisions of this subpart which apply to the rating he seeks.

61.125 AERONAUTICAL KNOWLEDGE.

An applicant for a commercial pilot certificate must have logged ground instruction from an authorized instructor, or must present evidence showing that he has satisfactorily completed a course of instruction or home study, in at least the following areas of aeronautical knowledge appropriate to the category of aircraft for which a rating is sought.
  (a) **Airplanes.** (1) The regulations of this chapter governing the operations, privileges, and limitations of a commercial pilot, and the accident reporting requirements of the National Transportation Board;
    (2) Basic aerodynamics and the principles of flight which apply to airplanes; and

(3) Airplane operations, including the use of flaps, retractable landing gears, controllable propellers, high altitude operation with and without pressurization, loading and balance computations, and the significance and use of airplane performance speeds.

(b) **Rotorcraft.** (1) The regulations of this chapter which apply to the operations, privileges, and limitations of a commercial rotorcraft pilot, and the accident reporting requirements of the National Transportation Safety Board;

(2) Meteorology, including the characteristics of air masses and fronts, elements of weather forecasting, and the procurement and use of aeronautical weather reports and forecasts;

(3) The use of aeronautical charts and the magnetic compass for pilotage and dead reckoning, and the use of radio aids for VFR navigation; and

(4) The safe and efficient operation of helicopters or gyroplanes, as appropriate to the rating sought.

(c) **Gliders.** (1) The regulations of this chapter pertinent to commercial glider pilot operations, privileges, and limitations and the accident reporting requirements of the National Transportation Safety Board;

(2) Glider navigation, including the use of aeronautical charts and the magnetic compass, and radio orientation;

(3) The recognition of weather situations of concern to the glider pilot from the ground and in flight, and the procurement and use of aeronautical weather reports and forecasts; and

(4) The safe and efficient operation of gliders, including ground and aero tow procedures, signals, critical sailplane performance speeds, and safety precautions.

(d) **Airships.** (1) The regulations of this chapter pertinent to airship operations, VFR and IFR, including the privileges and limitations of a commercial airship pilot;

(2) Airship navigation, including pilotage, dead reckoning, and the use of radio aids for VFR and IFR navigation, and IFR approaches;

(3) The use and limitations of the required flight instruments;

(4) ATC procedures for VFR and IFR operations, and the use of IFR charts and approach plates;

(5) Meteorology, including the characteristics of air masses and fronts, and the procurement and use of aeronautical weather reports and forecasts;

(6) Airship ground and flight instruction procedures; and

(7) Airship operating procedures and emergency operations, including free ballooning procedures.

(e) **Free balloons.** (1) The regulations of this chapter pertinent to commercial free balloon piloting privileges, limitations, and flight operations;

(2) The use of aeronautical charts and the magnetic compass for free balloon navigation;

(3) The recognition of weather conditions significant to free balloon flight operations, and the procurement and use of aeronautical weather reports and forecasts appropriate to free ballooning;

(4) Free balloon flight and ground instruction procedures; and

(5) Operating principles and procedures for free balloons, including emergency procedures such as crowd control and protection, high wind and water landings, and operations in proximity to buildings and power lines.

61.127 FLIGHT PROFICIENCY.

The applicant for a commercial pilot certificate must have logged instruction from an authorized flight instructor in at least the following pilot operations. In addition, his logbook must contain an endorsement by an authorized flight instructor who has given him the instruction certifying that he has found the applicant prepared to perform each of those operations competently as a commercial pilot.

(a) **Airplanes.** (1) Preflight duties, including load and balance determination, line inspection, and aircraft servicing;

(2) Flight at critically slow airspeeds, recognition of imminent stalls, and recovery from stalls with and without power;

(3) Normal and crosswind takeoffs and landings, using precision approaches, flaps, power as appropriate, and specified approach speeds;

(4) Maximum performance takeoffs and landings, climbs, and descents;

(5) Operation of an airplane equipped with a retractable landing gear, flaps, and controllable propeller(s), including normal and emergency operations; and

(6) Emergency procedures, such as coping with power loss or equipment malfunctions, fire in flight, collision avoidance precautions, and engine-out procedures if a multiengine airplane is used.

(b) **Helicopters.** (1) Preflight duties, including line inspection and helicopter servicing;

(2) Straight and level flight, climbs, turns, and descents;

(3) Air taxiing, hovering, and maneuvering by ground references;

(4) Normal and crosswind takeoffs and landings;

(5) Rapid descent with power and recovery;

(6) Airport and traffic pattern operations, including collision avoidance precautions and radio communications;

(7) Cross-country flight operations; and

(8) Emergency operations, including landing on slopes, high altitude takeoffs and roll-on landings, operations on confined areas and pinnacles, autorotational descents, partial power failures, and rapid decelerations.

(c) **Gyroplanes.** (1) Preflight operations, including line inspection and gyroplane servicing;

(2) Straight and level flight, turns, climbs, and descents;

(3) Flight maneuvering by ground references;

(4) Maneuvering at critically slow airspeeds, and the recognition of and recovery from high rates of descent at slow airspeeds;

(5) Normal and crosswind takeoffs and landings;

(6) Airport and traffic pattern operations, including collision avoidance precautions and radio communications;

(7) Cross-country flight operations; and

(8) Emergency procedures, such as power failures, equipment malfunctions, maximum performance takeoffs and landings and simulated

liftoffs at low airspeed and high angles of attack.

(d) **Gliders.** (1) Preflight duties, including glider assembly and preflight inspection;

(2) Glider launches by ground (auto or winch) or by aero tows (the applicant's certificate is limited to the kind of tow selected);

(3) Precision maneuvering, including straight glides, turns to headings, steep turns, and spirals in both directions;

(4) The correct use of sailplane performance speeds, flight at critically slow airspeeds, and the recognition of and recovery from stalls entered from straight flight and from turns; and

(5) Accuracy approaches and landings, with the nose of the glider coming to rest short of and within 100 feet of a line or mark.

(e) **Airships.** (1) Ground handling, mooring, and preflight operations;

(2) Straight and level flight, turns, climbs, and descents, under VFR and simulated IFR conditions;

(3) Takeoffs and landings with positive and with negative static lift;

(4) Turns and figure eights;

(5) Precision turns to headings under simulated IFR conditions;

(6) Preparing and filing IFR flight plans, and complying with IFR clearances;

(7) IFR radio navigation and instrument approach procedures;

(8) Cross-country flight operations, using pilotage, dead reckoning, and radio aids; and

(9) Emergency operations, including engine-out operations, free ballooning an airship and ripcord procedures (may be simulated).

(f) **Free balloons.** (1) Inflating, rigging, and mooring a free balloon;

(2) Ground and flight crew briefing;

(3) Ascents;

(4) Descents;

(5) Landings;

(6) Operation of airborne heater, if balloon is so equipped; and

(7) Emergency operations, including the use of the ripcord (may be simulated), and recovery from a terminal velocity descent if a balloon with an airborne heater is used.

61.129 AIRPLANE RATING: AERONAUTICAL EXPERIENCE.

(a) **General.** An applicant for a commercial pilot certificate with an airplane rating must hold a private pilot certificate with an airplane rating. If he does not hold that certificate and rating he must meet the flight experience requirements for a private pilot certificate and airplane rating and pass the applicable written and practical test prescribed in Subpart D of this Part. In addition, the applicant must hold an instrument rating (airplane), or the commercial pilot certificate that is issued is endorsed with a limitation prohibiting the carriage of passengers for hire in airplanes on crosscountry flights of more than 50 nautical miles, or at night.

(b) **Flight time as pilot.** An applicant for a commercial pilot certificate with an airplane rating must have a total of at least 250 hours of flight time as pilot, which may include not more than 50 hours of instruction from an authorized instructor in a ground trainer acceptable to the Administrator.

The total flight time as pilot must include—

(1) 100 hours in powered aircraft, including at least—

(i) 50 hours in airplanes; and

(ii) 10 hours of flight instruction and practice given by an authorized flight instructor in an airplane having a retractable landing gear, flaps, and a controllable pitch propeller; and

(2) 50 hours of flight instruction given by an authorized flight instructor, including—

(i) 10 hours of instrument instruction, of which at least 5 hours must be in flight in airplanes; and

(ii) 10 hours of instruction in preparation for the commercial pilot flight test; and

(3) 100 hours of pilot in command time, including at least—

(i) 50 hours in airplanes; and

(ii) 50 hours of cross-country flights, each flight with a landing at a point more than 50 nautical miles from the point of departure, including a flight with landings at three points each of which is more than 200 nautical miles from the other two points, except that those flights conducted in Hawaii may be made with landings at points which are 100 nautical miles apart; and

(iii) 5 hours of night flying including at least 10 takeoffs and landings as sole manipulator of the controls.

61.131 ROTORCRAFT RATINGS: AERONAUTICAL EXPERIENCE.

(a) **Helicopter.** An applicant for a commercial pilot certificate with a helicopter rating must have a total of at least 150 hours of flight time as pilot, including—

(1) 100 hours in powered aircraft and at least 50 hours in helicopters;

(2) 100 hours of pilot in command time, including a cross-country flight with landings at three points, each of which is more than 50 nautical miles from each of the other points;

(3) 40 hours of flight instruction from an authorized flight instructor, including 15 hours in helicopters; and

(4) 10 hours as pilot in command in helicopters, including—

(i) Five takeoffs and landings at night; and

(ii) Takeoffs and landings at three different airports which serve both airplanes and helicopters; and

(iii) Takeoffs and landings at three points other than airports.

(b) **Gyroplanes.** An applicant for a commercial pilot certificate with a gyroplane rating must have a total of at least 200 hours of flight time as pilot, including—

(1) 100 hours in powered aircraft;

(2) 100 hours as pilot in command, including a cross-country flight with landings at three points, each of which is more than 50 nautical miles from each of the other two points;

(3) 75 hours as pilot in command in gyroplanes, including—

(i) Flights with takeoffs and landings at three different paved airports and three unpaved airports; and

(ii) Three flights with takeoffs and landings at an airport with an operating control tower; and

(4) Twenty hours of flight instruction in gyroplanes, including 5 hours in preparation for the commercial pilot flight test.

61.133 GLIDER RATING: AERONAUTICAL EXPERIENCE.

An applicant for a commercial pilot certificate with a glider rating must meet either of the following aeronautical experience requirements:

(a) A total of at least 25 hours of pilot time in aircraft, including 20 hours in gliders, and a total of 100 glider flights as pilot in command, including 25 flights during which 360° turns were made; or

(b) A total of 200 hours of pilot time in heavier-than-air aircraft, including 20 glider flights as pilot in command during which 360° turns were made.

61.135 AIRSHIP RATING: AERONAUTICAL EXPERIENCE.

An applicant for a commercial pilot certificate with an airship rating must have a total of at least 200 hours of flight time as pilot, including—

(a) Fifty hours of flight time as pilot in airships;

(b) 30 hours of flight time performing the duties of pilot in command in airships, including—

(1) 10 hours of cross-country flight; and

(2) 10 hours of night flight; and

(c) 40 hours of instrument time, of which at least 20 hours must be in flight with 10 hours of that flight time in airships.

61.137 FREE BALLOON RATING: AERONAUTICAL EXPERIENCE.

An applicant for a commercial pilot certificate with a free balloon rating must have the following flight time as pilot:

(a) If a gas balloon or a hot air balloon with an airborne heater is used, a total of at least 35 hours of flight time as pilot including—

(1) 20 hours in free balloons; and

(2) 10 flights in free balloons, including—

(i) Six flights under the supervision of a commercial free balloon pilot;

(ii) Two solo flights;

(iii) Two flights of at least 2 hours duration if a gas balloon is used, or at least 1 hour duration if a hot air balloon with an airborne heater is used; and

(iv) One ascent under control to more than 10,000 feet above the takeoff point if a gas balloon is used or 5,000 feet above the takeoff point if a hot air balloon with an airborne heater is used.

(b) If a hot air balloon without an airborne heater is used, 10 flights in free balloons including—

(1) Six flights under the supervision of a commercial free balloon pilot; and

(2) Two solo flights.

61.139 COMMERCIAL PILOT PRIVILEGES AND LIMITATIONS: GENERAL.

The holder of a commercial pilot certificate may:

(a) Act as pilot in command of an aircraft carrying persons or property for compensation or hire;

(b) Act as pilot in command of an aircraft for compensation or hire; and

(c) Give flight instruction in an airship if he holds a lighter-than-air category and an airship class rating, or in a free balloon if he holds a free balloon class rating.

61.141 AIRSHIP AND FREE BALLOON RATINGS: LIMITATIONS.

(a) If the applicant for a free balloon class rating takes his flight test in a hot air balloon without an airborne heater, his pilot certificate contains an endorsement restricting the exercise of the privileges of that rating to hot air balloons without airborne heaters. The restriction may be deleted when the holder of the certificate obtains the pilot experience and passes the test required for a rating on a free balloon with an airborne heater or a gas balloon.

(b) If the applicant for a free balloon class rating takes his flight test in a hot air balloon with an airborne heater, his pilot certificate contains an endorsement restricting the exercise of the privileges of that rating to hot air balloons with airborne heaters. The restriction may be deleted when the holder of the certificate obtains the pilot experience required for a rating on a gas balloon.

Subpart F—Airline Transport Pilots

61.151 ELIGIBILITY REQUIREMENTS: GENERAL.

To be eligible for an airline transport pilot certificate, a person must—

(a) Be at least 23 years of age;

(b) Be of good moral character;

(c) Be able to read, write, and understand the English language and speak it without accent or impediment of speech that would interfere with two-way radio conversation;

(d) Be a high school graduate, or its equivalent in the Administrator's opinion, based on the applicant's general experience and aeronautical experience, knowledge, and skill;

(e) Have a first-class medical certificate issued under Part 67 of this chapter within the 6 months before the date he applies; and

(f) Comply with the sections of this Part that apply to the rating he seeks.

61.153 AIRPLANE RATING: AERONAUTICAL KNOWLEDGE.

An applicant for an airline transport pilot certificate with an airplane rating must, after meeting the requirements of 61.151 (except paragraph (a) thereof) and 61.155, pass a written test on—

(a) The sections of this Part relating to airline transport pilots and Part 121, Subpart C of Part 65, and §§ 91.1 through 91.9 and Subpart B of Part 91 of this chapter, and so much of Parts 21 and 25 of this chapter as relate to the operations of air carrier aircraft;

(b) The fundamentals of air navigation and use of formulas, instruments, and other navigational aids, both in aircraft and on the ground, that are necessary for navigating aircraft by instruments;

(c) The general system of weather collection and dissemination;

(d) Weather maps, weather forecasting, and weather sequence abbreviations, symbols, and nomenclature;

(e) Elementary meteorology, including knowledge of cyclones as associated with fronts;

(f) Cloud forms;

(g) "National Weather Service Federal Meteorological Handbook No. 1," as amended;

(h) Weather conditions, including icing conditions and upper-air winds, that affect aeronautical activities;

(i) Air navigation facilities used on Federal airways, including rotating beacons, course lights, radio ranges, and radio marker beacons;

(j) Information from airplane weather observations and meteorological data reported from observations made by pilots on air carrier flights;

(k) The influence of terrain on meteorological conditions and developments, and their relation to air carrier flight operations;

(l) Radio communication procedure in aircraft operations; and

(m) Basic principles of loading and weight distribution and their effect on flight characteristics.

61.155 AIRPLANE RATING: AERONAUTICAL EXPERIENCE.

(a) An applicant for an airline transport pilot certificate with an airplane rating must hold a commercial pilot certificate or a foreign airline transport pilot or commercial pilot license without limitations, issued by a member state of ICAO, or he must be a pilot in an Armed Force of the United States whose military experience qualifies him for a commercial pilot certificate under 61.73 of this Part.

(b) An applicant must have had—

(1) At least 250 hours of flight time as pilot in command of an airplane, or as copilot of an airplane performing the duties and functions of a pilot in command under the supervision of a pilot in command, or any combination thereof, at least 100 hours of which were cross-country time and 25 hours of which were night flight time; and

(2) At least 1500 hours of flight time as a pilot including at least—

(i) 500 hours of cross-country flight time;

(ii) 100 hours of night flight time; and

(iii) 75 hours of actual or simulated instrument time, at least 50 hours of which were in actual flight.

Flight time used to meet the requirements of subparagraph (1) of this paragraph may also be used to meet the requirements of subparagraph (2) of this paragraph. Also, an applicant who has made at least 20 night takeoffs and landings to a full stop may substitute one additional night takeoff and landing to a full stop for each hour of night flight time required by subparagraph (2)(ii) of this paragraph. However, not more than 25 hours of night flight time may be credited in this manner.

(c) If an applicant with less than 150 hours of pilot-in-command time otherwise meets the requirements of paragraph (b)(1) of this section, his certificate will be endorsed "Holder does not meet the pilot-in-command flight experience requirements of ICAO", as prescribed by Article 39 of the "Convention on International Civil Aviation." Whenever he presents satisfactory written evidence that he has accumulated the 150 hours of pilot-in-command time, he is entitled to a new certificate without the endorsement.

(d) A commercial pilot may credit toward the 1500 hours total flight time requirement of paragraph (b)(2) of this section the following flight time in operations conducted under Part 121 of this chapter:

(1) All second-in-command time acquired in airplanes required to have more than one pilot by their approved Aircraft Flight Manuals or airworthiness certificates; and

(2) Flight engineer time acquired in airplanes required to have a flight engineer by their approved Aircraft Flight Manuals, while participating at the same time in an approved pilot training program approved under Part 121 of this chapter.

However, the applicant may not credit under subparagraph (2) of this paragraph more than 1 hour for each 3 hours of flight engineer flight time so acquired, nor more than a total of 500 hours.

(e) If an applicant who credits second-in-command or flight engineer time under paragraph (d) of this section toward the 1500 hours total flight time requirement of paragraph (b)(2) of this section—

(1) Does not have at least 1200 hours of flight time as a pilot including no more than 50 percent of his second-in-command time and none of his flight engineer time; but

(2) Otherwise meets the requirements of paragraph (b)(2) of this section, his certificate will be endorsed "Holder does not meet the pilot flight experience requirements of ICAO," as prescribed by Article 39 of the "Convention on International Civil Aviation." Whenever he presents satisfactory evidence that he has accumulated 1200 hours of flight time as a pilot including no more than 50 percent of his second-in-command time and none of his flight engineer time, he is entitled to a new certificate without the endorsement.

61.157 AIRPLANE RATING: AERONAUTICAL SKILL.

(a) An applicant for an airline transport pilot certificate with a single-engine or multiengine class rating or an additional type rating must pass a practical test that includes the items set forth in Appendix A of this Part. The FAA inspector or designated examiner may modify any required maneuver where necessary for the reasonable and safe operation of the airplane being used and, unless specifically prohibited in Appendix A, may combine any required maneuvers and may permit their performance in any convenient sequence.

(b) Whenever an applicant for an airline transport pilot certificate does not already have an instrument rating he shall, as part of the oral part of the practical test, comply with 61.65(g), and, as part of the flight part, perform each additional maneuver required by 61.65(g) that is appropriate to the airplane type and not required in Appendix A of this Part.

(c) Unless the Administrator requires certain or all maneuvers to be performed, the person giving a flight test for an airline transport pilot certificate or additional airplane class or type rating may, in his discretion, waive any of the maneuvers for which a specific waiver authority is contained in Appendix A of this part if a pilot being checked—

(1) Is employed as a pilot by a Part 121 certificate holder; and

(2) Within the preceding 6 calendar months, has successfully completed that certificate holder's approved training program for the airplane type involved.

(d) The items specified in paragraph (a) of this section may be performed in the airplane simulator or other training device specified in Appendix A to this part for the particular item if—

(1) The airplane simulator or other training device meets the requirements of 121.407 of this chapter; and

(2) In the case of items preceded by an asterisk (*) in Appendix A, the applicant has successfully completed the training set forth in 121.424(d) of this chapter. However, the FAA inspector or designated examiner may require Items II(d), V(f), or V(g) of Appendix A to this Part to be performed in the airplane if he determines that action is necessary to determine the applicant's competence with respect to that maneuver.

61.159 ROTORCRAFT RATING: AERONAUTICAL KNOWLEDGE.

(a) An applicant for an airline transport pilot certificate with a rotorcraft category and a gyroplane class rating, or a rotorcraft category and a helicopter class rating limited to VFR only must pass a written test on—

(1) So much of this chapter as relates to air carrier rotorcraft operations;

(2) Rotorcraft design, components, systems and performance limitations;

(3) Basic principles of loading and weight distribution and their effect on rotorcraft flight characteristics;

(4) Air traffic control systems and procedures relating to rotorcraft;

(5) Procedures for operating rotorcraft in potentially hazardous meteorological conditions; and

(6) Flight theory as applicable to rotorcraft.

(b) In addition to the requirements of paragraph (a) of this section, an applicant for an airline transport pilot certificate with a rotorcraft category and helicopter class rating not limited to VFR must pass a written test on the items listed under paragraphs (b) through (m) of 61.153.

61.161 ROTORCRAFT RATING: AERONAUTICAL EXPERIENCE.

(a) An applicant for an airline transport pilot certificate with a rotorcraft rating must hold a commercial pilot certificate, or its equivalent as determined by the Administrator.

(b) In addition, such an applicant must have had at least 1200 hours of flight time as a pilot within the 8 years before the date he applies including at least—

(1) 5 hours in rotorcraft within the 60 days before that date;

(2) 500 hours of cross-country flight time;

(3) 100 hours at night, including at least 15 hours in rotorcraft; and

(4) 200 hours in rotorcraft, including at least 75 hours as pilot in command or as second in command performing the duties and functions of a pilot in command under the supervision of a pilot in command, or any combination thereof.

(c) In addition to the requirements of paragraphs (a) and (b) of this section, an applicant for an airline transport pilot certificate with a rotorcraft category and a helicopter class rating not limited to VFR must have at least 75 hours of instrument time under actual or simulated instrument conditions of which at least 50 hours were completed in flight with at least 25 hours in helicopters as pilot in command, or as second in command performing the duties and functions of a pilot in command under the supervision of a pilot in command, or any combination thereof.

61.163   ROTORCRAFT RATING: AERONAUTICAL SKILL.

(a) An applicant for an airline transport pilot certificate with a rotorcraft category and a gyroplane class rating or a rotorcraft category and helicopter class rating limited to VFR must show his ability to satisfactorily pilot rotorcraft by performing at least the following:

(1) Normal takeoffs and landings, crosswind landings, climbs and climbing turns, steep turns, maneuvering at minimum speed, rapid descent, and quick stops;

(2) Simulated emergency procedures, including failure of an engine or other component or system, fire, ditching, evacuation, and operating emergency equipment;

(3) Approach and landing with simulated one engine inoperative in multiengine helicopters or in autorotation in single engine helicopters; and

(4) Any other maneuvers considered necessary to show his ability.

(b) An applicant for an airline transport pilot certificate with a rotorcraft category and a helicopter class rating not limited to VFR must perform the maneuvers set forth in this paragraph and if he has not obtained a certificate under paragraph (a) of this section, must perform any additional maneuvers required in that paragraph:

(1) Equipment test (oral). (2) Preflight check. (3) Taxiing, or sailing and docking. (4) Runups. (5) Takeoffs. (6) Climbs and climbing turns (not required if applicant holds a helicopter instrument rating and a certificate under paragraph (a) of this section). (7) Maneuvers at slow speed. (8) Airport traffic pattern. (9) Accuracy approaches and spot landings (single-engine rating only). (10) Landing technique. (11) Crosswind takeoff. (12) Traffic control procedure. (13) Steep turns. (14) Timed turns (not required if applicant holds a helicopter instrument rating). (15) Recovery from unusual attitudes. (16) Use of radio equipment. (17) Orientation. (18) Beam bracketing. (19) Cone (station) identification. (20) Instrument approach procedures. (21) Missed approach procedures. (22) Use of directional radio. (23) Rapid descent. (24) Engine(s)-out procedure (multiengine rating only). (25) Maneuvering with engine(s)-out (multiengine rating only). (26) Maneuvering for landing at weather minimums. (27) Takeoff and landing with simulated engine(s) failure (multiengine rating only). (28) Emergencies. (29) Smoothness and coordination. (30) Judgment.

The maneuvers described in subparagraphs (6), (7), (13), (14), (15), (17), (18), (19), (20), (21), (22), (23), and (25) of this paragraph must be performed solely by reference to instruments. The FAA flight inspector conducting the test may require the maneuvers described in subparagraphs (6), (14), and (15) to be performed on a partial panel.

(c) The holder of an airline transport pilot certificate with a rotorcraft category and helicopter class rating who applies for an additional helicopter type rating must show his ability to satisfactorily pilot the type helicopter for which he seeks a rating by performing the maneuvers listed in paragraph (a) of this section for a rating limited to VFR only, or the maneuvers listed in paragraph (b) of this section for a rating not limited to VFR.

(d) Any maneuver required by this section may be modified by the examining inspector as necessary for the reasonable and safe operations of the rotorcraft being used.

61.165   ADDITIONAL CATEGORY RATINGS.

(a) **Rotorcraft category and gyroplane class rating or helicopter class rating limited to VFR only.** The holder of an airline transport pilot certificate (airplane rating) who applies for a rotorcraft category and gyroplane class rating, or a rotorcraft category and helicopter class rating limited to VFR only must meet the applicable requirements of 61.159 and 61.163 and—

(1) Have at least 100 hours, including at least 15 hours at night, of rotorcraft flight time as pilot in command or as second in command performing the duties and functions of a pilot in command under the supervision of a pilot in command who holds an airline transport pilot certificate with an appropriate rotorcraft rating, or any combination thereof; or

(2) Complete a training program conducted by a certificated air carrier or other approved agency requiring at least 75 hours of rotorcraft flight time as pilot in command, second in command, or as flight instruction from an appropriately rated FAA certificated flight instructor or an airline transport pilot, or any combination thereof, including at least 15 hours of night flight time.

(b) **Rotorcraft category and helicopter class rating not limited to VFR.** The holder of an airline transport pilot certificate (airplane rating) who applies for a rotorcraft category and helicopter class rating not limited to VFR must meet the applicable requirements of 61.159, 61.161, and 61.163.

(c) **Airplane rating.** The holder of an airline transport pilot certificate (rotorcraft rating) who applies for an airplane rating, must comply with 61.153 through 61.157 and—

(1) Have at least 100 hours, including at least 15 hours at night, of airplane flight time as pilot in command or as second in command performing the duties and functions of a pilot in command under the supervision of a pilot in command who holds an airline transport pilot certificate with an appropriate airplane rating, or any combination thereof; or

(2) Complete a training program conducted by a certificated air carrier or other approved agency requiring at least 75 hours of airplane flight time as pilot in command, second in command, or as flight instruction from an

appropriately rated FAA certificated flight instructor or an airline transport pilot, or any combination thereof, including at least 15 hours of night flight time.

61.167 TESTS.

(a) Each applicant for an airline transport pilot certificate must pass each practical and theoretical test to the satisfaction of the Administrator. The minimum passing grade in each subject is 70 percent. Each flight maneuver is graded separately. Other tests are graded as a whole.

(b) Information collected incidentally to such a test shall be treated as a confidential matter by the persons giving the test and by employees of the FAA.

61.169 INSTRUCTION IN AIR TRANSPORTATION SERVICE.

An airline transport pilot may instruct other pilots in air transportation service in aircraft of the category, class, and type for which he is rated. However, he may not instruct for more than 8 hours in one day nor more than 36 hours in any 7-day period. He may instruct under this section only in aircraft with functioning dual controls. Unless he has a flight instructor certificate, an airline transport pilot may instruct only as provided in this section.

61.171 GENERAL PRIVILEGES AND LIMITATIONS.

An airline transport pilot has the privileges of a commercial pilot with an instrument rating. The holder of a commercial pilot certificate who qualifies for an airline transport pilot certificate retains the ratings on his commercial pilot certificate, but he may exercise only the privileges of a commercial pilot with respect to them.

Subpart G—Flight Instructors

61.181 APPLICABILITY.

This subpart prescribes the requirements for the issuance of flight instructor certificates and ratings, the conditions under which those certificates and ratings are necessary, and the limitations upon these certificates and ratings.

61.183 ELIGIBILITY REQUIREMENTS: GENERAL.

To be eligible for a flight instructor certificate a person must—
  (a) Be at least 18 years of age;
  (b) Read, write, and converse fluently in English;
  (c) Hold—
    (1) A commercial or airline transport pilot certificate with an aircraft rating appropriate to the flight instructor rating sought, and
    (2) An instrument rating, if the person is applying for an airplane or an instrument instructor rating;
  (d) Pass a written test on the subjects in which ground instruction is required by 61.185; and
  (e) Pass an oral and flight test on those items in which instruction is required by 61.187.

61.185 AERONAUTICAL KNOWLEDGE.

(a) Present evidence showing that he has satisfactorily completed a course of instruction in at least the following subjects:

(1) The learning process.
(2) Elements of effective teaching.
(3) Student evaluation, quizzing, and testing.
(4) Course development.
(5) Lesson planning.
(6) Classroom instructing techniques.

(b) Have logged ground instruction from an authorized ground or flight instructor in all of the subjects in which ground instruction is required for a private and commercial pilot certificate, and for an instrument rating, if an airplane or instrument instructor rating is sought.

61.187 FLIGHT PROFICIENCY.

(a) An applicant for a flight instructor certificate must have received flight instruction, appropriate to the instructor rating sought, in the subjects listed in this paragraph by a person authorized in paragraph (b) of this section. In addition, his logbook must contain an endorsement by the person who has given him the instruction certifying that he has found the applicant competent to pass a practical test on the following subjects:

(1) Preparation and conduct of lesson plans for students with varying backgrounds and levels of experience and ability.
(2) The evaluation of student flight performance.
(3) Effective preflight and postflight instruction.
(4) Flight instructor responsibilities and certifying procedures.
(5) Effective analysis and correction of common student pilot flight errors.
(6) Performance and analysis of standard flight training procedures and maneuvers appropriate to the flight instructor rating sought.

(b) The flight instruction required by paragraph (a) of this section must be given by a person who has held a flight instructor certificate during the 24 months immediately preceding the date the instruction is given, who meets the general requirements for a flight instructor certificate prescribed in 61.183, and who has given at least 200 hours of flight instruction, or 80 hours in the case of glider instruction, as a certificated flight instructor.

61.189 FLIGHT INSTRUCTOR RECORDS.

(a) Each certificated flight instructor shall sign the logbook of each person to whom he has given flight or ground instruction and specify in that book the amount of the time and the date on which it was given. In addition, he shall maintain a record in his flight instructor logbook, or in a separate document containing the following:

(1) The name of each person whose logbook or student pilot certificate he has endorsed for solo flight privileges. The record must include the type and date of each endorsement.
(2) The name of each person for whom he has signed a certification for a written, flight, or practical test, including the kind of test, date of his

certification, and the result of the test.

(b) The record required by this section shall be retained by the flight instructor separately or in his logbook for at least 3 years.

61.191 ADDITIONAL FLIGHT INSTRUCTOR RATINGS.

The holder of a flight instructor certificate who applies for an additional rating on that certificate must—

(a) Hold an effective pilot certificate with ratings appropriate to the flight instructor rating sought.

(b) Have had at least 15 hours as pilot in command in the category and class of aircraft appropriate to the rating sought; and

(c) Pass the written and practical test prescribed in this subpart for the issuance of a flight instructor certificate with the rating sought.

61.193 FLIGHT INSTRUCTOR AUTHORIZATIONS.

(a) The holder of a flight instructor certificate is authorized, within the limitations of his instructor certificate and ratings, to give—

(1) In accordance with his pilot ratings, the flight instruction required by this Part for a pilot certificate or rating;

(2) Ground instruction or a home study course required by this Part for a pilot certificate and rating;

(3) Ground and flight instruction required by this subpart for a flight instructor certificate and rating, if he meets the requirements prescribed in 61.187 for the issuance of a flight instructor certificate;

(4) The flight instruction required for an initial solo or cross-country flight; and

(5) The flight review required in 61.157(a).

(b) The holder of a flight instructor certificate is authorized within the limitations of his instructor certificate to endorse—

(1) In accordance with 61.87(d)(1) and 61.93(c)(1), the pilot certificate of a student pilot he has instructed authorizing the student to conduct solo or solo cross-country flights, or act as pilot-in-command of an airship requiring more than one flight crewmember;

(2) In accordance with 61.87(d)(1), the logbook of a student pilot he has instructed authorizing single or repeated solo flights;

(3) In accordance with 61.93(c)(2), the logbook of a student pilot whose preparation and preflight planning for a solo cross-country flight he has reviewed and found adequate for a safe flight under the conditions he has listed in the logbook;

(4) The logbook of a pilot or flight instructor he has examined certifying that the pilot or flight instructor is prepared for a written or flight test required by this Part; and

(5) In accordance with 61.187, the logbook of an applicant for a flight instructor certificate certifying that he has examined the applicant and found him competent to pass the practical test required by this Part.

(c) A flight instructor with a rotorcraft and helicopter rating or an airplane single-engine rating may also endorse the pilot certificate and logbook of a student pilot he has instructed authorizing the student to conduct solo and cross-country flights in a single-place gyroplane.

61.195 FLIGHT INSTRUCTOR LIMITATIONS.

The holder of a flight instructor certificate is subject to the following limitations:

(a) **Hours of instruction.** He may not conduct more than eight hours of flight instruction in any period of 24 consecutive hours.

(b) **Ratings.** He may not conduct flight instruction in any aircraft for which he does not hold a category, class, and type rating, if appropriate, on his pilot and flight instructor certificate. However, the holder of a flight instructor certificate effective on November 1, 1973, may continue to exercise the privileges of that certificate until it expires, but not later than November 1, 1975.

(c) **Endorsement of student pilot certificate.** He may not endorse a student pilot certificate for initial solo or solo cross-country flight privileges, unless he has given that student pilot flight instruction required by this Part for the endorsement, and considers that the student is prepared to conduct the flight safely with the aircraft involved.

(d) **Logbook endorsement.** He may not endorse a student pilot's logbook for solo flight unless he has given that student flight instruction and found him prepared for solo flight in the type of aircraft involved, or for a cross-country flight, unless he has reviewed the student's flight preparation, planning, equipment, and proposed procedures and found them to be adequate for the flight proposed under existing circumstances.

(e) **Solo flights.** He may not authorize any student pilot to make a solo flight unless he possesses a valid student pilot certificate endorsed for solo in the make and model aircraft to be flown. In addition, he may not authorize any student pilot to make a solo cross-country flight unless he possesses a valid student pilot certificate endorsed for solo cross-country flight in the category of aircraft to be flown.

(f) **Instruction in multiengine airplane or helicopter.** He may not give flight instruction required for the issuance of a certificate or a category, or class rating, in a multiengine airplane or a helicopter, unless he has at least 5 hours of experience as pilot in command in the make and model of that airplane or helicopter, as the case may be.

61.197 RENEWAL OF FLIGHT INSTRUCTOR CERTIFICATES.

The holder of a flight instructor certificate may have his certificate renewed for an additional period of 24 months if he passes the practical test for a flight instructor certificate and the rating involved, or those portions of that test that the Administrator considers necessary to determine his competency as a flight instructor. His certificate may be renewed without taking the practical test if—

(a) His record of instruction shows that he is a competent flight instructor;

(b) He has a satisfactory record as a company check pilot, chief flight instructor, pilot in command of an aircraft operated under Part 121 of this chapter, or other activity involving the regular evaluation of pilots, and passes any oral test that may be necessary to determine that instructor's knowledge of current pilot training and certification requirements and standards; or

(c) He has successfully completed, within 90 days before the application for the renewal of his certificate, an approved flight instructor refresher course consisting of not less than 24 hours of ground or flight instruction, or both.

61.199 EXPIRED FLIGHT INSTRUCTOR CERTIFICATES AND RATINGS.

(a) **Flight instructor certificates.** The holder of an expired flight instructor certificate may exchange that certificate for a new certificate by passing the practical test prescribed in § 61.187.

(b) **Flight instructor ratings.** A flight instructor rating or a limited flight instructor rating on a pilot certificate is no longer valid and may not be exchanged for a similar rating or a flight instructor certificate. The holder of either of those ratings is issued a flight instructor certificate only if he passes the written and practical test prescribed in this subpart for the issue of that certificate.

61.201 CONVERSION TO NEW SYSTEM OF INSTRUCTOR RATINGS.

(a) **General.** The holder of a flight instructor certificate that does not bear any of the new class or instrument ratings listed in 61.5(c)(2), (3), or (4) for an instructor certificate, may not exercise the privileges of that certificate after November 1, 1975. Before that date he may exchange a certificate which has not expired for a flight instructor certificate with the appropriate new ratings in accordance with the provisions of this section. The holder of a flight instructor certificate with a glider rating need not convert that rating to a new class rating to exercise the privileges of that certificate and rating.

(b) **Airplane—single-engine.** An airplane—single-engine rating may be issued to the holder of an effective flight instructor certificate with an airplane rating who has passed the flight instructor practical test in a single-engine airplane, or who has given at least 20 hours of flight instruction in single-engine airplanes as a certificated flight instructor.

(c) **Airplane—multiengine.** An airplane—multiengine class rating may be issued to the holder of an effective flight instructor certificate with an airplane rating who has passed the flight instructor practical test in a multiengine airplane, or who has given at least 20 hours of flight instruction in multiengine airplanes as a certificated flight instructor.

(d) **Rotorcraft—helicopter.** A rotorcraft—helicopter class rating may be issued to the holder of an effective flight instructor certificate with a rotorcraft rating who has passed the flight instructor practical test in a helicopter, or who has given at least 20 hours of flight instruction in helicopters as a certificated flight instructor.

(e) **Rotorcraft—gyroplane.** A rotorcraft—gyroplane class rating may be issued to the holder of an effective flight instructor certificate with a rotorcraft rating who has passed the flight instructor practical test in a gyroplane, or who has given at least 20 hours of flight instruction in gyroplanes as a certificated flight instructor.

(f) **Instrument—airplane.** An instrument—airplane instructor rating may be issued to the holder of an effective flight instructor certificate with an instrument rating who has passed the instrument instructor practical test in an airplane, or who has given at least 20 hours of instrument instruction in an airplane as a certificated flight instructor.

(g) **Instrument—helicopter.** An instrument—helicopter rating may be issued to the holder of an effective flight instructor certificate with an instrument rating who has passed the instrument instructor practical test in a helicopter, or who has given at least 20 hours of instrument flight instruction in helicopters as a certificated flight instructor.

Part 67

Medical Standards and Certification

CONTENTS

SUBPART A—GENERAL

Subpart A – General

67.1 APPLICABILITY.

This subpart prescribes the medical standards for issuing medical certificates for airmen.

67.11 ISSUE.

An applicant who meets the medical standards prescribed in this Part, based on medical examination and evaluation of his history and condition is entitled to an appropriate medical certificate.

67.13 FIRST-CLASS MEDICAL CERTIFICATE.

(a) To be eligible for a first-class medical certificate, an applicant must meet the requirements of paragraphs (b) through (f) of this section.

(b) **Eye:**

(1) Distant visual acuity of 20/20 or better in each eye separately, without correction: or of at least 20/100 in each eye separately corrected to 20/20 or better with corrective lenses (glasses or contact lenses) in which case the applicant may be qualified only on the condition that he wears those corrective lenses while exercising the privileges of his airman certificate.

(2) Near vision of at least v=1.00 at 18 inches with each eye separately, with or without corrective glasses.

(3) Normal color vision.

(4) Normal fields of vision.

(5) No acute or chronic pathological condition of either eye or adenexae that might interfere with its proper function, might progress to that degree, or might be aggravated by flying.

(6) Bifoveal fixation and vergencephoria relationships sufficient to prevent a break in fusion under conditions that may reasonably occur in performing airman duties.

Tests for the factors named in subparagraph (6) of this paragraph are not required except for applicants found to have more than one prism diopter of hyperphoria, six prism diopters of esophoria, or six prism diopters of exophoria. If these values are exceeded, the Federal Air Surgeon may require the applicant to be examined by a qualified eye specialist to determine if there is bifoveal fixation and adequate vergencephoria relationship. However, if the applicant is otherwise qualified, he is entitled to a medical certificate pending the results of the examination.

(c) **Ear, nose, throat, and equilibrium:**

(1) Ability to—

(i) Hear the whispered voice at a distance of at least 20 feet with each ear separately; or

(ii) Demonstrate a hearing acuity of at least 50 percent of normal in each ear throughout the effective speech and radio range as shown by a standard audiometer.

(2) No acute or chronic disease of the middle or internal ear.

(3) No disease of the mastoid.

(4) No unhealed (unclosed) perforation of the eardrum.

(5) No disease or malformation of the nose or throat that might interfere with, or be aggravated by, flying.

(6) No disturbance in equilibrium.

(d) **Mental and neurologic—(1) Mental.** (i) No established medical history or clinical diagnosis of any of the following:

(a) A personality disorder that is severe enough to have repeatedly manifested itself by overt acts.

(b) A psychosis.

(c) Alcoholism. As used in this section, "alcoholism" means a condition in which a person's intake of alcohol is great enough to damage his physical health or personal or social functioning, or when alcohol has become a prerequisite to his normal functioning.

(d) Drug dependence. As used in this section, "drug dependence" means a condition in which a person is addicted to or dependent on drugs other than alcohol, tobacco, or ordinary caffeine-containing beverages, as evidenced by habitual use or a clear sense of need for the drug.

(ii) No other personality disorder, neurosis, or mental condition that the Federal Air Surgeon finds—

(a) Makes the applicant unable to safely perform the duties or exercise the privileges of the airman certificate that he holds or for which he is applying; or

(b) May reasonably be expected, within 2 years after the finding, to make him unable to perform those duties or exercise those privileges; and the findings are based on the case history and appropriate, qualified, medical judgment relating to the condition involved.

(2) **Neurologic.** (i) No established medical history or clinical diagnosis of either of the following:

(a) Epilepsy.

(b) A disturbance of consciousness without satisfactory medical explanation of the cause.

(ii) No other convulsive disorder, disturbance of consciousness, or neurologic condition that the Federal Air Surgeon finds—

(a) Makes the applicant unable to safely perform the duties or exercise the privileges of the airman certificate that he holds or for which he is applying; or

(b) May reasonably be expected, within 2 years after the finding, to make him unable to perform those duties or exercise those privileges; and the findings are based on the case history and appropriate, qualified, medical judgment relating to the condition involved.

(e) **Cardiovascular:**

(1) No established medical history or clinical diagnosis of—

(i) Myocardial infarction; or

(ii) Angina pectoris or other evidence of coronary heart disease that the Federal Air Surgeon finds may reasonably be expected to lead to myocardial infarction.

(2) If the applicant has passed his thirty-fifth birthday but not his fortieth, he must, on the first examination after his thirty-fifth birthday, show an absence of myocardial infarction on electrocardiographic examination.

(3) If the applicant has passed his fortieth birthday, he must annually show an absence of myocardial infarction on electrocardiographic examination.

(4) Unless the adjusted maximum readings apply, the applicant's reclining blood pressure may not be more than the maximum reading for his age group in the following table:

Age Group	Maximum readings (reclining blood pressure in mm)		Adjusted maximum readings (reclining blood pressure in mm)[1]	
	Systolic	Diastolic	Systolic	Diastolic
20–29	140	88	—	—
30–39	145	92	155	98
40–49	155	96	165	100
50 and over	160	98	170	100

[1] For an applicant at least 30 years of age whose reclining blood pressure is more than the maximum reading for his age group and whose cardiac and kidney conditions, after complete cardiovascular examination, are found to be normal.

(5) If the applicant is at least 40 years of age, he must show a degree of circulatory efficiency that is compatible with the safe operation of aircraft at high altitudes.

An electrocardiogram, made according to acceptable standards and techniques within the 90 days before an examination for a first-class certificate, is accepted at the time of the physical examination as meeting the requirements of subparagraph (2) and (3) of this paragraph.

(f) **General medical condition:**

(1) No established medical history or clinical diagnosis of diabetes mellitus that requires insulin or any other hypoglycemic drug for control.

(2) No other organic, functional, or structural disease, defect, or limitation that the Federal Air Surgeon finds—

(i) Makes the applicant unable to safely perform the duties or exercise the privileges of the airman certificate that he holds or for which he is applying; or

(ii) May reasonably be expected, within two years after the finding, to make him unable to perform those duties or exercise those privileges; and the findings are based on the case history and appropriate, qualified, medical judgment relating to the condition involved.

67.15 SECOND-CLASS MEDICAL CERTIFICATE

(a) To be eligible for a second-class medical certificate, an applicant must meet the requirements of paragraphs (b) through (f) of this section.

(b) **Eye:**

(1) Distant visual acuity of 20/20 or better in each eye separately, without correction; or of at least 20/100 in each eye separately corrected to 20/20 or better with corrective lenses (glasses or contact lenses) in which case the applicant may be qualified only on the condition that he wears corrective lenses while exercising the privileges of his airman certificate.

(2) Enough accommodation to pass a test prescribed by the Administrator based primarily on ability to read official aeronautical maps.

(3) Normal fields of vision.

(4) No pathology of the eye.

(5) Ability to distinguish aviation signal red, aviation signal green, and white.

(6) Bifoveal fixation and vergencephoria relationship sufficient to prevent a break in fusion under conditions that may reasonably occur in performing airman duties.

Tests for the factors named in subparagraph (6) of this paragraph are not required except for applicants found to have more than one prism diopter of hyperphoria, six prism diopters of esophoria, or six prism diopters of exophoria. If these values are exceeded, the Federal Air Surgeon may require the applicant to be examined by a qualified eye specialist to determine if there is bifoveal fixation and adequate vergencephoria relationship. However, if the applicant is otherwise qualified, he is entitled to a medical certificate pending the results of the examination.

(c) **Ear, nose, throat, and equilibrium:**

(1) Ability to hear the whispered voice at 8 feet with each ear separately.

(2) No acute or chronic disease of the middle or internal ear.

(3) No disease of the mastoid.

(4) No unhealed (unclosed) perforation of the eardrum.

(5) No disease or malformation of the nose or throat that might interfere with, or be aggravated by, flying.

(6) No disturbance in equilibrium.

(d) **Mental and neurologic**—(1) **Mental.** (i) No established medical history or clinical diagnosis of any of the following:

(*a*) A personality disorder that is severe enough to have repeatedly manifested itself by overt acts.

(*b*) A psychosis.

(*c*) Alcoholism. As used in this section, "alcoholism" means a condition in which a person's intake of alcohol is great enough to damage his physical health or personal or social functioning, or when alcohol has become a prerequisite to his normal functioning.

(*d*) Drug dependence: As used in this section, "drug dependence" means a condition in which a person is addicted to or dependent on drugs other than alcohol, tobacco, or ordinary caffeine-containing beverages, as evidenced by habitual use or a clear sense of need for the drug.

(ii) No other personality disorder, neurosis, or mental condition that the Federal Air Surgeon finds—

(*a*) Makes the applicant unable to safely perform the duties or exercise the privileges of the airman certificate that he holds or for which he is applying; or

(*b*) May reasonably be expected, within two years after the finding, to make him unable to perform those duties or exercise those privileges; and the findings are based on the case history and appropriate, qualified, medical judgment relating to the condition involved.

(2) **Neurologic:** (i) No established medical history or clinical diagnosis of either of the following:

(*a*) Epilepsy.

(*b*) A disturbance of consciousness without satisfactory medical explanation of the cause.

(ii) No other convulsive disorder, disturbance of consciousness, or neurologic condition that the Federal Air Surgeon finds—

(a) Makes the applicant unable to safely perform the duties or exercise the privileges of the airman certificate that he holds or for which he is applying; or

(b) May reasonably be expected, within two years after the finding, to make him unable to perform those duties or exercise those privileges; and the findings are based on the case history and appropriate, qualified, medical judgment relating to the condition involved.

(e) **Cardiovascular:**

(1) No established medical history or clinical diagnosis of—

(i) Myocardial infarction; or

(ii) Angina pectoris or other evidence of coronary heart disease that the Federal Air Surgeon finds may reasonably be expected to lead to myocardial infarction.

(f) **General medical condition:**

(1) No established medical history or clinical diagnosis of diabetes mellitus that requires insulin or any other hypoglycemic drug for control.

(2) No other organic, functional, or structural disease, defect, or limitation that the Federal Air Surgeon finds—

(i) Makes the applicant unable to safely perform the duties or exercise the privileges of the airman certificate that he holds or for which he is applying; or

(ii) May reasonably be expected, within 2 years after the finding to make him unable to perform those duties or exercise those privileges; and the findings are based on the case history and appropriate, qualified, medical judgment relating to the condition involved.

67.17 THIRD-CLASS MEDICAL CERTIFICATE.

(a) To be eligible for a third-class medical certificate, an applicant must meet the requirements of paragraphs (b) through (f) of this section.

(b) **Eye:**

(1) Distant visual acuity of 20/50 or better in each eye separately, without correction; or if the vision in either or both eyes is poorer than 20/50 and is corrected to 20/30 or better in each eye with corrective lenses (glasses or contact lenses), the applicant may be qualified on the condition that he wears those corrective lenses while exercising the privileges of his airman certificate.

(2) No serious pathology of the eye.

(3) Ability to distinguish aviation signal red, aviation signal green, and white.

(c) **Ears, nose, throat, and equilibrium:**

(1) Ability to hear the whispered voice at 3 feet.

(2) No acute or chronic disease of the internal ear.

(3) No disease or malformation of the nose or throat that might interfere with, or be aggravated by, flying.

(4) No disturbance in equilibrium.

(d) **Mental and neurologic**—(1) **Mental.** (i) No established medical history or clinical diagnosis of any of the following:

(*a*) A personality disorder that is severe enough to have repeatedly manifested itself by overt acts.

(*b*) A psychosis.

(*c*) Alcoholism: As used in this section, "alcoholism" means a condition in which a person's intake of alcohol is great enough to damage his physical health or personal or social functioning, or when alcohol has become a prerequisite to his normal functioning.

(*d*) Drug dependence: As used in this section, "drug dependence" means a condition in which a person is addicted to or dependent on drugs other than alcohol, tobacco, or ordinary caffeine-containing beverages, as evidenced by habitual use or a clear sense of need for the drug.

(ii) No other personality disorder, neurosis, or mental condition that the Federal Air Surgeon finds—

(*a*) Makes the applicant unable to safely perform the duties or exercise the privileges of the airman certificate that he holds or for which he is applying; or

(*b*) May reasonably be expected, within 2 years after the finding, to make him unable to perform those duties or exercise those privileges; and the findings are based on the case history and appropriate, qualified, medical judgment relating to the condition involved.

(2) **Neurologic.** (i) No established medical history or clinical diagnosis of either of the following:

(*a*) Epilepsy.

(*b*) A disturbance of consciousness without satisfactory medical explanation of the cause.

(ii) No other convulsive disorder, disturbance of consciousness, or neurologic condition that the Federal Air Surgeon finds—

(*a*) Makes the applicant unable to safely perform the duties or exercise the privileges of the airman certificate that he holds or for which he is applying; or

(*b*) May reasonably be expected, within 2 years after the finding, to make him unable to perform those duties or exercise those privileges; and the findings are based on the case history and appropriate, qualified, medical judgment relating to the condition involved.

(e) **Cardiovascular:**

(1) No established medical history or clinical diagnosis of—

(i) Myocardial infarction; or

(ii) Angina pectoris or other evidence of coronary heart disease that the Federal Air Surgeon finds may reasonably be expected to lead to myocardial infarction.

(f) **General medical condition:**

(1) No established medical history or clinical diagnosis of diabetes mellitus that requires insulin or any other hypoglycemic drug for control;

(2) No other organic, functional or structural disease, defect, or limitation that the Federal Air Surgeon finds—

(i) Makes the applicant unable to safely perform the duties or exercise the privileges of the airman certificate that he holds or for which he is applying; or

(ii) May reasonably be expected, within 2 years after the finding, to make him unable to perform those duties or exercise those privileges; and the findings are based on the case history and appropriate, qualified, medical judgment relating to the condition involved.

67.19 SPECIAL ISSUE: OPERATIONAL LIMITATIONS.

(a) A medical certificate of the appropriate class may be issued to an applicant who does not meet the medical standards of this Part, under the following procedures:

(1) The Federal Air Surgeon may in his discretion find that a special medical flight or practical test, or special medical evaluation, should be conducted to determine whether the applicant can perform his duties under the airman certificate he holds, or for which he is applying, in a manner that will not endanger safety in air commerce during the period the certificate would be in force. Upon such a finding, the Federal Air Surgeon authorizes the conduct of that test or evaluation. The Federal Air Surgeon may also consider the applicant's operational experience for this purpose.

(2) If the Federal Air Surgeon authorizes a procedure under subparagraph (1) of this paragraph, the applicant must show to the satisfaction of the Federal Air Surgeon, by the prescribed procedure, that he can perform those duties in the manner referred to in subparagraph (1). Upon such a showing, the Federal Air Surgeon issues to the applicant a medical certificate of the appropriate class.

(b) Any operational limitation on, or limit on the duration of, a certificate issued under this section that the Federal Air Surgeon determines is needed for safety shall be specified on the airman or medical certificate held by, or issued to, the applicant.

(c) An applicant who has taken a practical or flight test for a medical certificate under this section, and who has had a medical certificate issued to him under this section as a result of that test, need not take the test again during later physical examinations unless the Federal Air Surgeon determines that his physical deficiency has become enough more pronounced to require such an additional test.

(d), Except for air traffic control tower operators, this section does not apply to an applicant who fails to meet the requirements of 67.13 (d)(1)(i), (d)(2)(i), (e)(1), or (f)(1), 67.15 (d)(1)(i), (d)(2)(i), (e), or (f)(1), or 67.17 (d)(1)(i), (d)(2)(i), (e), or (f)(1). A medical certificate issued to an air traffic control tower operator who does not meet the requirements of any of those sections is valid only for performing air traffic control tower operator duties.

(e) The authority exercised by the Federal Air Surgeon under paragraphs (a), (b), and (c) of this section is also exercised by the Chief, Aeromedical Certification Branch, Civil Aeromedical Institute, and each Regional Flight Surgeon.

67.20 APPLICATIONS, CERTIFICATES, LOGBOOKS, REPORTS AND RECORDS: FALSIFICATION, REPRODUCTION, OR ALTERATION.

(a) No person may make or cause to be made—

(1) Any fraudulent or intentionally false statement on any application for a medical certificate under this Part;

(2) Any fraudulent or intentionally false entry in any logbook, record, or report that is required to be kept, made, or used, to show compliance with any requirement for any medical certificate under this Part;

(3) Any reproduction, for fraudulent purpose, of any medical certificate under this Part;

(4) Any alteration of any medical certificate under this Part.

(b) The commission by any person of an act prohibited under paragraph (a) of this section is a basis for suspending or revoking any airman, ground instructor, or medical certificate or rating held by that person.

Subpart B — Certification Procedures

67.21 APPLICABILITY.

This subpart prescribes the general procedures that apply to the issue of medical certificates for airmen.

67.23 MEDICAL EXAMINATIONS: WHO MAY GIVE.

(a) **First class.** Any aviation medical examiner who is specifically designated for the purpose may give the examination for the first class certificate. Any interested person may obtain a list of these aviation medical examiners, in any area, from the FAA Regional Director of the region in which the area is located.

(b) **Second class and third class.** Any aviation medical examiner may give the examination for the second or third class certificate. Any interested person may obtain a list of aviation medical examiners, in any area, from the FAA Regional Director of the region in which the area is located.

67.25 DELEGATION OF AUTHORITY.

(a) The authority of the Administrator, under section 602 of the Federal Aviation Act of 1958 (49 U.S.C. 1422), to issue or deny medical certificates is delegated to the Federal Air Surgeon, to the extent necessary to—

(1) Examine applicants for and holders of medical certificates for compliance with applicable medical standards; and

(2) Issue, renew, or deny medical certificates to applicants and holders based upon compliance or noncompliance with applicable medical standards. Subject to limitations in this chapter, the authority delegated in subparagraphs (1) and (2) of this paragraph is also delegated to aviation medical examiners and to authorized representatives of the Federad Air Surgeon within the FAA.

(b) The authority of the Administrator, under subsection 314(b) of the Federal Aviation Act of 1958 (49 U.S.C. 1355(b)), to reconsider the action of an aviation medical examiner is delegated to the Federal Air Surgeon, the Chief, Aeromedical Certification Branch, Civil Aeromedical Institute, and each Regional Flight Surgeon. Except where the applicant does not meet the standards of 67.13(d)(1)(i), (d)(2)(i), (e)(1), or (f)(1), 67.15(d)(1)(i), (d)(2)(i), (e), or (f)(1), or 67.17(d)(1)(i), (d)(2)(i), (e) or (f)(i), any action taken under this paragraph other than by the Federal Air Surgeon is subject to reconsideration by the Federal Air Surgeon. A certificate issued by an aviation medical examiner is considered to be affirmed as issued unless an FAA official named in this paragraph on his own initiative reverses that issuance within 60 days after the date of issuance. However, if within 60 days after the date of issuance that official requests the certificate holder to submit additional medical information, he may on his own initiative reverse the issuance within 60 days after he receives the requested information.

(c) The authority of the Administrator, under section 609 of the Federal Aviation Act of 1958 (49 U.S.C. 1429), to re-examine any civil airman, to the extent necessary to determine an airman's qualification to continue to hold an airman medical certificate, is delegated to the Federal Air Surgeon and his authorized representatives within the FAA.

67.27 DENIAL OF MEDICAL CERTIFICATE.

(a) Any person who is denied a medical certificate by an aviation medical examiner may, within 30 days after the date of the denial, apply in writing and in duplicate to the Federal Air Surgeon, Attention: Chief, Aeromedical Certification Brach, Civil Aeromedical Institute, Federal Aviation Administration, Post Office Box 25082, Oklahoma City, Okla., 73125, for reconsideration of that denial. If he does not apply for reconsideration during the 30 day period after the date of the denial, he is considered to have withdrawn his application for a medical certificate.

(b) The denial of a medical certificate—

(1) By an aviation medical examiner is not a denial by the Administrator under section 602 of the Federal Aviation Act of 1958 (49 U.S.C. 1422);

(2) By the Federal Air Surgeon is considered to be a denial by the Administrator under that section of the Act; and

(3) By the Chief, Aeromedical Certification Branch, Civil Aeromedical Institute, or a Regional Flight Surgeon is considered to be a denial by the Administrator under that section of the Act where the applicant does not meet the standards of 67.13(d)(1)(i), (d)(2)(i), (e)(1), or (f)(1), 67.15(d)(1)(i), (d)(2)(i), (e), or (f)(1), or 67.17(d)(1)(i), (d)(2)(i), (e), or (f)(1). Any action taken under 67.25(b) that wholly or partly reverses the issue of a medical certificate by an aviation medical examiner is the denial of a medical certificate under this paragraph (b).

(c) If the issue of a medical certificate is wholly or partly reversed upon reconsideration by the Federal Air Surgeon, the Chief, Aeromedical Certification Branch, Civil Aeromedical Institute, or a Regional Flight Surgeon, the person holding that certificate shall surrender it, upon request of the FAA.

67.29 MEDICAL CERTIFICATES BY SENIOR FLIGHT SURGEONS OF ARMED FORCES.

(a) The FAA has designated senior flight surgeons of the Armed Forces on specified military posts, stations, and facilities, as aviation medical examiners.

(b) An aviation medical examiner described in paragraph (a) of this section may give physical examinations to applicants for FAA medical certificates who are on active duty or who are, under Department of Defense medical programs, eligible for FAA medical certification as civil airmen. In addition, such an examiner may issue or deny an appropriate FAA medical certificate in accordance with the regulations of this chapter and the policies of the FAA.

(c) Any interested person may obtain a list of the military posts, stations, and facilities at which a senior flight surgeon has been designated as an aviation medical examiner, from the Surgeon General of the armed force concerned or from the Chief, Aeromedical Certification Branch, AC–130, Department of Transportation, Federal Aviation Administration, Civil Aeromedical Institute, Post Office Box 25082, Oklahoma City, Ok. 73125.

67.31 MEDICAL RECORDS.

Whenever the Administrator finds that additional medical information or history is necessary to determine whether an applicant for or the holder of a medical certificate meets the medical standards for it, he requests that person to furnish that information or authorize any clinic, hospital, doctor, or other person to release to the Administrator any available information or records concerning that history. If the applicant, or holder, refuses to provide the requested medical information or history or to authorize the release so requested, the Administrator may suspend, modify, or revoke any medical certificate that he holds or may, in the case of an applicant, refuse to issue a medical certificate to him.

Part 91
General Operating and Flight Rules
CONTENTS

SUBPART A—GENERAL

SUBPART E—OPERATING NOISE LIMITS*

Subpart A – General

91.1 APPLICABILITY.

(a) Except as provided in paragraph (b) of this section, this Part prescribes rules governing the operation of aircraft (other than moored balloons, kites, unmanned rockets, and unmanned free balloons) within the United States.

(b) Each person operating a civil aircraft of U.S. registry outside of the United States shall—

(1) When over the high seas, comply with Annex 2 (Rules of the Air) to the Convention on International Civil Aviation and with §§ 91.70(c) and 91.90 of Subpart B;

(2) When within a foreign country, comply with the regulations relating to the flight and maneuver of aircraft there in force;

(3) Except for §§ 91.15(b), 91.17, 91.38, and 91.43, comply with Subparts A, C, and D of this Part so far as they are not inconsistent with applicable regulations of the foreign country where the aircraft is operated or Annex 2 to the Convention on International Civil Aviation; and

(4) When over the North Atlantic within airspace designated as Minimum Navigation Performance Specifications airspace, comply with § 91.20.

(c) Annex 2 to the Convention on International Civil Aviation, Sixth Edition—September 1970, with amendments through Amendment 20 effective August 1976, to which reference is made in this Part is incorporated into this Part and made a part hereof as provided in 5 U.S.C. 552 and pursuant to 1 CFR Part 51. Annex 2 (including a complete historic file of changes thereto) is available for public inspection at the Rules Docket, AGC-24, Federal Aviation Administration, 800 Independence Avenue, S.E., Washington, D.C. 20591. In addition, Annex 2 may be purchased from the International Civil Aviation Organization (Attention: Distribution Officer), P.O. Box 400, Succursale; Place de L'Aviation Internationale, 1000 Sherbrooke Street West, Montreal, Quebec, Canada H3A 2R2.

91.2 CERTIFICATE OF AUTHORIZATION FOR CERTAIN CATEGORY II OPERATIONS.

The Administrator may issue a certificate of authorization authorizing deviations from the requirements of §§ 91.6, 91.33(f), and 91.34 of this subpart for the operation of small airplanes identified as Category A aircraft in § 97.3 of this chapter in Category II operations, if he finds that the proposed operation can be safely conducted under the terms of the certificate. Such authorization does not permit operation of the aircraft carrying persons or property for compensation or hire.

91.3 RESPONSIBILITY AND AUTHORITY OF THE PILOT IN COMMAND.

(a) The pilot in command of an aircraft is directly responsible for, and is the final authority as to, the operation of that aircraft.

(b) In an emergency requiring immediate action, the pilot in command may deviate from any rule of this subpart or of Subpart B to the extent required to meet that emergency.

(c) Each pilot in command who deviates from a rule under paragraph (b) of this section shall, upon the request of the Administrator, send a written report of that deviation to the Administrator.

91.4 PILOT IN COMMAND OF AIRCRAFT REQUIRING MORE THAN ONE REQUIRED PILOT.

No person may operate an aircraft that is type certificated for more than one required pilot flight crewmember unless the pilot flight crew consists of a pilot in command who meets the requirements of § 61.58 of this chapter.

91.5 PREFLIGHT ACTION.

Each pilot in command shall, before beginning a flight, familiarize himself with all available information concerning that flight. This information must include:

(a) For a flight under IFR or a flight not in the vicinity of an airport, weather reports and forecasts, fuel requirements, alternatives available if the planned flight cannot be completed, and any known traffic delays of which he has been advised by ATC.

(b) For any flight, runway lengths at airports of intended use, and the following takeoff and landing distance information:

(1) For civil aircraft for which an approved airplane or rotorcraft flight manual containing takeoff and landing distance data is required, the takeoff and landing distance data contained therein; and

(2) For civil aircraft other than those specified in subparagraph (1) of this paragraph, other reliable information appropriate to the aircraft, relating to aircraft performance under expected values of airport elevation and runway slope, aircraft gross weight, and wind and temperature.

91.6 CATEGORY II OPERATION: GENERAL OPERATING RULES.

91.7 FLIGHT CREWMEMBERS AT STATIONS.

(a) During takeoff and landing, and while en route, each required flight crewmember shall—

(1) Be at his station unless his absence is necessary in the performance of his duties in connection with the operation of the aircraft or in connection with his physiological needs; and

(2) Keep his seat belt fastened while at his station.

(b) After July 18, 1978, each flight crewmember of a U.S. registered civil airplane shall, during takeoff and landing, keep the shoulder harness fastened while at his station. This paragraph does not apply if—

346

(1) The seat at the crewmember's station is not equipped with a shoulder harness; or

(2) The crewmember would be unable to perform his required duties with the shoulder harness fastened.

91.8 PROHIBITION AGAINST INTERFERENCE WITH CREWMEMBERS.

No person may assault, threaten, intimidate, or interfere with a crewmember in the performance of the crewmember's duties aboard an aircraft being operated.

91.9 CARELESS OR RECKLESS OPERATION.

No person may operate an aircraft in a careless or reckless manner so as to endanger the life or property of another.

91.10 CARELESS OR RECKLESS OPERATION OTHER THAN FOR THE PURPOSE OF AIR NAVIGATION.

No person may operate an aircraft other than for the purpose of air navigation, on any part of the surface of an airport used by aircraft for air commerce (including areas used by those aircraft for receiving or discharging persons or cargo), in a careless or reckless manner so as to endanger the life or property of another.

91.11 LIQUOR AND DRUGS.

(a) No person may act as a crewmember of a civil aircraft—

(1) Within 8 hours after the consumption of any alcoholic beverage;

(2) While under the influence of alcohol; or

(3) While using any drug that affects his faculties in any way contrary to safety.

(b) Except in an emergency, no pilot of a civil aircraft may allow a person who is obviously under the influence of intoxicating liquors or drugs (except a medical patient under proper care) to be carried in that aircraft.

91.12 CARRIAGE OF NARCOTIC DRUGS, MARIJUANA, AND DEPRESSANT OR STIMULANT DRUGS OR SUBSTANCES.

(a) Except as provided in paragraph (b) of this section, no person may operate a civil aircraft within the United States with knowledge that narcotic drugs, marijuana, and depressant or stimulant drugs or substances as defined in Federal or State statutes are carried in the aircraft.

(b) Paragraph (a) of this section does not apply to any carriage of narcotic drugs, marijuana, and depressant or stimulant drugs or substances authorized by or under any Federal or State statute or by any Federal or State agency.

91.13 DROPPING OBJECTS.

No pilot in command of a civil aircraft may allow any object to be dropped from that aircraft in flight that creates a hazard to persons or property.

However, this section does not prohibit the dropping of any object if reasonable precautions are taken to avoid injury or damage to persons or property.

[§ 91.14 USE OF SAFETY BELTS.

(a) Unless otherwise authorized by the Administrator—

(1) No pilot may take off a U.S. registered civil aircraft (except a free balloon that incorporates a basket or gondola and an airship) unless the pilot in command of that aircraft ensures that each person on board is briefed on how to fasten and unfasten that person's safety belt.

(2) No pilot may take off or land a U.S. registered civil aircraft (except free balloons that incorporate baskets or gondolas and airships) unless the pilot in command of that aircraft ensures that each person on board has been notified to fasten his safety belt.

(3) During the takeoff and landing of U.S. registered civil aircraft (except free balloons that incorporate baskets or gondolas and airships) each person on board that aircraft must occupy a seat or berth with a safety belt properly secured about him. However, a person who has not reached his second birthday may be held by an adult who is occupying a seat or berth, and a person on board for the purpose of engaging in sport parachuting may use the floor of the aircraft as a seat.

(b) This section does not apply to operations conducted under Parts 121, 123, or 127 of this chapter. Subparagraph (a)(3) of this section does not apply to persons subject to § 91.7.]

91.15 PARACHUTES AND PARACHUTING.

(a) No pilot of a civil aircraft may allow a parachute that is available for emergency use to be carried in that aircraft unless it is an approved type and—

(1) If a chair type (canopy in back), it has been packed by a certificated and appropriately rated parachute rigger within the preceding 120 days; or

(2) If any other type, it has been packed by a certificated and appropriately rated parachute rigger—

(i) Within the preceding 120 days, if its canopy, shrouds, and harness are composed exclusively of nylon, rayon, or other similar synthetic fiber or materials that are substantial resistant to damage from mold, mildew, or other fungi and other rotting agents propagated in a moist environment; or

(ii) Within the preceding 60 days, if any part of the parachute is composed of silk, pongee, or other natural fiber, or materials not specified in subdivision (i) of this subparagraph.

(b) Except in an emergency, no pilot in command may allow, and no person may make, a parachute jump from an aircraft within the United States except in accordance with Part 105.

(c) Unless each occupant of the aircraft is wearing an approved parachute, no pilot of a civil aircraft carrying any person (other than a crewmember) may execute any intentional maneuver that exceeds—

(1) A bank of 60° relative to the horizon; or

(2) A nose-up or nose-down attitude of 30° relative to the horizon.

(d) Paragraph (c) of this section does not apply to—

(1) Flight tests for pilot certification or rating; or

(2) Spins and other flight maneuvers required by the regulations for any certificate or rating when given by—

(i) A certificated flight instructor; or

(ii) An airline transport pilot instructing in accordance with § 61.169 of this chapter.

(e) For the purpose of this section, "approved parachute" means—

(1) A parachute manufactured under a type certificate or a technical standard order (C-23 series); or

(2) A personnel-carrying military parachute identified by an NAF, AAF, or AN drawing number, an AAF order number, or any other military designation or specification number.

91.17 TOWING: GLIDERS.

(a) No person may operate a civil aircraft towing a glider unless:

(1) The pilot in command of the towing aircraft is qualified under § 61.69 of this chapter.

(2) The towing aircraft is equipped with a tow hitch of a kind, and installed in a manner, approved by the Administrator.

(3) The towline used has a breaking strength not less than 80 percent of the maximum certificated operating weight of the glider, and not more than twice this operating weight. However, the towline used may have a breaking strength more than twice the maximum certificated operating weight of the glider if—

(i) A safety link is installed at the point of attachment of the towline to the glider, with a breaking strength not less than 80 percent of the maximum certificated operating weight of the glider, and not greater than twice this operating weight; and

(ii) A safety link is installed at the point of attachment of the towline to the towing aircraft with a breaking strength greater, but not more than 25 percent greater, than that of the safety link at the towed glider end of the towline, and not greater than twice the maximum certificated operating weight of the glider.

(4) Before conducting any towing operations within a control zone, or before making each towing flight within a control zone if required by ATC, the pilot in command notifies the control tower if one is in operation in that control zone. If such a control tower is not in operation, he must notify the FAA flight service station serving the control zone before conducting any towing operations in that control zone.

(5) The pilots of the towing aircraft and the glider have agreed upon a general course of action including takeoff and release signals, airspeeds, and emergency procedures for each pilot.

(b) No pilot of a civil aircraft may intentionally release a towline, after release of a glider, in a manner so as to endanger the life or property of another.

91.18 TOWING: OTHER THAN UNDER 91.17.

(a) No pilot of a civil aircraft may tow anything with that aircraft (other than under § 91.17) except in accordance with the terms of a certificate of waiver issued by the Administrator.

(b) An application for certificate of waiver under this section is made on a form and in a manner prescribed by the Administrator and must be submitted to the nearest Flight Standards District Office.

91.19 PORTABLE ELECTRONIC DEVICES.

(a) Except as provided in paragraph (b) of this section, no person may operate, nor may any operator or pilot in command of an aircraft allow the operation of, any portable electronic device on any of the following U.S. registered civil aircraft:

    (1) Aircraft operated by an air carrier or commercial operator; or

    (2) Any other aircraft while it is operated under IFR.

(b) Paragraph (a) of this section does not apply to:

    (1) Portable voice recorders;

    (2) Hearing aids;

    (3) Heart pacemakers;

    (4) Electric shavers; or

    (5) Any other portable electronic device that the operator of the aircraft has determined will not cause interference with the navigation or communication system of the aircraft on which it is to be used.

(c) In the case of an aircraft operated by an air carrier or commercial operator, the determination required by paragraph (b)(5) of this section shall be made by the air carrier or commercial operator of the aircraft on which the particular device is to be used. In the case of other aircraft, the determination may be made by the pilot in command or other operator of the aircraft.

[91.20 OPERATIONS WITHIN THE NORTH ATLANTIC MINIMUM NAVIGATION PERFORMANCE SPECIFICATIONS AIRSPACE.

Unless otherwise authorized by the Administrator, no person may operate a civil aircraft of U.S. registry in North Atlantic (NAT) airspace designated as Minimum Navigation Performance Specifications (MNPS) airspace unless that aircraft has approved navigation performance capability which complies with the requirements of Appendix C to this Part. The Administrator authorizes deviations from the requirements of this section in accordance with Section 3 of Appendix C to this Part.]

91.21 FLIGHT INSTRUCTION; SIMULATED INSTRUMENT FLIGHT AND CERTAIN FLIGHT TESTS.

(a) No person may operate a civil aircraft (except a manned free balloon) that is being used for flight instruction unless that aircraft has fully functioning dual controls. [However, instrument flight instruction may be given in a single-engine airplane equipped with a single, functioning throwover control wheel, in place of fixed, dual controls of the elevator and ailerons, when:

(1) The instructor has determined that the flight can be conducted safely; and

(2) The person manipulating the controls has at least a private pilot certificate with appropriate category and class ratings.

(b) No person may operate a civil aircraft in simulated instrument flight unless—

(1) An appropriately rated pilot occupies the other control seat as safety pilot;

(2) The safety pilot has adequate vision forward and to each side of the aircraft, or a competent observer in the aircraft adequately supplements the vision of the safety pilot; and

(3) Except in the case of lighter-than-air aircraft, that aircraft is equipped with fully functioning dual controls. However, simulated instrument flight may be conducted in a single-engine airplane, equipped with a single, functioning, throwover control wheel, in place of fixed, dual controls of the elevator and ailerons, when—

(i) The safety pilot has determined that the flight can be conducted safely; and

(ii) The person manipulating the control has at least a private pilot certificate with appropriate category and class ratings.]

(c) No person may operate a civil aircraft that is being used for a flight test for an airline transport pilot certificate or a class or type rating on that certificate, or for a Federal Aviation Regulation Part 121 proficiency test, unless the pilot seated at the controls, other than the pilot being checked, is fully qualified to act as pilot in command of the aircraft.

[91.22 FUEL REQUIREMENTS FOR FLIGHT UNDER VFR.

(a) No person may begin a flight in an airplane under VFR unless (considering wind and forecast weather conditions) there is enough fuel to fly to the first point of intended landing and, assuming normal cruising speed—

(1) During the day, to fly after that for at least 30 minutes; or

(2) At night, to fly after that for at least 45 minutes.

(b) No person may begin a flight in a rotorcraft under VFR unless (considering wind and forecast weather conditions) there is enough fuel to fly to the first point of intended landing and, assuming normal cruising speed, to fly after that for at least 20 minutes]

91.23 FUEL REQUIREMENTS FOR FLIGHT IN IFR CONDITIONS.

[(a) Except as provided in paragraph (b) of this section, no person may operate a civil aircraft in IFR conditions unless it carries enough fuel (considering weather reports and forecasts, and weather conditions) to—

(1) Complete the flight to the first airport of intended landing;

(2) Fly from that airport to the alternate airport; and

(3) Fly after that for 45 minutes at normal cruising speed.

(b) Paragraph (a)(2) of this section does not apply if—

(1) Part 97 of this subchapter prescribes a standard instrument approach procedure for the first airport of intended landing; and

(2) For at least 1 hour before and 1 hour after the estimated time of arrival at the airport, the weather reports or forecasts or any combination of them, indicate—

(i) The ceiling will be at least 2,000 feet above the airport elevation; and

(ii) Visibility will be at least 3 miles.]

91.24 ATC TRANSPONDER [AND ALTITUDE REPORTING] EQUIPMENT AND USE.

(a) **All airspace: U.S. registered civil aircraft.** For operations not conducted under Parts 121, 123, 127, or 135 of this chapter, ATC transponder equipment installed after January 1, 1974, in U.S. registered civil aircraft not previously equipped with an ATC transponder, and all ATC transponder equipment used in U.S. registered civil aircraft after July 1, 1975, must meet the performance and environmental requirements of any class of TSO-C74b or any class of TSO-C74c as appropriate, except that the Administrator may approve the use fo TSO-C74 or TSO-C74a equipment after July 1, 1975, if the applicant submits data showing that such equipment meets the minimum performance standards of the appropriate class of TOS-C74c and environmental conditions of the TSO under which it was manufactured.

(b) **Controlled airspace: all aircraft.** Except for persons operating helicopters in terminal control areas at or below 1,000 feet AGL under the terms of a letter of agreement, and except for persons operating gliders above 12,500 feet m.s.l. but below the floor of the positive control area, no person may operate an aircraft in the controlled airspace prescribed in subparagraphs (b)(1) through (b)(4) of this paragraph, unless that aircraft is equipped with an operable coded radar beacon transponder having a mode 3/A 4096 code capability, replying to mode 3/A interrogation with the code specified by ATC, and is equipped with automatic pressure altitude reporting equipment having a mode C capability that automatically replies to mode C interrogations by transmitting pressure altitude information in 100-foot increments. This requirement applies—

(1) In Group I Terminal Control Areas governed by §91.90(a);

(2) In Group II Terminal Control Areas

(3) In Group III Terminal Control Areas governed by § 91.90(c), except as provided therein; and

(4) In all controlled airspace of the 48 contiguous States and the District of Columbia, above 12,500 feet m.s.l., excluding the airspace at and below 2,500 feet a.g.l.

(c) **ATC authorized deviations.** ATC may authorize deviations from paragraph (b) of this section—

(1) Immediately, to allow an aircraft with an inoperative transponder to continue to the airport of ultimate destination, including any intermediate stops, or to proceed to a place where suitable repairs can be made, or both;

(2) Immediately, for operations of aircraft with an operating transpon-

der but without operating automatic pressure altitude reporting equipment having a Mode C capability and

(3) On a continuing basis, or for individual flights, for operations of aircraft without a transponder, in which case the request for a deviation must be submitted to the ATC facility having jurisdiction over the airspace concerned at least 4 hours before the proposed operation.

91.25   VOR EQUIPMENT CHECK FOR IFR OPERATIONS.

(a) No person may operate a civil aircraft under IFR using the VOR system of radio navigation unless the VOR equipment of that aircraft—

(1) Is maintained, checked, and inspected under an approved procedure; or

(2) Has been operationally checked within the preceding [30] days and was found to be within the limits of the permissible indicated bearing error set forth in paragraph (b) or (c) of this section.

(b) Except as provided in paragraph (c) of this section, each person conducting a VOR check under paragraph (a)(2) of this section shall—

(1) Use, at the airport of intended departure, an FAA operated or approved test signal or a test signal radiated by a certificated and appropriately rated radio repair station or, outside the United States, a test signal operated or approved by appropriate authority, to check the VOR equipment (the maximum permissible indicated bearing error is plus or minus 4 degrees);

(2) If a test signal is not available at the airport of intended departure, use a point on an airport surface designated as a VOR system checkpoint by the Administrator or, outside the United States, by appropriate authority (the maximum permissible bearing error is plus or minus 4 degrees);

(3) If neither a test signal nor a designated checkpoint on the surface is available, use an airborne checkpoint designated by the Administrator or, outside the United States, by appropriate authority (the maximum permissible bearing error is plus or minus 6 degrees); or

(4) If no check signal or point is available while in flight:

(i) Select a VOR radial that lies along the centerline of an established VOR airway;

(ii) Select a prominent ground point along the selected radial preferably more than 20 miles from the VOR ground facility and maneuver the aircraft directly over the point at a reasonably low altitude; and

(iii) Note the VOR bearing indicated by the receiver when over the ground point (the maximum permissible variation between the published radial and the indicated bearing is 6 degrees).

(c) If dual system VOR (units independent of each other except for the antenna) is installed in the aircraft, the person checking the equipment may check one system against the other in place of the check procedures specified in paragraph (b) of this section. He shall tune both systems to the same VOR ground facility and note the indicated bearings to that station. The maximum permissible variation between the two indicated bearings is 4 degrees.

[(d) Each person making the VOR operational check as specified in paragraph (b) or (c) of this section shall enter the date, place, bearing error, and sign the aircraft log or other record. In addition, if a test signal radiated by a repair station, as specified in paragraph (b)(1) of this section, is used, an entry must be made in the aircraft log or other record by the repair station certificate holder or the certificate holder's representative certifying to the bearing transmitted by the repair station for the check and the date of transmission.]

91.27 CIVIL AIRCRAFT: CERTIFICATIONS REQUIRED.

(a) Except as provided in §91.28, no person may operate a civil aircraft unless it has within it the following:

(1) An appropriate and current airworthiness certificate. Each U.S. airworthiness certificate used to comply with this subparagraph (except a special flight permit, a copy of the applicable operations specifications issued under § 21.197(c) of this chapter, appropriate sections of the air carrier manual required by Parts 121 and 127 of this chapter containing that portion of the operations specifications issued under § 21.197(c), or an authorization under § 91.45), must have on it the registration number assigned to the aircraft under Part 47 of this chapter. However, the airworthiness certificate need not have on it an assigned special identification number before 10 days after that number is first affixed to the aircraft. A revised airworthiness certificate having on it an assigned special identification number, that has been affixed to an aircraft, may only be obtained upon application to an FAA Flight Standards District Office.

(2) A registration certificate issued to its owner.

(b) No person may operate a civil aircraft unless the airworthiness certificate required by paragraph (a) of this section or a special flight authorization issued under § 91.28 is displayed at the cabin or cockpit entrance so that it is legible to passengers or crew.

91.28 SPECIAL FLIGHT AUTHORIZATIONS FOR FOREIGN CIVIL AIRCRAFT.

91.29 CIVIL AIRCRAFT AIRWORTHINESS.

(a) No person may operate a civil aircraft unless it is in an airworthy condition.

(b) The pilot in command of a civil aircraft is responsible for determining whether that aircraft is in condition for safe flight. He shall discontinue the flight when unairworthy mechanical or structural conditions occur.

[91.30 INOPERABLE INSTRUMENTS AND EQUIPMENT FOR MULTI ENGINE AIRCRAFT.

(a) No person may take off a multi engine civil aircraft with inoperable instruments or equipment installed unless the following conditions are met:

(1) An approved Minimum Equipment List exists for that aircraft.

(2) The aircraft has within it a letter of authorization, issued by the FAA Flight Standards Office having jurisdiction over the area in which the operator is located, authorizing operation of the aircraft under the Minimum

Equipment List. The letter of authorization may be obtained by written request of the airworthiness certificate holder. The Minimum Equipment List and the letter of authorization constitute a supplemental type certificate for the aircraft.

(3) The approved Minimum Equipment List must:

(i) Be prepared in accordance with the limitations specified in paragraph (b) of this section.

(ii) Provide for the operation of the aircraft with the instruments and equipment in an inoperable condition.

(4) The aircraft records available to the pilot must include an entry describing the inoperable instruments and equipment.

(5) The aircraft is operated under all applicable conditions and limitations contained in the Minimum Equipment List and the letter authorizing the use of the list.

(b) The following instruments and equipment may not be included in a Minimum Equipment List:

(1) Instruments and equipment that are either specifically or otherwise required by the airworthiness requirements under which the aircraft is type certificated and which are essential for safe operations under all operating conditions.

(2) Instruments and equipment required by an airworthiness directive to be in operable condition unless the airworthiness directive provides otherwise.

(3) Instruments and equipment required for specific operations by this Part.

(c) A person authorized to use an approved Minimum Equipment List issued under Part 121 or 135 for a specific aircraft may use that Minimum Equipment List in connection with operations conducted with that aircraft under this Part.

(d) Notwithstanding any other provision of this section, an aircraft with inoperable instruments or equipment may be operated under a special flight permit issued in accordance with §§ 21.197 and 21.199 of this chapter. (EDITOR'S NOTE: At press time, FAA was considering modifying § 91.30)]

91.31 CIVIL AIRCRAFT OPERATING LIMITATIONS AND MARKING REQUIREMENTS.

(a) Except as provided in paragraph (d) of this section, no person may operate a civil aircraft without compliance with the operating limitations for that aircraft prescribed by the certificating authority of the country of registry.

(b) No person may operate a U.S. registered civil aircraft—

(1) For which an Airplane or Rotorcraft Flight Manual is required by § 21.5 unless there is available in the aircraft a current approved Airplane or Rotorcraft Flight Manual or the manual provided for in § 121.141(b); and

(2) For which an Airplane or Rotorcraft Flight Manual is not required by § 21.5, unless there is available in the aircraft a current approved Airplane

or Rotorcraft Flight Manual, approved manual material, markings, and placards, or any combination thereof.

(c) No person may operate a U.S. registered civil aircraft unless that aircraft is identified in accordance with Part 45 of this chapter.

(d) Any person taking off or landing a helicopter certificated under Part 29 of this chapter at a heliport constructed over water may make such momentary flight as is necessary for takeoff or landing through the prohibited range of the limiting height-speed envelope established for that helicopter if that flight through the prohibited range takes place over water on which a safe ditching can be accomplished, and if the helicopter is amphibious or is equipped with floats or other emergency flotation gear adequate to accomplish a safe emergency ditching on open water.

(e) The Airplane or Rotorcraft Flight Manual, or manual material, markings and placards required by paragraph (b) of this section must contain each operating limitation prescribed for that aircraft by the Administrator, including the following:

(1) Powerplant (e.g., r.p.m., manifold pressure, gas temperature, etc.).

(2) Airspeeds (e.g., normal operating speed, flaps extended speed, etc.).

(3) Aircraft weight, center of gravity, and weight distribution, including the composition of the useful load in those combinations and ranges intended to ensure that the weight and center of gravity position will remain within approved limits (e.g., combinations and ranges of crew, oil, fuel, and baggage).

(4) Minimum flight crew.

(5) Kinds of operation.

(6) Maximum operating altitude.

(7) Maneuvering flight load factors.

(8) Rotor speed (for rotorcraft).

(9) Limiting height-speed envelope (for rotorcraft).

91.32 SUPPLEMENTAL OXYGEN.

(a) **General.** No person may operate a civil aircraft of U.S. registry—

(1) At cabin pressure altitudes above 12,500 feet (MSL) up to and including 14,000 feet (MSL), unless the required minimum flight crew is provided with and uses supplemental oxygen for that part of the flight at those altitudes that is of more than 30 minutes duration;

(2) At cabin pressure altitudes above 14,000 feet (MSL) unless the required minimum flight crew is provided with and uses supplemental oxygen during the entire flight time at those altitudes; and

(3) At cabin pressure altitudes above 15,000 feet (MSL), unless each occupant of the aircraft is provided with supplemental oxygen.

(b) **Pressurized cabin aircraft.**

(1) No person may operate a civil aircraft of U.S. registry with a pressurized cabin—

(i) At flight altitudes above flight level 250, unless at least a 10-minute supply of supplemental oxygen, in addition to any oxygen required to satisfy paragraph (a) of this section, is available for each occupant of the aircraft for use in the event that a descent is necessitated by loss of cabin pressurization; and

(ii) At flight altitudes above flight level 350, unless one pilot at the controls of the airplane is wearing and using an oxygen mask that is secured and sealed, and that either supplies oxygen at all times or automatically supplies oxygen whenever the cabin pressure altitude of the airplane exceeds 14,000 feet (MSL) except that the one pilot need not wear and use an oxygen mask while at or below flight level 410 if there are two pilots at the controls and each pilot has a quick-donning type of oxygen mask that can be placed on the face with one hand from the ready position within five seconds, supplying oxygen and properly secured and sealed.

(2) Notwithstanding subparagraph (1)(ii) of this paragraph, if for any reason at any time it is necessary for one pilot to leave his station at the controls of the aircraft when operating at flight altitudes above flight level 350, the remaining pilot at the controls shall put on and use his oxygen mask until the other pilot has returned to his station.

91.33 POWERED CIVIL AIRCRAFT WITH STANDARD CATEGORY U.S. AIRWORTHINESS CERTIFICATES: INSTRUMENT AND EQUIPMENT REQUIREMENTS.

(a) **General.** Except as provided in paragraphs (c)(3) and (e) of this section, no person may operate a powered civil aircraft with a standard category U.S. airworthiness certificate in any operation described in paragraphs (b) through (f) of this section unless that aircraft contains the instruments and equipment specified in those paragraphs (or FAA-approved equivalents) for that type of operation, and those instruments and items of equipment are in operable condition.

(b) **Visual flight rules (day).** For VFR flight during the day the following instruments and equipment are required:

(1) Airspeed indicator.

(2) Altimeter.

(3) Magnetic direction indicator.

(4) Tachometer for each engine.

(5) Oil pressure gauge for each engine using pressure system.

(6) Temperature gauge for each liquid-cooled engine.

(7) Oil temperature gauge for each air-cooled engine.

(8) Manifold pressure gauge for each altitude engine.

(9) Fuel gauge indicating the quantity of fuel in each tank.

(10) Landing gear position indicator, if the aircraft has a retractable landing gear.

(11) If the aircraft is operated for hire over water and beyond power-off gliding distance from shore, approved flotation gear readily available to each occupant, and at least one pyrotechnic signaling device.

(12) Except as to airships, approved safety belts for all occupants who have reached their second birthday. [After December 4, 1980, each safety belt must be equipped with an approved metal to metal latching device.] The rated strength of each safety belt shall not be less than that corresponding with the ultimate load factors specified in the current applicable aircraft

airworthiness requirements considering the dimensional characteristics of the safety belt arrangement. The webbing of each safety belt shall be replaced as required by the Administrator.

(13) For small civil airplanes manufactured after July 18, 1978, an approved shoulder harness for each front seat. The shoulder harness must be designed to protect the occupant from serious head injury when the occupant experiences the ultimate inertia forces specified in § 23.561(b)(2) of this chapter. Each shoulder harness installed at a flight crewmember station must permit the crewmember, when seated and with his safety belt and shoulder harness fastened, to perform all functions necessary for flight operations. For purposes of this paragraph—(i) The date of manufacture of an airplane is the date the inspection acceptance records reflect that the airplane is complete and meets the FAA Approved Type Design Data; and (ii) A front seat is a seat located at a flight crewmember station or any seat located alongside such a seat.

(c) **Visual flight rules (night).** For VFR flight at night the following instruments and equipment are required:

(1) Instruments and equipment specified in paragraph (b) of this section.

(2) Approved position lights.

(3) An approved aviation red or aviation white anticollision light system on all U.S. registered civil aircraft. Anticollision light systems initially installed after August 11, 1971, on aircraft for which a type certificate was issued or applied for before August 11, 1971, must at least meet the anticollision light standards of Parts 23, 25, 27, or 29, as applicable, that were in effect on August 10, 1971, except that the color may be either aviation red or aviation white. In the event of failure of any light of the anticollision light system, operations with the aircraft may be continued to a stop where repairs or replacement can be made.

(4) If the aircraft is operated for hire, one electric landing light.

(5) An adequate source of electrical energy for all installed electrical and radio equipment.

(6) One spare set of fuses, or three spare fuses of each kind required.

(d) **Instrument flight rules.** For IFR flight the following instruments and equipment are required:

(1) Instruments and equipment specified in paragraph (b) of this section and for night flight, instruments and equipment specified in paragraph (c) of this section.

(2) Two way radio communications system and navigational equipment appropriate to the ground facilities to be used.

(3) Gyroscopic rate-of-turn indicator, except on the following aircraft:

(i) Large airplanes with a third attitude instrument system useable through flight attitudes of 360 degrees of pitch and roll and installed in accordance with § 121.305(j) of this chapter; and

(ii) Rotorcraft, type certificated under Part 29 of this chapter, with a third attitude instrument system useable through flight attitudes of ± 80 degrees of pitch and ± 120 degrees of roll and installed in accordance with § 29.1303(g) of this chapter.

(4) Slip-skid indicator.

(5) Sensitive altimeter adjustable for barometric pressure.

(6) A clock displaying hours, minutes, and seconds with a sweep-second pointer or digital presentation.

(7) Generator of adequate capacity.

(8) Gyroscopic bank and pitch indicator (artificial horizon).

(9) Gyroscopic direction indicator (directional gyro or equivalent).

(e) **Flight at and above 24,000 feet MSL.** If VOR navigational equipment is required under subparagraph (d)(2) of this section, no person may operate a U.S. registered civil aircraft within the 50 states or the District of Columbia, at or above 24,000 feet MSL, unless that aircraft is equipped with an approved distance measuring equipment (DME). When DME required by this paragraph fails at and above 24,000 feet MSL, the pilot in command of the aircraft shall notify ATC immediately, and may then continue operations at and above 24,000 feet MSL to the next airport of intended landing at which repairs or replacement of the equipment can be made.

(f) **Category II operations.**

91.34 CATEGORY II MANUAL.

91.35 FLIGHT RECORDERS AND COCKPIT VOICE RECORDERS.

91.36 DATA CORRESPONDENCE BETWEEN AUTOMATICALLY REPORTED PRESSURE ALTITUDE DATA AND THE PILOT'S ALTITUDE REFERENCE.

No person may operate any automatic pressure altitude reporting equipment associated with a radar beacon transponder—

(a) When deactivation of that equipment is directed by ATC;

(b) Unless, as installed, that equipment was tested and calibrated to transmit altitude data corresponding within 125 feet (on a 95-percent probability basis) of the indicated or calibrated datum of the altimeter normally used to maintain flight altitude, with that altimeter referenced to 29.92 inches of mercury [for altitudes from sea level to the maximum operating altitude of the aircraft; or]

(c) After September 1, 1979, unless the altimeters and digitizers in that equipment meet the standards in TSO–C10b and TSO–C88, respectively.

91.37 TRANSPORT CATEGORY CIVIL AIRPLANE WEIGHT LIMITATIONS.

91.38 INCREASED MAXIMUM CERTIFICATED WEIGHTS FOR CERTAIN AIRPLANES OPERATED IN ALASKA.

91.39 RESTRICTED CATEGORY CIVIL AIRCRAFT; OPERATING LIMITATIONS.

(a) No person may operate a restricted category civil aircraft—

(1) For other than the special purpose for which it is certificated; or

(2) In an operation other than one necessary for the accomplishment of the work activity directly associated with that special purpose.

For the purposes of this paragraph, the operation of a restricted category civil aircraft to provide flight crewmember training in a special purpose operation for which the aircraft is certificated is considered to be an operation for that special purpose.

(b) No person may operate a restricted category civil aircraft carrying persons or property for compensation or hire. For the purposes of this paragraph, a special purpose operation involving the carriage of persons or materials necessary for the accomplishment of that operation such as crop dusting, seeding, spraying, and banner towing (including the carrying of required persons or materials to the location of that operation), and an operation for the purpose of providing flight crewmember training in a special purpose operation, are not considered to be the carrying of persons or property for compensation or hire.

(c) No person may be carried on a restricted category civil aircraft unless—

(1) He is a flight crewmember;

(2) He is a flight crewmember trainee;

(3) He performs an essential function in connection with a special purpose operation for which the aircraft is certificated; or

(4) He is necessary for the accomplishment of the work activity directly associated with that special purpose.

(d) Except when operating in accordance with the terms and conditions of a certificate of waiver or special operating limitations issued by the Administrator, no person may operate a restricted category civil aircraft within the United States—

(1) Over a densely populated area;

(2) In a congested airway; or

(3) Near a busy airport where passenger transport operations are conducted.

(e) An application for a certificate of waiver under paragraph (d) of this section is made on a form and in a manner prescribed by the Administrator and must be submitted to the Flight Standards District Office having jurisdiction over the area in which the applicant is located.

(f) After December 9, 1977, this section does not apply to non-passenger-carrying civil rotorcraft external-load operations conducted under Part 133 of this chapter.

(g) No person may operate a small restricted category civil airplane, manufactured after July 18, 1978, unless an approved shoulder harness is installed for each front seat. The shoulder harness must be designed to protect each occupant from serious head injury when the occupant experiences the ultimate inertia forces specified in § 23.561(b)(2) of this chapter. The shoulder harness installation at each flight crewmember station must permit the crewmember, when seated and with his safety belt and shoulder harness fastened, to perform all functions necessary for flight operations. For purposes of this paragraph—

(1) The date of manufacture of an airplane is the date the inspection

acceptance records reflect that the airplane is complete and meets the FAA Approved Type Design Data; and

(2) A front seat is a seat located at a flight crewmember station or any seat located alongside such a seat.

91.40 LIMITED CATEGORY CIVIL AIRCRAFT; OPERATING LIMITATIONS.

No person may operate a limited category civil aircraft carrying persons or property for compensation or hire.

91.41 PROVISIONALLY CERTIFICATED CIVIL AIRCRAFT; OPERATING LIMITATIONS.

(a) No person may operate a provisionally certificated civil aircraft unless he is eligible for a provisional airworthiness certificate under § 21.213 of this chapter.

(b) No person may operate a provisionally certificated civil aircraft outside the United States unless he has specific authority to do so from the Administrator and each foreign country involved.

(c) Unless otherwise authorized by the Director, Flight Standards Service, no person may operate a provisionally certificated civil aircraft in air transportation.

(d) Unless otherwise authorized by the Administrator, no person may operate a provisionally certificated civil aircraft except—

(1) In direct conjunction with the type or supplemental type certification of that aircraft;

(2) For training flight crews, including simulated air carrier operations;

(3) Demonstration flights by the manufacturer for prospective purchasers;

(4) Market surveys by the manufacturer;

(5) Flight checking of instruments, accessories, and equipment, that do not affect the basic airworthiness of the aircraft; or

(6) Service testing of the aircraft.

(e) Each person operating a provisionally certificated civil aircraft shall operate within the prescribed limitations displayed in the aircraft or set forth in the provisional aircraft flight manual or other appropriate document. However, when operating in direct conjunction with the type or supplemental type certification of the aircraft, he shall operate under the experimental aircraft limitations of § 21.191 of this chapter and when flight testing, shall operate under the requirements of § 91.93 of this chapter.

(f) Each person operating a provisionally certificated civil aircraft shall establish approved procedures for—

(1) The use and guidance of flight and ground personnel in operating under this section; and

(2) Operating in and out of airports where takeoffs or approaches over populated areas are necessary.

No person may operate that aircraft except in compliance with the approved procedures.

(g) Each person operating a provisionally certificated civil aircraft shall ensure that each flight crewmember is properly certificated and has adequate knowledge of, and familiarity with, the aircraft and procedures to be used by that crewmember.

(h) Each person operating a provisionally certificated civil aircraft shall maintain it as required by applicable regulations and as may be specially prescribed by the Administrator.

(i) Whenever the manufacturer, or the Administrator, determines that a change in design, construction or operation is necessary to ensure safe operation, no person may operate a provisionally certificated civil aircraft until that change has been made and approved. Section 21.99 of this chapter applies to operations under this section.

(j) Each person operating a provisionally certificated civil aircraft—

(1) May carry in that aircraft only persons who have a proper interest in the operations allowed by this section or who are specifically authorized by both the manufacturer and the Administrator; and

(2) Shall advise each person carried that the aircraft is provisionally certificated.

(k) The Administrator may prescribe additional limitations or procedures that he considers necessary, including limitations on the number of persons who may be carried in the aircraft.

91.42 AIRCRAFT HAVING EXPERIMENTAL CERTIFICATES; OPERATING LIMITATIONS.

(a) No person may operate an aircraft that has an experimental certificate:

(1) For other than the purpose for which the certificate was issued; or

(2) Carrying persons or property for compensation or hire.

(b) No person may operate an aircraft that has an experimental certificate outside of an area assigned by the Administrator until it is shown that:

(1) The aircraft is controllable throughout its normal range of speeds and throughout all the maneuvers to be executed; and

(2) The aircraft has no hazardous operating characteristics or design features.

(c) Unless otherwise authorized by the Administrator in special operating limitations, no person may operate an aircraft that has an experimental certificate over a densely populated area or in a congested airway. The Administrator may issue special operating limitations for particular aircraft to permit takeoffs and landings to be conducted over a densely populated area or in a congested airway, in accordance with terms and conditions specified in the authorization in the interest of safety in air commerce.

(d) Each person operating an aircraft that has an experimental certificate shall:

(1) Advise each person carried of the experimental nature of the aircraft;

(2) Operate under VFR, day only, unless otherwise specifically authorized by the Administrator; and

(3) Notify the control tower of the experimental nature of the aircraft

when operating the aircraft into or out of airports with operating control towers.

(e) The Administrator may prescribe additional limitations that he considers necessary, including limitations on the persons that may be carried in the aircraft.

91.43 SPECIAL RULES FOR FOREIGN CIVIL AIRCRAFT.

91.45 AUTHORIZATION FOR FERRY FLIGHT WITH ONE ENGINE INOPERATIVE BY AIR CARRIERS AND COMMERCIAL OPERATORS OF LARGE AIRCRAFT.

91.47 EMERGENCY EXITS FOR AIRPLANES CARRYING PASSENGERS FOR HIRE.

91.49 AURAL SPEED WARNING DEVICE.

91.50 TRANSPORT CATEGORY AIRPLANES—PITOT HEAT INDICATION SYSTEMS.

91.51 ALTITUDE ALERTING SYSTEM OR DEVICE; TURBO-JET POWERED CIVIL AIRPLANES.

91.52 EMERGENCY LOCATOR TRANSMITTERS.

(a) Except as provided in paragraphs (e) and (f) of this section, no person may operate a U.S. registered civil airplane unless it meets the applicable requirements of paragraphs (b), (c), and (d) of this section.

(b) To comply with paragraph (a) of this section, each U.S. registered civil airplane must be equipped as follows:

(1) For operations governed by the supplemental air carrier and commercial operator rules of Part 121 of this chapter, or the air travel club rules of Part 123 of this chapter, there must be attached to the airplane an automatic type emergency locator transmitter that is in operable condition and meets the applicable requirements of § 37.200 of this chapter;

(2) For charter flights governed by the domestic and flag air carrier rules of Part 121 of this chapter, there must be attached to the airplane an automatic type emergency locator transmitter that is in operable condition and meets the applicable requirements of § 37.200 of this chapter;

(3) For operations governed by Part 135 of this chapter, there must be attached to the airplane an automatic type emergency locator transmitter that is in operable condition and meets the applicable requirements of § 37.200 of this chapter; and

(4) For operations other than those specified in subparagraphs (1), (2), and (3) of this paragraph, there must be attached to the airplane a personnel type or an automatic type emergency locator transmitter that is in operable condition and meets the applicable requirements of § 37.200 of this chapter.

(c) Each emergency locator transmitter required by paragraphs (a) and (b) of this section must be attached to the airplane in such a manner that the probability of damage to the transmitter, in the event of crash impact, is minimized. Fixed and deployable automatic type transmitters must be attached to the airplane as far aft as practicable.

(d) Batteries used in the emergency locator transmitters required by paragraphs (a) and (b) of this section must be replaced (or recharged, if the battery is rechargeable)—

(1) When the transmitter has been in use for more than one cumulative hour; or

(2) When 50 percent of their useful life (or, for rechargeable batteries, 50 percent of their useful life of charge), as established by the transmitter manufacturer under § 37.200(g)(2) of this chapter, has expired.

The new expiration date for the replacement (or recharge) of the battery must be legibly marked on the outside of the transmitter and entered in the aircraft maintenance record. Subparagraph (2) of this paragraph does not apply to batteries (such as water-activated batteries) that are essentially unaffected during probable storage intervals.

(e) Notwithstanding paragraphs (a) and (b) of this section, a person may—

(1) Ferry a newly acquired airplane from the place where possession of it was taken to a place where the emergency locator transmitter is to be installed; and

(2) Ferry an airplane with an inoperative emergency locator transmitter from a place where repairs or replacement cannot be made to a place where they can be made.

No persons other than required crewmembers may be carried aboard an airplane being ferried pursuant to paragraph (e) of this section.

(f) Paragraphs (a) and (b) of this section do not apply to—

(1) Turbojet-powered aircraft;

(2) Aircraft while engaged in scheduled flights by scheduled air carriers certificated by the Civil Aeronautics Board;

(3) Aircraft while engaged in training operations conducted entirely within a 50-mile radius of the airport from which such local flight operations began;

(4) Aircraft while engaged in flight operations incident to design and testing;

(5) New aircraft while engaged in flight operations incident to their manufacture, preparation, and delivery;

(6) Aircraft while engaged in flight operations incident to the aerial application of chemicals and other substances for agricultural purposes;

(7) Aircraft certificated by the Administrator for research and development purposes;

(8) Aircraft while used for showing compliance with regulations, crew training, exhibition, air racing, or market surveys;

(9) Aircraft equipped to carry not more than one person; and

(10) An aircraft during any period for which the transmitter has been temporarily removed for inspection, repair, modification or replacement, subject to the following:

364

(i) No person may operate the aircraft unless the aircraft records contain an entry which includes the date of initial removal, the make, model, serial number and reason for removal of the transmitter, and a placard is located in view of the pilot to show 'ELT not installed."

(ii) No person may operate the aircraft more than 90 days after the ELT is initially removed from the aircraft.

91.53 (RESERVED.)

91.54 TRUTH IN LEASING CLAUSE REQUIREMENT IN LEASES AND CONDITIONAL SALES CONTRACTS.

(a) Except as provided in paragraph (b) of this section, the parties to a lease or contract of conditional sale involving a United States registered large civil aircraft and entered into after January 2, 1973, shall execute a written lease or contract and include therein a written truth in leasing clause as a concluding paragraph in large print, immediately preceding the space for the signature of the parties, which contains the following with respect to each such aircraft:

(1) Identification of the Federal Aviation Regulations under which the aircraft has been maintained and inspected during the 12 months preceding the execution of the lease or contract of conditional sale; and certification by the parties thereto regarding the aircraft's status of compliance with applicable maintenance and inspection requirements in this Part for the operation to be conducted under the lease or contract of conditional sale.

(2) [The name and address (printed or typed) and the signature of the person responsible for operational control of the aircraft under the lease or contract of conditional sale, and certification that each person understands that person's responsibilities for compliance with applicable Federal Aviation Regulations.]

(3) A statement that an explanation of factors bearing on operational control and pertinent Federal Aviation Regulations can be obtained from the nearest FAA Flight Standards District Office, General Aviation District Office, or Air Carrier District Office.

(b) The requirements of paragraph (a) of this section do not apply—

(1) To a lease or contract of conditional sale when:

(i) The party to whom the aircraft is furnished is a foreign air carrier or certificate holder under Part 121, 123, 127, 135, or 141 of this chapter; or

(ii) The party furnishing the aircraft is a foreign air carrier, certificate holder under Part 121, 123, 127, or 141 of this chapter, or a certificate holder under Part 135 of this chapter having appropriate authority to engage in air taxi operations with large aircraft.

(2) To a contract of conditional sale, when the aircraft involved has not been registered anywhere prior to the execution of the contract, except as a new aircraft under a dealer's aircraft registration certificate issued in accordance with § 47.61 of this chapter.

(c) No person may operate a large civil aircraft of U.S. registry that is subject to a lease or contract of conditional sale to which paragraph (a) of this section applies, unless—

(1) The lessee or conditional buyer, or the registered owner if the lessee is not a citizen of the United States, has mailed a copy of the lease or contract that complies with the requirements of paragraph (a) of this section, within 24 hours of its execution, to the Flight Standards Technical Division, Post Office Box 25724, Oklahoma City, OK 73125;

(2) A copy of the lease or contract that complies with the requirements of paragraph (a) of this section is carried in the aircraft. The copy of the lease or contract shall be made available for review upon request by the Administrator; and

(3) The lessee or conditional buyer, or the registered owner if the lessee is not a citizen of the United States, has notified by telephone or in person, the FAA Flight Standards District Office, General Aviation District Office, Air Carrier District Office, or International Field Office nearest the airport where the flight will originate. Unless otherwise authorized by that office, the notification shall be given at least 48 hours prior to takeoff in the case of the first flight of that aircraft under that lease or contract and inform the FAA of—

(i) The location of the airport of departure;

(ii) The departure time; and

(iii) The registration number of the aircraft involved.

(d) The copy of the lease or contract furnished to the FAA under paragraph (c) of this section is commercial or financial information obtained from a person. It is, therefore, privileged and confidential, and will not be made available by the FAA for public inspection or copying under 5 U.S.C. 552(b)(4), unless recorded with the FAA under Part 49 of this chapter.

(e) For purpose of this section, a lease means any agreement by a person to furnish an aircraft to another person for compensation or hire, whether with or without flight crewmembers, other than an agreement for the sale of an aircraft and a contract of conditional sale under Section 101 of the Federal Aviation Act of 1958. The person furnishing the aircraft is referred to as the lessor and the person to whom it is furnished the lessee.

91.55 CIVIL AIRCRAFT SONIC BOOM.

[91.57 AVIATION SAFETY REPORTING PROGRAM; PROHIBITION AGAINST USE OF REPORTS FOR ENFORCEMENT PURPOSES.

The Administrator of the FAA will not use reports submitted to the National Aeronautics and Space Administration under the Aviation Safety Reporting Program (or information derived therefrom) in any enforcement action, except information concerning criminal offenses or accidents which are wholly excluded from the Program.]

[91.58 MATERIALS FOR COMPARTMENT INTERIORS.

No person may operate an airplane that conforms to an amended or supplemental type certificate issued in accordance with SFAR NO. 41 for a maximum certificated takeoff weight in excess of 12,500 pounds, unless within one year after issuance of the initial airworthiness certificate under that SFAR, the airplane meets the compartment requirements set forth in § 25.853(a), (b), (b-1), (b-2), and (b-3) of this chapter in effect on September 26, 1978.]

Subpart B — Flight Rules

General

91.61 APPLICABILITY.

This subpart prescribes flight rules governing the operation of aircraft within the United States.

91.63 WAIVERS.

(a) The Administrator may issue a certificate of waiver authorizing the operation of aircraft in deviation of any rule of this subpart if he finds that the proposed operation can be safely conducted under the terms of that certificate of waiver.

(b) An application for a certificate of waiver under this section is made on a form and in a manner prescribed by the Administrator and may be submitted to any FAA office.

(c) A certificate of waiver is effective as specified in that certificate.

91.65 OPERATING NEAR OTHER AIRCRAFT.

(a) No person may operate an aircraft so close to another aircraft as to create a collision hazard.

(b) No person may operate an aircraft in formation flight except by arrangement with the pilot in command of each aircraft in the formation.

(c) No person may operate an aircraft, carrying passengers for hire, in formation flight.

(d) Unless otherwise authorized by ATC, no person operating an aircraft may operate his aircraft in accordance with any clearance or instruction that has been issued to the pilot of another aircraft for radar Air Traffic Control purposes.

91.67 RIGHT-OF-WAY RULES; EXCEPT WATER OPERATIONS.

(a) **General.** When weather conditions permit, regardless of whether an operation is conducted under Instrument Flight Rules or Visual Flight Rules, vigilance shall be maintained by each person operating an aircraft so as to see and avoid other aircraft in compliance with this section. When a rule of this section gives another aircraft the right of way, he shall give way to that aircraft and may not pass over, under, or ahead of it, unless well clear.

(b) **In distress.** An aircraft in distress has the right of way over all other air traffic.

(c) **Converging.** When aircraft of the same category are converging at approximately the same altitude (except head-on, or nearly so) the aircraft to the other's right has the right of way. If the aircraft are of different categories—

(1) A balloon has the right of way over any other category of aircraft;

(2) A glider has the right of way over an airship, airplane or rotorcraft; and

(3) An airship has the right of way over an airplane or rotorcraft.
However, an aircraft towing or refueling other aircraft has the right of way over all other engine-driven aircraft.

(d) **Approaching head-on.** When aircraft are approaching each other head-on, or nearly so, each pilot of each aircraft shall alter course to the right.

(e) **Overtaking.** Each aircraft that is being overtaken has the right of way and each pilot of an overtaking aircraft shall alter course to the right to pass well clear.

(f) **Landing.** Aircraft, while on final approach to land, or while landing, have the right of way over other aircraft in flight or operating on the surface. When two or more aircraft are approaching an airport for the purpose of landing, the aircraft at the lower altitude has the right of way, but it shall not take advantage of this rule to cut in front of another which is on final approach to land, or to overtake that aircraft.

(g) **Inapplicability.** This section does not apply to the operation of an aircraft on water.

91.69 RIGHT-OF-WAY RULES; WATER OPERATIONS.

(a) **General.** Each person operating an aircraft on the water shall, insofar as possible, keep clear of all vessels and avoid impeding their navigation, and shall give way to any vessel or other aircraft that is given the right of way by any rule of this section.

(b) **Crossing.** When aircraft, or an aircraft and a vessel are on crossing courses, the aircraft or vessel to the other's right has the right of way.

(c) **Approaching head-on.** When aircraft, or an aircraft and a vessel, are approaching head-on or nearly so, each shall alter its course to the right to keep well clear.

(d) **Overtaking.** Each aircraft or vessel that is being overtaken has the right of way, and the one overtaking shall alter course to keep well clear.

(e) **Special circumstances.** When aircraft, or an aircraft and a vessel, approach so as to involve risk of collision, each aircraft or vessel shall proceed with careful regard to existing circumstances including the limitations of the respective craft.

91.70 AIRCRAFT SPEED.

(a) Unless otherwise authorized by the Administrator, no person may operate an aircraft below 10,000 feet MSL at an indicated airspeed of more than 250 knots (288 m.p.h.).

(b) Unless otherwise authorized or required by ATC, no person may operate an aircraft within an airport traffic area at an indicated airspeed of more than—

(1) In the case of a reciprocating engine aircraft, 156 knots (180 m.p.h.); or

(2) In the case of a turbine-powered aircraft, 200 knots (230 m.p.h.).

Paragraph (b) of this section does not apply to any operations within a Terminal Control Area. Such operations shall comply with paragraph (a) of this section.

(c) No person may operate an aircraft in the airspace underlying a Terminal Control Area, or in a VFR corridor designated through a Terminal Control Area, at an indicated airspeed of more than 200 knots (230 m.p.h.).

However, if the minimum safe airspeed for any particular operation is greater than the maximum speed prescribed in this section, the aircraft may be operated at that minimum speed.

91.71 ACROBATIC FLIGHT.

No person may operate an aircraft in acrobatic flight—

(a) Over any congested area of a city, town or settlement;

(b) Over an open air assembly of persons;

(c) Within a control zone or Federal airway;

(d) Below an altitude of 1,500 feet above the surface; or

(e) When flight visibility is less than three miles.

For the purposes of this section, acrobatic flight means an intentional maneuver involving an abrupt change in an aircraft's attitude, an abnormal attitude, or abnormal acceleration, not necessary for normal flight.

91.73 AIRCRAFT LIGHTS.

No person may, during the period from sunset to sunrise (or, in Alaska, during the period a prominent unlighted object cannot be seen from a distance of three statute miles or the sun is more than six degrees below the horizon)—

(a) Operate an aircraft unless it has lighted position lights;

(b) Park or move an aircraft in, or in dangerous proximity to, a night flight operations area of an airport unless the aircraft—

(1) Is clearly illuminated;

(2) Has lighted position lights; or

(3) Is in an area which is marked by obstruction lights.

(c) Anchor an aircraft unless the aircraft—

(1) Has lighted anchor lights; or

(2) Is in an area where anchor lights are not required on vessels; or

(d) Operate an aircraft, required by § 91.33(c)(3) to be equipped with an anticollision light system, unless it has approved and lighted aviation red or aviation white anticollision lights. However, the anticollision lights need not be lighted when the pilot in command determines that, because of operating conditions, it would be in the interest of safety to turn the lights off.

91.75 COMPLIANCE WITH ATC CLEARANCES AND INSTRUCTIONS.

(a) When an ATC clearance has been obtained, no pilot in command may deviate from that clearance, except in an emergency, unless he obtains an amended clearance. However, except in positive controlled airspace, this paragraph does not prohibit him from cancelling an IFR flight plan if he is operating in VFR weather conditions. If a pilot is uncertain of the meaning of an ATC clearance, he shall immediately request clarification from ATC.

(b) Except in an emergency, no person may, in an area in which air traffic control is exercised, operate an aircraft contrary to an ATC instruction.

(c) Each pilot in command who deviates, in an emergency, from an ATC clearance or instruction shall notify ATC of that deviation as soon as possible.

(d) Each pilot in command who (though not deviating from a rule of this subpart) is given priority by ATC in an emergency, shall, if requested by ATC, submit a detailed report of that emergency within 48 hours to the chief of that ATC facility.

91.77 ATC LIGHT SIGNALS.

ATC light signals have the meaning shown in the following table.

Color and type of signal	Meaning with respect to aircraft on the surface	Meaning with respect to aircraft in flight
Steady green	Cleared for takeoff	Cleared to land.
Flashing green	Cleared to taxi	Return for landing (to be followed by steady green at proper time).
Steady red	Stop	Give way to other aircraft and continue circling.
Flashing red	Taxi clear of runway in use.	Airport unsafe—do not land.
Flashing white	Return to starting point on airport.	Not applicable.
Alternating red and green	Exercise extreme caution.	Exercise extreme caution.

91.79 MINIMUM SAFE ALTITUDES; GENERAL.

Except when necessary for takeoff or landing, no person may operate an aircraft below the following altitudes:

(a) **Anywhere.** An altitude allowing, if a power unit fails, an emergency landing without undue hazard to persons or property on the surface.

(b) **Over congested areas.** Over any congested area of a city, town, or settlement, or over any open air assembly of persons, an altitude of 1,000 feet above the highest obstacle within a horizontal radius of 2,000 feet of the aircraft.

(c) **Over other than congested areas.** An altitude of 500 feet above the surface, except over open water or sparsely populated areas. In that case, the aircraft may not be operated closer than 500 feet to any person, vessel, vehicle, or structure.

(d) **Helicopters.** Helicopters may be operated at less than the minimums prescribed in paragraph (b) and (c) of this section if the operation is conducted without hazard to persons or property on the surface. In addition, each person operating a helicopter shall comply with routes or altitudes specifically prescribed for helicopters by the Administrator.

91.81 ALTIMETER SETTINGS.

(a) Each person operating an aircraft shall maintain the cruising altitude or flight level of that aircraft, as the case may be, by reference to an altimeter that is set, when operating—

(1) Below 18,000 feet MSL, to—

(i) The current reported altimeter setting of a station along the route and within 100 nautical miles of the aircraft;

(ii) If there is no station within the area prescribed in subdivision (i) of this subparagraph, the current reported altimeter setting of an appropriate available station; or

(iii) In the case of an aircraft not equipped with a radio, the elevation of the departure airport or an appropriate altimeter setting available before departure; or

(2) At or above 18,000 feet MSL, to 29.92″ Hg.

(b) The lowest usable flight level is determined by the atmospheric pressure in the area of operation, as shown in the following table:

CURRENT ALTIMETER SETTING	LOWEST USABLE FLIGHT LEVEL
29.92 (or higher)	180
29.91 through 29.42	185
29.41 through 28.92	190
28.91 through 28.42	195
28.41 through 27.92	200
27.91 through 27.42	205
27.41 through 26.92	210

(c) To convert minimum altitude prescribed under §§ 91.79 and 91.119 to the minimum flight level, the pilot shall take the flight-level equivalent of the minimum altitude in feet and add the appropriate number of feet specified below, according to the current reported altimeter setting:

CURRENT ALTIMETER SETTING	ADJUSTMENT FACTOR
29.92 (or higher)	None
29.91 through 29.42	500 feet
29.41 through 28.92	1,000 feet
28.91 through 28.42	1,500 feet
28.41 through 27.92	2,000 feet
27.91 through 27.42	2,500 feet
27.41 through 26.92	3,000 feet

91.83 FLIGHT PLAN; INFORMATION REQUIRED.

(a) Unless otherwise authorized by ATC, each person filing an IFR or VFR flight plan shall include in it the following information:

(1) The aircraft identification number and, if necessary, its radio call sign.

(2) The type of the aircraft or, in the case of a formation flight, the type of each aircraft and the number of aircraft, in the formation.

(3) The full name and address of the pilot in command or, in the case of a formation flight, the formation commander.

(4) The point and proposed time of departure.

(5) The proposed route, cruising altitude (or flight level), and true airspeed at that altitude.

(6) The point of first intended landing and the estimated elapsed time until over that point.

(7) The radio frequencies to be used.

(8) The amount of fuel on board (in hours).

(9) In the case of an IFR flight plan, an alternate airport, except as provided in paragraph (b) of this section.

(10) The number of persons in the aircraft [except where that information is otherwise readily available to the FAA.]

(11) Any other information the pilot in command or ATC believes is necessary for ATC purposes.

[(b) **Exceptions to applicability of paragraph (a)(9) of this section.** Paragraph (a)(9) of this section does not apply if Part 97 of this subchapter prescribes a standard instrument approach procedure for the first airport of intended landing and, for at least one hour before and one hour after the estimated time of arrival, the weather reports or forecasts or any combination of them, indicate—

(1) The ceiling will be at least 2,000 feet above the airport elevation; and

(2) Visibility will be at least 3 miles.]

(c) **IFR alternate airport weather minimums.**

Unless otherwise authorized by the Administrator, no person may include an alternate airport in an IFR flight plan unless current weather forecasts indicate that, at the estimated time of arrival at the alternate airport, the ceiling and visibility at that airport will be at or above the following alternate airport weather minimums:

(1) If an instrument approach procedure has been published in Part 97 of this chapter for that airport, the alternate airport minimums specified in that procedure or, if none are so specified, the following minimums:

(i) Precision approach procedure: Ceiling 600 feet and visibility 2 statute miles.

(ii) Nonprecision approach procedure: Ceiling 800 feet and visibility 2 statute miles.

(2) If no instrument approach procedure has been published in Part 97 of this chapter for that airport, the ceiling and visibility minimums are those allowing descent from the MEA, approach, and landing, under basic VFR.

(d) **Cancellation.** When a flight plan has been activated, the pilot in command, upon canceling or completing the flight under the flight plan, shall notify an FAA Flight Service Station or ATC facility.

91.84   FLIGHTS BETWEEN MEXICO OR CANADA AND THE UNITED STATES.

Unless otherwise authorized by ATC, no person may operate a civil aircraft between Mexico or Canada and the United States without filing an IFR or VFR flight plan, as appropriate.

91.85   OPERATING ON OR IN THE VICINITY OF AN AIRPORT; GENERAL RULES.

(a) Unless otherwise required by Part 93 of this chapter, each person operating an aircraft on or in the vicinity of an airport shall comply with the requirements of this section and of §§ 91.87 and 91.89.

(b) Unless otherwise authorized or required by ATC, no person may operate an aircraft within an airport traffic area except for the purpose of landing at, or taking off from, an airport within that area. ATC authorizations may be given as individual approval of specific operations or may be contained in written agreements between airport users and the tower concerned.

(c) After March 28, 1977, except when necessary for training or certification, the pilot in command of a civil turbojet-powered airplane shall use, as a final landing flap setting, the minimum certificated landing flap setting set forth in the approved performance information in the Airplane Flight Manual for the applicable conditions. However, each pilot in command has the final authority and responsibility for the safe operation of his airplane, and he may use a different flap setting approved for that airplane if he determines that it is necessary in the interest of safety.

91.87 OPERATION AT AIRPORTS WITH OPERATING CONTROL TOWERS.

(a) **General.** Unless otherwise authorized or required by ATC, each person operating an aircraft to, from, or on an airport, with an operating control tower shall comply with the applicable provisions of this section.

(b) **Communications with control towers operated by the United States.** No person may, within an airport traffic area, operate an aircraft to, from, or on an airport having a control tower operated by the United States unless two-way radio communications are maintained between that aircraft and the control tower. However, if the aircraft radio fails in flight, he may operate that aircraft and land if weather conditions are at or above basic VFR weather minimums, he maintains visual contact with the tower, and he receives a clearance to land. If the aircraft radio fails while in flight under IFR, he must comply with § 91.127.

(c) **Communications with other control towers.** No person may, within an airport traffic area, operate an aircraft to, from, or on an airport having a control tower that is operated by any person other than the United States unless—

(1) If that aircraft's radio equipment so allows, two-way radio communications are maintained between the aircraft and the tower; or

(2) If that aircraft's radio equipment allows only reception from the tower, the pilot has the tower's frequency monitored.

(d) **Minimum altitudes.** When operating to an airport with an operating control tower, each pilot of—

(1) A turbine-powered airplane or a large airplane shall, unless otherwise required by the applicable distance from cloud criteria, enter the airport traffic area at an altitude of at least 1,500 feet above the surface of the airport and maintain at least 1,500 feet within the airport traffic area, including the traffic pattern, until further descent is required for a safe landing;

(2) A turbine-powered airplane or a large airplane approaching to land on a runway being served by an ILS, shall, if the airplane is ILS equipped, fly that airplane at an altitude at or above the glide slope between the outer marker (or the point of interception with the glide slope, if compliance with the applicable distance from clouds criteria requires interception closer in) and the middle marker; and

(3) An airplane approaching to land on a runway served by a visual approach slope indicator, shall maintain an altitude at or above the glide slope until a lower altitude is necessary for a safe landing.

However, subparagraphs (2) and (3) of this paragraph do not prohibit normal bracketing maneuvers above or below the glide slope that are conducted for the purpose of remaining on the glide slope.

(e) **Approaches.** When approaching to land at an airport with an operating control tower, each pilot of—

(1) An airplane, shall circle the airport to the left; and

(2) A helicopter, shall avoid the flow of fixed-wing aircraft.

(f) **Departures.** No person may operate an aircraft taking off from an airport with an operating control tower except in compliance with the following:

(1) Each pilot shall comply with any departure procedures established for that airport by the FAA.

(2) Unless otherwise required by the departure procedure or the applicable distance from clouds criteria, each pilot of a turbine-powered airplane and each pilot of a large airplane shall climb to an altitude of 1,500 feet above the surface as rapidly as practicable.

(g) **Noise abatement runway system.** When landing or taking off from an airport with an operating control tower, and for which a formal runway use program has been established by the FAA, each pilot of a turbine-powered airplane and each pilot of a large airplane, assigned a noise abatement runway by ATC, shall use that runway. [However, consistent with the final authority of the pilot in command concerning the safe operation of the aircraft as prescribed in § 91.3(a), ATC may assign a different runway if requested by the pilot in the interest of safety.]

(h) **Clearances required.** No person may, at any airport with an operating control tower, operate an aircraft on a runway or taxiway, or takeoff or land an aircraft, unless an appropriate clearance is received from ATC. A clearance to "taxi to" the takeoff runway assigned to the aircraft is not a clearance to cross that assigned takeoff runway, or to taxi on that runway at any point, but is a clearance to cross other runways that intersect the taxi route to that assigned takeoff runway. A clearance to "taxi to" any point other than an assigned takeoff runway is a clearance to cross all runways that intersect the taxi route to that point.

91.89 OPERATION AT AIRPORTS WITHOUT CONTROL TOWERS.

(a) Each person operating an aircraft to or from an airport without an operating control tower shall—

(1) In the case of an airplane approaching to land, make all turns of that airplane to the left unless the airport displays approved light signals or visual markings indicating that turns should be made to the right, in which case the pilot shall make all turns to the right;

(2) In the case of a helicopter approaching to land, avoid the flow of fixed-wing aircraft; and

(3) In the case of an aircraft departing the airport, comply with any FAA traffic pattern for that airport.

91.90 TERMINAL CONTROL AREAS.

(a) **Group I Terminal Control Areas—**

(1) **Operating rules.** No person may operate an aircraft within a Group I Terminal Control Area designated in Part 71 of this chapter except in compliance with the following rules:

(i) No person may operate an aircraft within a Group I Terminal Control Area unless he has received an appropriate authorization from ATC prior to the operation of that aircraft in that area.

(ii) Unless otherwise authorized by ATC, each person operating a large turbine engine powered airplane to or from a primary airport shall operate at or above the designated floors while within the lateral limits of the Terminal Control Area.

(2) **Pilot requirements.** The pilot in command of a civil aircraft may not land or take off that aircraft from an airport within a Group I Terminal Control Area unless he holds at least a private pilot certificate.

(3) **Equipment requirements.** Unless otherwise authorized by ATC in the case of in-flight VOR, TACAN, or two-way radio failure; or unless otherwise authorized by ATC in the case of a transponder failure occurring at any time, no person may operate an aircraft within a Group I Terminal Control Area unless that aircraft is equipped with—

(i) An operable VOR or TACAN receiver (except in the case of helicopters);

(ii) An operable two-way radio capable of communicating with ATC on appropriate frequencies for that Terminal Control Area; and

(iii) The applicable equipment specified in § 91.24.

(b) **Group II Terminal Control Areas—**

(1) **Operating rules.** No person may operate an aircraft within a Group II Terminal Control Area designated in Part 71 of this chapter except in compliance with the following rules:

(i) No person may operate an aircraft within a Group II Terminal Control Area unless he has received an appropriate authorization from ATC prior to operation of that aircraft in that area, and unless two-way radio communications are maintained, within that area, between that aircraft and the ATC facility.

(ii) Unless otherwise authorized by ATC, each person operating a large turbine engine powered airplane to or from a primary airport shall operate at or above the designated floors while within the lateral limits of the Terminal Control Area.

(2) **Equipment requirements.** Unless otherwise authorized by ATC in the case of in-flight VOR, TACAN, or two-way radio failure; or unless otherwise authorized by ATC in the case of a transponder failure occurring at any time, no person may operate an aircraft within a Group II Terminal Control Area unless that aircraft is equipped with—

(i) An operable VOR or TACAN receiver (except in the case of helicopters);

(ii) An operable two-way radio capable of communicating with ATC on the appropriate frequencies for that terminal control area; and

(iii) The applicable equipment specified in § 91.24, except that automatic pressure altitude reporting equipment is not required for any operation within the Terminal Control Area, and a transponder is not required for IFR flights operating to or from an airport outside of but in close proximity to the Terminal Control Area, when the commonly used transition, approach, or departure procedures to such airport require flight within the Terminal Control Area.

(c) **Group III Terminal Control Areas.** No person may operate an aircraft within a Group III Terminal Control Area designated in Part 71 unless the applicable provisions of § 91.24(b) are complied with, except that such compliance is not required if two-way radio communications are maintained, within the TCA, between the aircraft and the ATC facility, and the pilot provides position, altitude, and proposed flight path prior to entry.

91.91 TEMPORARY FLIGHT RESTRICTIONS.

(a) Whenever the Administrator determines it to be necessary in order to prevent an unsafe congestion of sightseeing aircraft above an incident or event which may generate a high degree of public interest, or to provide a safe environment for the operation of disaster relief aircraft, a Notice to Airmen will be issued designating an area within which temporary flight restrictions apply.

(b) When a Notice to Airmen has been issued under this Section, no person may operate an aircraft within the designated area unless—

(1) That aircraft is participating in disaster relief activities and is being operated under the direction of the agency responsible for relief activities;

(2) That aircraft is being operated to or from an airport within the area and is operated so as not to hamper or endanger relief activities;

(3) That operation is specifically authorized under an IFR ATC clearance;

(4) VFR flight around or above the area is impracticable due to weather, terrain, or other considerations, prior notice is given to the Air Traffic Service facility specified in the Notice to Airmen, and en route operation through the area is conducted so as not to hamper or endanger relief activities; or,

(5) That aircraft is carrying properly accredited news representatives, or persons on official business concerning the incident or event which generated the issuance of the Notice to Airmen; the operation is conducted in accordance with § 91.79; the operation is conducted above the altitudes being used by relief aircraft unless otherwise authorized by the agency responsible for relief activities; and further, in connection with this type of operation, prior to entering the area the operator has filed with the Air Traffic Service facility specified in the Notice to Airmen a flight plan that includes the following information:

(i) Aircraft identification, type and color.

(ii) Radio communications frequencies to be used.

(iii) Proposed times of entry and exit of the designated area.

(iv) Name of news media or purpose of flight.

(v) Any other information deemed necessary by ATC.

91.93 FLIGHT TEST AREAS.

No person may flight test an aircraft except over open water, or sparsely populated areas, having light air traffic.

91.95 RESTRICTED AND PROHIBITED AREAS.

(a) No person may operate an aircraft within a restricted area (designated in Part 73) contrary to the restrictions imposed, or within a prohibited area, unless he has the permission of the using or controlling agency, as appropriate.

(b) Each person conducting, within a restricted area, an aircraft operation (approved by the using agency) that creates the same hazards as the operations for which the restricted area was designated, may deviate from the rules of this subpart that are not compatible with his operation of the aircraft.

91.97 POSITIVE CONTROL AREAS AND ROUTE SEGMENTS.

(a) Except as provided in paragraph (b) of this section, no person may operate an aircraft within a positive control area, or positive control route segment designated in Part 71 of this chapter, unless that aircraft is—

(1) Operated under IFR at a specific flight level assigned by ATC;

(2) Equipped with instruments and equipment required for IFR operations;

(3) Flown by a pilot rated for instrument flight; and

(4) Equipped, when in a positive control area, with—

(i) The applicable equipment specified in § 91.24; and

(ii) A radio providing direct pilot/controller communication on the frequency specified by ATC for the area concerned.

(b) ATC may authorize deviations from the requirements of paragraph (a) of this section. In the case of an inoperative transponder, ATC may immediately approve an operation within a positive control area allowing flight to continue, if desired, to the airport of ultimate destination, including any intermediate stops, or to proceed to a place where suitable repairs can be made, or both. A request for authorization to deviate from a requirement of paragraph (a) of this section, other than for operation with an inoperative transponder as outlined above, must be submitted at least 4 days before the proposed operation, in writing, to the ATC center having jurisdiction over the positive control area concerned. ATC may authorize a deviation on a continuing basis or for an individual flight, as appropriate.

91.99 (RESERVED.)

91.101 OPERATIONS TO OR OVER CUBA.

No person may operate a civil aircraft from the United States to Cuba unless—

(a) Departure is from an international airport of entry designated in § 6.13 of the Air Commerce Regulations of the Bureau of Customs (19 CFR 6.13); and

(b) In the case of departure from any of the 48 contiguous states or the District of Columbia, the pilot in command of the aircraft has filed—

(1) A DVFR or IFR flight plan as prescribed in § 99.11 or § 99.13 of this chapter; and

(2) A written statement, within one hour before departure, with the office of Immigration and Naturalization Service at the airport of departure, containing—

(i) All information in the flight plan;

(ii) The name of each occupant of the aircraft;

(iii) The number of occupants of the aircraft; and

(iv) A description of the cargo, if any.

This section does not apply to the operation of aircraft by a scheduled air carrier over routes authorized in operations specifications issued by the Administrator.

91.102 FLIGHT LIMITATION IN THE PROXIMITY OF SPACE FLIGHT RECOVERY OPERATIONS.

No person may operate any aircraft of U.S. registry, or pilot any aircraft under the authority of an airman certificate issued by the Federal Aviation Administration within areas designated in a Notice to Airmen (NOTAM) for space flight recovery operations except when authorized by ATC, or operated under the control of the Department of Defense Manager for Manned Space Flight Support Operations.

91.103 OPERATION OF CIVIL AIRCRAFT OF CUBAN REGISTRY.

91.104 FLIGHT RESTRICTIONS IN THE PROXIMITY OF THE PRESIDENTIAL AND OTHER PARTIES.

No person may operate an aircraft over or in the vicinity of any area to be visited or traveled by the President, the Vice President, or other public figures contrary to the restrictions established by the Administrator and published in a Notice to Airmen (NOTAM).

Visual Flight Rules

91.105 BASIC VFR WEATHER MINIMUMS.

(a) Except as provided in § 91.107, no person may operate an aircraft under VFR when the flight visibility is less, or at a distance from clouds that is less, than that prescribed for the corresponding altitude in the following table:

Altitude	Flight visibility	Distance from clouds
1,200 feet or less above the surface (regardless of MSL altitude)—		
Within controlled airspace	3 statute miles	500 feet below. 1,000 feet above. 2,000 feet horizontal.
Outside controlled airspace	1 statute mile except as provided in § 91.105(b)	Clear of clouds.
More than 1,200 feet above the surface but less than 10,000 feet MSL—		
Within controlled airspace	3 statute miles	500 feet below. 1,000 feet above. 2,000 feet horizontal.

Outside controlled airspace . . . . 1 statute mile	{	500 feet below. 1,000 feet above. 2,000 feet horizontal.
More than 1,200 feet above the surface and at or above 10,000 feet MSL . . . . 5 statute miles	{	1,000 feet below. 1,000 feet above. 1 mile horizontal.

(b) When the visibility is less than one mile, a helicopter may be operated outside controlled airspace at 1,200 feet or less above the surface if operated at a speed that allows the pilot adequate opportunity to see any air traffic or other obstruction in time to avoid a collision.

(c) Except as provided in § 91.107, no person may operate an aircraft, under VFR, within a control zone beneath the ceiling when the ceiling is less than 1,000 feet.

(d) Except as provided in § 91.107, no person may take off or land an aircraft, or enter the traffic pattern of an airport, under VFR, within a control zone—

(1) Unless ground visibility at that airport is at least 3 statute miles; or

(2) If ground visibility is not reported at that airport, unless flight visibility during landing or takeoff, or while operating in the traffic pattern, is at least 3 statute miles.

(e) For the purposes of this section, an aircraft operating at the base altitude of a transition area or control area is considered to be within the airspace directly below that area.

91.107 SPECIAL VFR WEATHER MINIMUMS IN A CONTROL ZONE.

(a) Except as provided in § 93.113 of this chapter, when a person has received an appropriate ATC clearance, the special weather minimums of this section instead of those contained in § 91.105 apply to the operation of an aircraft by that person in a control zone under VFR.

(b) No person may operate an aircraft in a control zone under VFR except clear of clouds.

(c) No person may operate an aircraft (other than a helicopter) in a control zone under VFR unless flight visibility is at least one statute mile.

(d) No person may take off or land an aircraft (other than a helicopter) at any airport in a control zone under VFR—

(1) Unless ground visibility at that airport is at least one statute mile; or

(2) If ground visibility is not reported at that airport, unless flight visibility during landing or takeoff is at least one statute mile.

(e) No person may operate an aircraft (other than a helicopter) in a control zone under the special weather minimums of this section, between sunset and sunrise (or in Alaska, when the sun is more than 6 degrees below the horizon) unless:

(1) That person meets the applicable requirements for instrument flight

under Part 61 of this chapter; and

   (2) The aircraft is equipped as required in § 91.33(d).

91.109   VFR CRUISING ALTITUDE OR FLIGHT LEVEL.

Except while holding in a holding pattern of 2 minutes or less, or while turning, each person operating an aircraft under VFR in level cruising flight more than 3,000 feet above the surface shall maintain the appropriate altitude or flight level prescribed below, unless otherwise authorized by ATC:

   (a) When operating below 18,000 feet MSL and—

   (1) On a magnetic course of zero degrees through 179 degrees, any odd thousand foot MSL altitude +500 feet (such as 3,500, 5,500, or 7,500); or

   (2) On a magnetic course of 180 degrees through 359 degrees, any even thousand foot MSL altitude +500 feet (such as 4,500, 6,500, or 8,500).

   (b) When operating above 18,000 feet MSL to flight level 290 (inclusive), and—

   (1) On a magnetic course of zero degrees through 179 degrees, any odd flight level +500 feet (such as 195, 215, or 235); or

   (2) On a magnetic course of 180 degrees through 359 degrees, any even flight level +500 feet (such as 185, 205, or 225).

   (c) When operating above flight level 290 and—

   (1) On a magnetic course of zero degrees through 179 degrees, any flight level, at 4,000-foot intervals, beginning at and including flight level 300 (such as flight level 300, 340, or 380); or

   (2) On a magnetic course of 180 degrees through 359 degrees, any flight level, at 4,000-foot intervals, beginning at and including flight level 320 (such as flight level 320, 360, or 400).

Instrument Flight Rules

91.115   ATC CLEARANCE AND FLIGHT PLAN REQUIRED.

No person may operate an aircraft in controlled airspace under IFR unless—

   (a) He has filed an IFR flight plan; and

   (b) He has received an appropriate ATC clearance.

91.116   TAKEOFF AND LANDING UNDER IFR: GENERAL.

   (a) **Instrument approaches to civil airports.** Unless otherwise authorized by the Administrator (including ATC), each person operating an aircraft shall, when an instrument letdown to an airport is necessary, use a standard instrument approach procedure prescribed for that airport in Part 97 of this chapter.

   (b) **Landing minimums.** Unless otherwise authorized by the Administrator, no person operating an aircraft (except a military aircraft of the United States) may land that aircraft using a standard instrument approach procedure prescribed in Part 97 of this chapter unless the visibility is at or above the landing minimum prescribed in that Part for the procedure used. If the landing minimum in a standard instrument approach procedure prescribed in Part 97 of this chapter is stated in terms of ceiling and visibility, the visibility minimum applies. However, the ceiling minimum shall be added to the field elevation and that value observed as the MDA or DH, as appropriate to the procedure being executed.

(c) **Civil airport takeoff minimums.** Unless otherwise authorized by the Administrator, no person operating an aircraft under Part 121, 123, 129, or 135 of this chapter may take off from a civil airport under IFR unless weather conditions are at or above the weather minimums for IFR takeoff prescribed for that airport in Part 97 of this chapter. If takeoff minimums are not prescribed in Part 97 of this chapter, for a particular airport, the following minimums apply to takeoffs under IFR for aircraft operating under those Parts:

(1) Aircraft having two engines or less: One statute mile visibility.

(2) Aircraft having more than two engines: One-half statute mile visibility.

(d) **Military airports.** Unless otherwise prescribed by the Administrator, each person operating a civil aircraft under IFR into, or out of, a military airport shall comply with the instrument approach procedures and the takeoff and landing minimums prescribed by the military authority having jurisdiction on that airport.

(e) **Comparable values of RVR and ground visibility.**

(1) If RVR minimums for takeoff or landing are prescribed in an instrument approach procedure, but RVR is not reported for the runway of intended operation, the RVR minimum shall be converted to ground visibility in accordance with the table in subparagraph (2) of this paragraph and observed as the applicable visibility minimum for takeoff or landing on that runway.

(2)

RVR (feet)	Visibility (statute miles)
1,600	¼
2,400	½
3,200	⅝
4,000	¾
4,500	⅞
5,000	1
6,000	1¼

(f) **Operation on unpublished routes and use of radar in instrument approach procedures.** When radar is approved at certain locations for ATC purposes, it may be used not only for surveillance and precision radar approaches, as applicable, but also may be used in conjunction with instrument approach procedures predicated on other types of radio navigational aids. Radar vectors may be authorized to provide course guidance through the segments of an approach procedure to the final approach fix or position. When operating on an unpublished route or while being radar vectored, the pilot, when an approach clearance is received, shall, in addition to complying with § 91.119, maintain his last assigned altitude (1) unless a different altitude is assigned by ATC, or (2) until the aircraft is established on a segment of a published route or instrument approach procedure. After the aircraft is so established, published altitudes apply to descent within each succeeding route or approach segment unless a different altitude is assigned by ATC. Upon reaching the final approach fix or position, the pilot may either complete his instrument approach in accordance with the procedure approved for the facility, or may continue a surveillance or precision radar approach to a landing.

(g) **Use of low or medium frequency simultaneous radio ranges for ADF procedures.** Low frequency or medium frequency simultaneous radio ranges may be used as an ADF instrument approach aid if an ADF procedure for the airport concerned is prescribed by the Administrator, or if an approach is conducted using the same courses and altitudes for the ADF approach as those specified in the approved range procedure.

(h) **Limitations on procedure turns.** In the case of a radar initial approach to a final approach fix or position, or a timed approach from a holding fix, or where the procedure specifies "NOPT" or "FINAL," no pilot may make a procedure turn unless, when he receives his final approach clearance, he so advises ATC.

91.117   LIMITATIONS ON USE OF INSTRUMENT APPROACH PROCEDURES (OTHER THAN CATEGORY II).

(a) **General.** Unless otherwise authorized by the Administrator, each person operating an aircraft using an instrument approach procedure prescribed in Part 97 of this chapter shall comply with the requirements of this section. This section does not apply to the use of Category II approach procedures.

(b) **Descent below MDA or DH.** No person may operate an aircraft below the prescribed minimum descent altitude or continue an approach below the decision height unless—

(1) The aircraft is in a position from which a normal approach to the runway of intended landing can be made; and

(2) The approach threshold of that runway, or approach lights or other markings identifiable with the approach end of that runway, are clearly visible to the pilot.

If, upon arrival at the missed approach point or decision height, or at any time thereafter, any of the above requirements are not met, the pilot shall immediately execute the appropriate missed approach procedure.

(c) **Inoperative or unusable components and visual aids.** The basic ground components of an ILS are the localizer, glide slope, outer marker, and middle marker. The approach lights are visual aids normally associated with the ILS. In addition, if an ILS approach procedure in Part 97 of this chapter prescribes a visibility minimum of 1,800 feet or 2,000 feet RVR, high-intensity runway lights, touchdown zone lights, centerline lighting and marking and RVR are aids associated with the ILS for those minimums. Compass locator or precision radar may be substituted for the outer or middle marker. Surveillance radar may be substituted for the outer marker. Unless other specified by the Administrator, if a ground component, visual aid, or RVR is inoperative, or unusable, or not utilized, the straight-in minimums prescribed in any approach procedure in Part 97 of this chapter are raised in accordance with the following tables. Except as provided in subparagraph (5) of this paragraph or unless otherwise specified by the Administrator, if a ground component, visual aid, or RVR is inoperative, or unusable or not utilized, the straight-in minimums prescribed in any approach procedure in Part 97 of this chapter are raised in accordance with the following tables. If the related airborne equipment for a ground component is inoperative or not utilized, the increased minimums applicable to the related ground component shall be used. If more than one component or aid is inoperative, or unusable, or not utilized, each minimum is raised to the highest minimum required by any one of the components or aids which is inoperative, or unusable, or not utilized.

(1) ILS and PAR

Component or Aid	Increase Decision Height	Increase Visibility (Statute Miles)	*Approach Category
LOC[1]	ILS approach not authorized.	....	All.
GS	As specified in the procedure.	....	All.
OM[1], MM[1]	50 feet	None	ABC.
OM[1], MM[1]	50 feet	¼	D.
ALS	50 feet	¼	All.
SSALSR	50 feet	¼	ABC.
MALSR	50 feet	¼	ABC.

[1] Not applicable to PAR.

(2) ILS with visibility minimum of 1,800 or 2,000 feet RVR

Component or Aid	Increase Decision Height	Increase Visibility (Statute Miles)	* Approach Category
LOC	ILS approach not authorized.	....	All.
GS	As specified in the procedure.	....	All.
OM, MM	50 feet	To ½ mile.	ABC.
OM, MM	50 feet	To ¾ mile.	D.
ALS	50 feet	To ¾ mile.	All.
HIRL, TDZL, RCLS	None	To ½ mile.	All.
RCLM	As specified in the procedure.	....	All.
RVR	None	To ½ mile.	All.

(3) VOR, LOC, LDA, and ASR

Component or Aid	Increase MDA	Increase Visibility (Statute Miles)	* Approach Category
ALS, SSALSR, MALSR	None	½ mile	ABC.
SSALS, MALS, HIRL, REIL	None	¼ mile	ABC.

(4) NDB (ADF) and LFR

Component or Aid	Increase MDA	Increase Visibility (Statute Miles)	* Approach Category
ALS, SSALSR, MALSR	None	¼ mile	ABC.

* "Aircraft approach category" means a grouping of aircraft based on a speed of 1.3 V_{so} (at maximum certified landing weight) or on maximum certificated landing weight. V_{so} and the maximum certificated landing weight are those values as established for the aircraft by the certificating authority of the country of registry. If an aircraft falls into two categories, it is placed in the higher of the two. The categories are as follows:

Category A: Speed less than 91 knots; weight less than 30,001 pounds.

Category B: Speed 91 knots or more, but less than 121 knots; weight 30,001 pounds or more, but less than 60,001 pounds.

Category C: Speed 121 knots or more, but less than 141 knots; weight 60,001 pounds or more, but less than 150,001 pounds.

Category D: Speed 141 knots or more, but less than 166 knots; weight 150,001 pounds or more.

Category E: Speed 166 knots or more; any weight.

(5) The inoperative component tables in subparagraphs (1) through (4) of this paragraph do not apply to helicopter procedures. Helicopter procedure minimums are specified on each procedure for inoperative components.

91.119 MINIMUM ALTITUDES FOR IFR OPERATIONS.

(a) Except when necessary for takeoff or landing, or unless otherwise authorized by the Administrator, no person may operate an aircraft under IFR below—

(1) The applicable minimum altitudes prescribed in Parts 95 and 97 of this chapter; or

(2) If no applicable minimum altitude is prescribed in those Parts—

(i) In the case of operations over an area designated as a mountainous area in Part 95, an altitude of 2,000 feet above the highest obstacle within a horizontal distance of five statute miles from the course to be flown; or

(ii) In any other case, an altitude of 1,000 feet above the highest obstacle within a horizontal distance of five statute miles from the course to be flown.

However, if both a MEA and a MOCA are prescribed for a particular route or route segment, a person may operate an aircraft below the MEA down to, but not below, the MOCA, when within 25 statute miles of the VOR concerned (based on the pilot's reasonable estimate of that distance).

(b) **Climb.** Climb to a higher minimum IFR altitude shall begin immediately after passing the point beyond which that minimum altitude applies, except that, when ground obstructions intervene, the point beyond which the higher minimum altitude applies shall be crossed at or above the applicable MCA.

91.121 IFR CRUISING ALTITUDE OR FLIGHT LEVEL.

(a) **In controlled airspace.** Each person operating an aircraft under IFR in level cruising flight in controlled airspace shall maintain the altitude or flight level assigned that aircraft by ATC. However, if the ATC clearance assigns "VFR conditions-on-top," he shall maintain an altitude or flight level as prescribed by § 91.109.

(b) **In uncontrolled airspace.** Except while holding in a holding pattern of two minutes or less, or while turning, each person operating an aircraft under IFR in level cruising flight, in uncontrolled airspace, shall maintain an appropriate altitude as follows:

(1) When operating below 18,000 feet MSL and—

(i) On a magnetic course of zero degrees through 179 degrees, any odd thousand foot MSL altitude (such as 3,000, 5,000, or 7,000); or

(ii) On a magnetic course of 180 degrees through 359 degrees, any even thousand foot MSL altitude (such as 2,000, 4,000, or 6,000).

(2) When operating at or above 18,000 feet MSL, but below flight level 290, and—

(i) On a magnetic course of zero degrees through 179 degrees, any odd flight level (such as 190, 210, or 230); or

(ii) On a magnetic course of 180 degrees through 359 degrees, any even flight level (such as 180, 200, or 220).

(3) When operating at flight level 290 and above, and—

(i) On a magnetic coruse of zero degrees through 179 degrees, any flight level, at 4,000-foot intervals, beginning at and including flight level 290 (such as flight level 290, 330 or 370); or

(ii) On a magnetic course of 180 degrees through 359 degrees, any flight level, at 4,000-foot intervals, beginning at and including flight level 310 (such as flight level 310, 350, or 390).

91.123 COURSE TO BE FLOWN.

Unless otherwise authorized by ATC, no person may operate an aircraft within controlled airspace, under IFR, except as follows:

(a) On a Federal airway, along the centerline of that airway.

(b) On any other route, along the direct course between the navigational aids or fixes defining that route.

However, this section does not prohibit maneuvering the aircraft to pass well clear of other air traffic or the maneuvering of the aircraft, in VFR conditions, to clear the intended flight path both before and during climb or descent.

91.125 IFR, RADIO COMMUNICATIONS.

The pilot in command of each aircraft operated under IFR in controlled airspace shall have a continuous watch maintained on the appropriate frequency and shall report by radio as soon as possible—

(a) The time and altitude of passing each designated reporting point, or the reporting points specified by ATC, except that while the aircraft is under radar control, only the passing of those reporting points specifically requested by ATC need be reported;

(b) Any unforecast weather conditions encountered; and

(c) Any other information relating to the safety of flight.

91.127 IFR OPERATIONS; TWO-WAY RADIO COMMUNICATIONS FAILURE.

(a) **General.** Unless otherwise authorized by ATC, each pilot who has two-way radio communications failure when operating under IFR shall comply with the rules of this section.

(b) **VFR conditions.** If the failure occurs in VFR conditions, or if VFR conditions are encountered after the failure, each pilot shall continue the flight under VFR and land as soon as practicable.

(c) **IFR conditions.** If the failure occurs in IFR conditions, or if paragraph (b) of this section cannot be complied with, each pilot shall continue the flight according to the following:

(1) ROUTE.

(i) By the route assigned in the last ATC clearance received;

(ii) If being radar vectored, by the direct route from the point of radio failure to the fix, route, or airway specified in the vector clearance;

(iii) In the absence of an assigned route, by the route that ATC has advised may be expected in a further clearance; or

(iv) In the absense of an assigned route or a route that ATC has advised may be expected in a further clearance, by the route filed in the flight plan.

(2) ALTITUDE. At the highest of the following altitudes or flight levels for the route segment being flown:

(i) The altitude or flight level assigned in the last ATC clearance received;

(ii) The minimum altitude (converted, if appropriate, to minimum flight level as prescribed in § 91.81(c)) for IFR operations; or

(iii) The altitude or flight level ATC has advised may be expected in a further clearance.

(3) (Revoked.)

(4) LEAVE HOLDING FIX. If holding instructions have been received, leave the holding fix at the expect-further-clearance time received, or, if an expected approach clearance time has been received, leave the holding fix in order to arrive over the fix from which the approach begins as close as possible to the expected approach clearance time.

(5) DESCENT FOR APPROACH. Begin descent from the en route altitude or flight level upon reaching the fix from which the approach begins, but not before—

(i) The expect-approach-clearance time (if received); or

(ii) If no expect-approach-clearance time has been received, at the estimated time of arrival, shown on the flight plan, as amended with ATC.

91.129 OPERATION UNDER IFR IN CONTROLLED AIRSPACE; MALFUNCTION REPORTS.

(a) The pilot in command of each aircraft operated in controlled airspace under IFR, shall report immediately to ATC any of the following malfunctions of equipment occurring in flight:

(1) Loss of VOR, TACAN, ADF, or low frequency navigation receiver capability.

(2) Complete or partial loss of ILS receiver capability.

(3) Impairment of air/ground communications capability.

(b) In each report required by paragraph (a) of this section, the pilot in command shall include the—

(1) Aircraft identification;

(2) Equipment affected;

(3) Degree to which the capability of the pilot to operate under IFR in the ATC system is impaired; and

(4) Nature and extent of assistance he desires from ATC.

Subpart C—Maintenance, Preventive Maintenance, and Alterations

91.161 APPLICABILITY.

(a) This subpart prescribes rules governing the maintenance, preventive maintenance, and alteration of U.S. registered civil aircraft operating within or without the United States.

(b) Sections 91.165, 91.169, 91.170, 91.171, 91.173, and 91.174 of this subpart do not apply to an aircraft maintained in accordance with a continuous airworthiness maintenance program as provided in Part 121, 127, or 135 of this chapter.

91.163 GENERAL.

(a) The owner or operator of an aircraft is primarily responsible for maintaining that aircraft in an airworthy condition, including compliance with Part 39 of this chapter. (EDITOR'S NOTE—Part 39 details Airworthiness Directives.)

(b) No person may perform maintanance, preventive maintenance, or alterations on an aircraft other than as prescribed in this subpart and other applicable regulations, including Part 43.

(c) No person may operate a rotorcraft for which a Rotorcraft Maintenance Manual containing an "Airworthiness Limitations" section has been issued, unless the replacement times, inspection intervals, and related procedures specified in that section of the manual are complied with.

91.165 MAINTENANCE REQUIRED.

Each owner or operator of an aircraft shall have that aircraft inspected as prescribed in Subpart D or § 91.169 of this Part, as appropriate, and § 91.170 of this Part and shall, between required inspections, have defects repaired as prescribed in Part 43 of this chapter. In addition, he shall ensure that maintenance personnel make appropriate entries in the aircraft and maintenance records indicating the aircraft has been released to service.

91.167 CARRYING PERSONS OTHER THAN CREWMEMBERS AFTER REPAIRS OR ALTERATIONS.

(a) No person may carry any person (other than crewmembers) in an aircraft that has been repaired or altered in a manner that may have appreciably changed its flight characteritics, or substantially affected its operation in flight, until it has been approved for return to service in accordance with Part 43 and an appropriately rated pilot, with at least a private pilot's certificate, flies the aircraft, makes an operational check of the repaired or altered part, and logs the flight in the aircraft's records.

(b) Paragraph (a) of this section does not require that the aircraft be flown if ground tests or inspections, or both, show conclusively that the repair or alteration has not appreciably changed the flight characteristics, or subtantially affected the flight operation of the aircraft.

91.169 INSPECTIONS.

(a) Except as provided in paragraph (c) of this section, no person may operate an aircraft unless, within the preceding 12 calendar months, it has had—(1) an annual inspection in accordance with Part 43 of this chapter and has been approved for return to service by a person authorized by § 43.7 of this chapter; or (2) an inspection for the issue of an airworthiness certificate.

No inspection performed under paragraph (b) of the section may be substituted for any inspection required by this paragraph unless it is performed by a person authorized to perform annual inspections, and is entered as an 'annual' inspection in the required maintenance records.

(b) Except as provided in paragraph (c) of this section, no person may operate an aircraft carrying any person (other than a crewmember) for hire, and no person may give flight instruction for hire in an aircraft which that person provides, unless within the preceding 100 hours of time in service it has received an annual or 100-hour inspection and been approved for return to service in accordance with Part 43 of this chapter, or received an inspection for the issuance of an airworthiness certificate in accordance with Part 21 of this chapter. The 100-hour limitation may be exceeded by not more than 10 hours if necessary to reach a place at which the inspection can be done. The excess time, however, is included in computing the next 100 hours of time in service.

(c) Paragraphs (a) and (b) of this section do not apply to—(1) any aircraft for which its registered owner or operator complies with the progressive inspection requirements of § 91.171 and Part 43 of this chapter; (2) an aircraft that carries a special flight permit or a current experimental or provisional certificate; (3) any airplane operated by an air travel club that is inspected in accordance with Part 123 of this chapter and the operator's manual and operations specifications; (4) an aircraft inspected in accordance with an approved aircraft inspection program under Part 135 of this chapter and so identified by the registration number in the operations specifications of the certificate holder having the approved inspection program; or (5) any large airplane, or a turbojet- or turbopropeller-powered multiengine airplane, that is inspected in accordance with an inspection program authorized under Subpart D of this Part.

91.170 ALTIMETER SYSTEM TESTS AND INSPECTIONS.

(a) No person may operate an airplane in controlled airspace under IFR unless, within the preceding 24 calendar months, each static pressure system and each altimeter instrument has been tested and inspected and found to comply with Appendix E of Part 43 of this chapter. The static pressure system and altimeter instrument tests and inspections may be conducted by—

(1) The manufacturer of the airplane on which the tests and inspections are to be performed;

(2) A certificated repair station properly equipped to perform these functions and holding—

(i) An instrument rating, Class I;

(ii) A limited instrument rating appropriate to the make and model altimeter to be tested;

(iii) A limited rating appropriate to the test to be performed;

(iv) An airframe rating appropriate to the airplane to be tested; or

(v) A limited rating for a manufacturer issued for the altimeter in accordance with § 145.101(b)(4) of this chapter; or

(3) A certificated mechanic with an airframe rating (static pressure system tests and inspections only).

(b) (Revoked.)

(c) No person may operate an airplane in controlled airspace under IFR at an altitude above the maximum altitude to which an altimeter of that airplane has been tested.

91.171 PROGRESSIVE INSPECTION.

(a) Each registered owner or operator of an aircraft desiring to use the progressive inspection must submit a written request to the Flight Standards District Office having jurisdiction over the area in which the applicant is located, and shall provide—

(1) A certificated mechanic holding an inspection authorization, a certificated airframe repair station, or the manufacturer of the aircraft, to supervise or conduct the progressive inspection;

(2) A current inspection procedures manual available and readily

understandable to pilot and maintenance personnel containing, in detail—

 (i) An explanation of the progressive inspection, including the continuity of inspection responsibility, the making of reports, and the keeping of records and technical reference material;

 (ii) An inspection schedule, specifying the intervals in hours or days when routine and detailed inspections will be performed and including instructions for exceeding an inspection interval by not more than 10 hours while enroute and for changing an inspection interval because of service experience;

 (iii) Sample routine and detailed inspection forms and instructions for their use; and

 (iv) Sample reports and records, and instructions for their use;

 (3) Enough housing and equipment for necessary disassembly and proper inspection of the aircraft; and

 (4) Appropriate current technical information for the aircraft.

(b) The frequency and detail of the progressive inspection shall provide for the complete inspection of the aircraft within each 12 calendar months and be consistent with the manufacturer's recommendations, field service experience, and the kind of operation in which the aircraft is engaged. The progressive inspection schedule must insure that the aircraft at all times will be airworthy and will conform to all applicable FAA aircraft specifications, type certificate data sheets, airworthiness directives, and other approved data.

(c) If the progressive inspection is discontinued, the owner or operator shall immediately notify the local General Aviation District Office, in writing, of the discontinuance. After that discontinuance, the first annual inspection under § 91.169(a) is due within 12 calendar months after the last complete inspection of the aircraft under the progressive inspection. The 100-hour inspection under § 91.169(b) is due within 100 hours after that complete inspection. A complete inspection of the aircraft, for the purpose of determining when the annual and 100-hour inspections are due, will require a detailed inspection of the aircraft and all its components in accordance with the progressive inspection. A routine inspection of the aircraft and a detailed inspection of several components is not considered to be a complete inspection.

91.173 MAINTENANCE RECORDS.

(a) Except for work performed in accordance with §§ 91.170 and 91.177, each registered owner or operator shall keep the following records for the periods specified in paragraph (b) of this section:

 (1) Records of the maintenance and alteration, and records of the 100-hour, annual, progressive, and other required or approved inspections, as appropriate for each aircraft (including the airframe) and each engine, propeller, rotor, and appliance of an aircraft. The records must include— (i) A description (or reference to data acceptable to the Administrator) of the work performed; (ii) The date of completion of the work performed; and (iii) The signature and certificate number of the person approving the aircraft for return to service.

(2) Records containing the following information: (i) The total time in service of the airframe. (ii) The current status of life-limited parts of each airframe, engine, propeller, rotor, and appliance. (iii) The time since last overhaul of all items installed on the aircraft which are required to be overhauled on a specified time basis. (iv) The identification of the current inspection status of the aircraft, including the times since the last inspections required by the inspection program under which the aircraft and its appliances are maintained. (v) The current status of applicable airworthiness directives (AD) including, for each, the method of compliance, the AD number, and revision date. If the AD involves recurring action, the time and date when the next action is required. (vi) A list of current major alterations to each airframe, engine, propeller, rotor, and appliance.

(b) The owner or operator shall retain the following records for the periods prescribed:

(1) The records specified in paragraph (a)(1) of this section shall be retained until the work is repeated or suspended by other work or for 1 year after the work is performed.

(2) The records specified in paragraph (a)(2) of this section shall be retained and transferred with the aircraft at the time the aircraft is sold.

(3) A list of defects furnished to a registered owner or operator under § 43.9 of this chapter, shall be retained until the defects are repaired and the aircraft is approved for return to service.

(c) The owner or operator shall make all maintenance records required to be kept by this section available for inspection by the Administrator or any authorized representative of the National Transportation Safety Board (NTSB).

91.174 TRANSFER OF MAINTENANCE RECORDS.

Any owner or operator who sells a U.S. registered aircraft shall transfer to the purchaser, at the time of sale, the following records of that aircraft, in plain language form or in coded form at the election of the purchaser, if the coded form provides for the preservation and retrieval of information in a manner acceptable to the Administrator:

(a) The records specified in § 91.173(a)(2).

(b) The records specified in § 91.173(a)(1) which are not included in the records covered by paragraph (a) of this section, except that the purchaser may permit the seller to keep physical custody of such records. However, custody of records in the seller does not relieve the purchaser of his responsibility under § 91.173(c), to make the records available for inspection by the Administrator or any authorized representative of the National Transportation Safety Board (NTSB).

91.175 REBUILT ENGINE MAINTENANCE RECORDS.

(a) The owner or operator may use a new maintenance record, without previous operating history, for an aircraft engine rebuilt by the manufacturer or by an agency approved by the manufacturer.

(b) Each manufacturer or agency that grants zero time to an engine rebuilt by it shall enter, in the new record—(1) A signed statement of the date the engine was rebuilt; (2) Each change made as required by Airworthiness Directives; and (3) Each change made in compliance with manufacturer's service bulletins, if the entry is specifically requested in that bulletin.

(c) For the purposes of this section, a rebuilt engine is a used engine that has been completely disassembled, inspected, repaired as necessary, reassembled, tested, and approved in the same manner and to the same tolerances and limits as a new engine with either new or used parts. However, all parts used in it must conform to the production drawing tolerances and limits for new parts or be of approved oversized or undersized dimensions for a new engine.

91.177 ATC TRANSPONDER TESTS AND INSPECTIONS.

(a) After January 1, 1976, no person may use an ATC transponder that is specified in §§ 91.24(a), 121.345(c), 127.123(b), or 135.143(c) of this chapter, unless, within the preceding 24 calendar months, that ATC transponder has been tested and inspected and found to comply with Appendix F of Part 43 of this chapter.

(b) The tests and inspections specified in paragraph (a) of this section may be conducted by—

(1) A certificated repair station properly equipped to perform those functions and holding—

(i) A radio rating, class III;

(ii) A limited radio rating appropriate to the make and model transponder to be tested;

(iii) A limited rating appropriate to the test to be performed; or

(iv) A limited rating for manufacturer issued for the transponder in accordance with § 145.101(b)(4) of this chapter; or

(2) A certificate holder authorized to perform maintenance in accordance with §§ 121.379 or 127.140 of this chapter; or

(3) The manufacturer of the aircraft on which the transponder to be tested is installed, if the transponder was installed by that manufacturer.

Subpart D—Large and Turbine-Powered Multiengine Airplanes

91.181 APPLICABILITY.

(a) Sections 91.181–91.215 prescribe operating rules, in addition to those prescribed in other subparts of this Part, governing the operation of large and of turbojet-powered multiengine civil airplanes of U.S. registry. The operating rules in this subpart do not apply to those airplanes when they are required to be operated under Parts 121, 123, 129, 135, and 137 of this chapter. Sections 91.217 and 91.219 prescribe an inspection program for large and for turbine-powered (turbojet and turboprop) multiengine airplanes of U.S. registry when they are operated under this subpart or Parts 129 or 137 and for small turbine-powered multiengine airplanes operated under Part 135 of this chapter.

(b) Operations that may be conducted under the rules in this subpart instead of those in Parts 121, 123, 129, 135, and 137 of this chapter, when common carriage is not involved, include—

(1) Ferry or training flights;

(2) Aerial work operations such as aerial photography or survey, or pipeline patrol, but not including firefighting operations;

(3) Flights for the demonstration of an airplane to prospective customers when no charge is made except for those specified in paragraph (d) of this section;

(4) Flights conducted by the operator of an airplane for his personal transportation, or the transportation of his guests when no charge, assessment, or fee is made for the transportation;

(5) The carriage of officials, employees, guests, and property of a company on an airplane operated by that company, or the parent or a subsidiary of that company or a subsidiary of the parent, when the carriage is within the scope of, and incidental to, the business of the company (other than transportation by air) and no charge, assessment or fee is made for the carriage in excess of the cost of owning, operating, and maintaining the airplane, except that no charge of any kind may be made for the carriage of a guest of a company, when the carriage is not within the scope of, and incidental to, the business of that company;

(6) The carriage of company officials, employees, and guests of the company on an airplane operated under a time sharing, interchange, or joint ownership agreement as defined in paragraph (c) of this section;

(7) The carriage of property (other than mail) on an airplane operated by a person in the furtherance of a business or employment (other than transportation by air) when the carriage is within the scope of, and incidental to, that business or employment and no charge, assessment, or fee is made for the carriage other than those specified in paragraph (d) of this section;

(8) The carriage on an airplane of an athletic team, sports group, choral group, or similar group having a common purpose or objective when there is no charge, assessment, or fee of any kind made by any person for that carriage; and

(9) The carriage of persons on an airplane operated by a person in the furtherance of a business (other than transportation by air) for the purpose of selling to them land, goods, or property, including franchises or distributorships, when the carriage is within the scope of, and incidental to, that business and no charge, assessment, or fee is made for that carriage.

(c) As used in this section—

(1) A "time sharing agreement" means an arrangement whereby a person leases his airplane with flight crew to another person, and no charge is made for the flights conducted under that arrangement other than those specified in paragraph (d) of this section;

(2) An "interchange agreement" means an arrangement whereby a person leases his airplane to another person in exchange for equal time, when needed, on the other person's airplane, and no charge, assessment, or fee is made, except that a charge may be made not to exceed the difference between the cost of owning, operating, and maintaining the two airplanes;

(3) A "joint ownership agreement" means an arrangement whereby one of the registered joint owners of an airplane employs and furnishes the flight crew for that airplane and each of the registered joint owners pays a

share of the charges specified in the agreement.

(d) The following may be charged, as expenses of a specific flight, for transportation as authorized by paragraphs (b) (3) and (7) and (c) (1) of this section:

(1) Fuel, oil, lubricants, and other additives.

(2) Travel expenses of the crew, including food, lodging, and ground transportation.

(3) Hangar and tie-down costs away from the aircraft's base of operations.

(4) Insurance obtained for the specific flight.

(5) Landing fees, airport taxes, and similar assessments.

(6) Customs, foreign permit, and similar fees directly related to the flight.

(7) Inflight food and beverages.

(8) Passenger ground transportation.

(9) Flight planning and weather contract services.

(10) An additional charge equal to 100 percent of the expenses listed in subparagraph (1) of this paragraph.

91.183 FLYING EQUIPMENT AND OPERATING INFORMATION.

(a) The pilot in command of an airplane shall insure that the following flying equipment and aeronautical charts and data, in current and appropriate form, are accessible for each flight at the pilot station of the airplane:

(1) A flashlight having at least two size D cells, or the equivalent, that is in good working order.

(2) A cockpit checklist containing the procedures required by paragraph (b) of this section.

(3) Pertinent aeronautical charts.

(4) For IFR, VFR over-the-top, or night operations, each pertinent navigational en route, terminal area, and approach and letdown chart.

(5) In the case of multiengine airplanes, one-engine inoperative climb performance data.

(b) Each cockpit checklist must contain the following procedures and shall be used by the flight crewmembers when operating the airplane:

(1) Before starting engines.

(2) Before takeoff.

(3) Cruise.

(4) Before landing.

(5) After landing.

(6) Stopping engines.

(7) Emergencies.

(c) Each emergency cockpit checklist procedure required by paragraph (b)(7) of this section must contain the following procedures, as appropriate:

(1) Emergency operation of fuel, hydraulic, electrical, and mechanical systems.

(2) Emergency operation of instruments and controls.

(3) Engine inoperative procedures.

(4) Any other procedures necessary for safety.

(d) The equipment, charts, and data prescribed in this section shall be used by the pilot in command and other members of the flight crew, when pertinent.

91.185 FAMILIARITY WITH OPERATING LIMITATIONS AND EMERGENCY EQUIPMENT.

(a) Each pilot in command of an airplane shall, before beginning a flight, familiarize himself with the airplane flight manual for that airplane, if one is required, and with any placards, listings, instrument markings, or any combination thereof, containing each operating limitation prescribed for that airplane by the Administrator, including those specified in § 91.31(b).

(b) Each required member of the crew shall, before beginning a flight, familiarize himself with the emergency equipment installed on the airplane to which he is assigned and with the procedures to be followed for the use of that equipment in an emergency situation.

91.187 EQUIPMENT REQUIREMENTS: OVER-THE-TOP, OR NIGHT VFR OPERATIONS.

No person may operate an airplane over-the-top, or at night under VFR unless that airplane is equipped with the instruments and equipment required for IFR operations under § 91.33(d) and one electric landing light for night operations. Each required instrument and item of equipment must be in operable condition.

91.189 SURVIVAL EQUIPMENT FOR OVERWATER OPERATIONS.

(a) No person may take off an airplane for a flight over water more than 50 nautical miles from the nearest shoreline, unless that airplane is equipped with a life preserver or an approved flotation means for each occupant of the airplane.

(b) No person may take off an airplane for a flight over water more than 30 minutes flying time or 100 nautical miles from the nearest shoreline, unless it has on board the following survival equipment:

(1) A life preserver equipped with an approved survival locator light, for each occupant of the airplane.

(2) Enough liferafts (each equipped with an approved survival locator light) of a rated capacity and buoyancy to accommodate the occupants of the airplane.

(3) At least one pyrotechnic signaling device for each raft.

(4) One self-buoyant, water-resistant, portable emergency radio signaling device, that is capable of transmission on the appropriate emergency frequency or frequencies, and not dependent upon the airplane power supply.

(5) After June 26, 1979, a lifeline stored in accordance with § 25.1411(g) of this chapter.

(c) The required liferafts, life preservers, and signaling devices must be installed in conspicuously marked locations and easily accessible in the event of a ditching without appreciable time for preparatory procedures.

(d) A survival kit, appropriately equipped for the route to be flown, must be attached to each required liferaft.

91.191 RADIO EQUIPMENT FOR OVERWATER OPERATIONS.

(a) Except as provided in paragraphs (c) and (d) of this section, no person may take off an airplane for a flight over water more than 30 minutes flying time or 100 nautical miles from the nearest shoreline, unless it has at least the following operable radio communication and navigational equipment appropriate to the facilities to be used and able to transmit to, and receive from, at any place on the route, at least one surface facility:

(1) Two transmitters.
(2) Two microphones.
(3) Two headsets or one headset and one speaker.
(4) Two independent receivers for navigation.
(5) Two independent receivers for communications.

However, a receiver that can receive both communications and navigational signals may be used in place of a separate communications receiver and a separate navigational signal receiver.

(b) For the purposes of paragraphs (a) (4) and (5) of this section, a receiver is independent if the function of any part of it does not depend on the functioning of any part of another receiver.

(c) Notwithstanding the provisions of paragraph (a) of this section, a person may operate an airplane on which no passengers are carried from a place where repairs or replacement cannot be made to a place where they can be made, if not more than one of each of the dual items of radio communication and navigation equipment specified in subparagraphs (1)-(5) of paragraph (a) of this section malfunctions or becomes inoperative.

(d) Notwithstanding the provisions of paragraph (a) of this section, when both VHF and HF communications equipment are required for the route and the airplane has two VHF transmitters and two VHF receivers for communications, only one HF transmitter and one HF receiver is required for communications.

91.193 EMERGENCY EQUIPMENT.

(a) No person may operate an airplane unless it is equipped with the emergency equipment listed in this section:

(b) Each item of equipment—

(1) Must be inspected in accordance with § 91.217 to insure its continued serviceability and immediate readiness for its intended purposes;
(2) Must be readily accessible to the crew;
(3) Must clearly indicate its method of operation; and
(4) When carried in a compartment or container, must have that compartment or container marked as to contents and date of last inspection.

(c) Hand fire extinguishers must be provided for use in crew, passenger, and cargo compartments in accordance with the following:

(1) The type and quantity of extinguishing agent must be suitable for the kinds of fires likely to occur in the compartment where the extinguisher is intended to be used.

(2) At least one hand fire extinguisher must be provided and located on or near the flight deck in a place that is readily accessible to the flight crew.

(3) At least one hand fire extinguisher must be conveniently located in the passenger compartment of each airplane accommodating more than six but less than 31 passengers, and at least two hand fire extinguishers must be conveniently located in the passenger compartment of each airplane accommodating more than 30 passengers.

(d) First aid kits for treatment of injuries likely to occur in flight or in minor accidents must be provided.

(e) Each airplane accommodating more than 19 passengers must be equippped with a crash ax.

(f) Each passenger-carrying airplane must have a portable battery-powered megaphone or megaphones readily accessible to the crewmembers assigned to direct emergency evacuation, installed as follows:

(1) One magaphone on each airplane with a seating capacity of more than 60 but less than 100 passengers, at the most rearward location in the passenger cabin where it would be readily accessible to a normal flight attendent seat. However, the Administrator may grant a deviation from the requirements of this subparagraph if he finds that a different location would be more useful for evacuation of persons during an emergency.

(2) Two megaphones in the passenger cabin on each airplane with a seating capacity of more than 99 passengers, one installed at the forward end and the other at the most rearward location where it would be readily accessible to a normal flight attendant seat.

91.195   FLIGHT ALTITUDE RULES.

(a) Notwithstanding § 91.79, and except as provided in paragraph (b) of this section, no person may operate an airplane under VFR at less than—

(1) One thousand feet above the surface, or 1,000 feet from any mountain, hill, or other obstruction to flight, for day operations; and

(2) The altitudes prescribed in § 91.119, for night operations.

(b) This section does not apply—

(1) During takeoff or landing;

(2) When a different altitude is authorized by a waiver to this section under § 91.63; or

(3) When a flight is conducted under the special VFR weather minimums of § 91.107 with an appropriate clearance from ATC.

91.197   SMOKING AND SAFETY BELT SIGNS.

(a) Except as provided in paragraph (b) of this section, no person may operate an airplane carrying passengers unless it is equipped with signs that are visible to passengers and cabin attendants to notify them when smoking is prohibited and when safety belts should be fastened. The signs must be so constructed that the crew can turn them on and off. They must be turned on for each takeoff and each landing and when otherwise considered to be necessary by the pilot in command.

(b) The pilot in command of an airplane that is not equipped as provided in paragraph (a) of this section shall insure that the passengers are orally notified each time that it is necessary to fasten their safety belts and when smoking is prohibited.

91.199 PASSENGER BRIEFING.

(a) Before each takeoff the pilot in command of an airplane carrying passengers shall ensure that all passengers have been orally briefed on:

(1) Smoking;

(2) Use of safety belts;

(3) Location and means for opening the passenger entry door and emergency exits;

(4) Location of survival equipment;

(5) Ditching procedures and the use of flotation equipment required under § 91.189 for a flight over water; and

(6) The normal and emergency use of oxygen equipment installed on the airplane.

(b) The oral briefing required by paragraph (a) of this section shall be given by the pilot in command or a member of the crew, but need not be given when the pilot in command determines that the passengers are familiar with the contents of the briefing. It may be supplemented by printed cards for the use of each passenger containing—

(1) A diagram of, and methods of operating, the emergency exits; and

(2) Other instructions necessary for use of emergency equipment.

Each card used under this paragraph must be carried in convenient locations on the airplane for use of each passenger and must contain information that is pertinent only to the type and model airplane on which it is used.

91.201 CARRY-ON BAGGAGE.

No pilot in command of an airplane having a seating capacity of more than 19 passengers may permit a passenger to stow his baggage aboard that airplane except—

(a) In a suitable baggage or cargo storage compartment, or as provided in § 91.203; or

(b) Under a passenger seat in such a way that it will not slide forward under crash impacts severe enough to induce the ultimate inertia forces specified in § 25.561(b)(3) of this chapter, or the requirements of the regulations under which the airplane was type certificated. [After December 4, 1979 restraining devices must also limit sideward motion of under-seat baggage and be designed to withstand crash impacts severe enough to induce sideward forces specified in § 25.561(b)(3) of this chapter.]

91.203 CARRIAGE OF CARGO.

(a) No pilot in command may permit cargo to be carried in any airplane unless—

(1) It is carried in an approved cargo rack, bin, or compartment installed in the airplane;

(2) It is secured by means approved by the Administrator; or

(3) It is carried in accordance with each of the following:

(i) It is properly secured by a safety belt or other tiedown having enough strength to eliminate the possibility of shifting under all normally anticipated flight and ground conditions.

(ii) It is packaged or covered to avoid possible injury to passengers.

(iii) It does not impose any load on seats or on the floor structure that exceeds the load limitation for those components.

(iv) It is not located in a position that restricts the access to or use of any required emergency or regular exit, or the use of the aisle between the crew and the passenger compartment.

(v) It is not carried directly above seated passengers.

(b) When cargo is carried in cargo compartments that are designed to require the physical entry of a crewmember to extinguish any fire that may occur during flight, the cargo must be loaded so as to allow a crewmember to effectively reach all parts of the compartment with the contents of a hand fire extinguisher.

91.205 TRANSPORT CATEGORY AIRPLANE WEIGHT LIMITATIONS.

No person may take off a transport category airplane, except in accordance with the weight limitations prescribed for that airplane in § 91.37.

91.207 [REVOKED]

91.209 OPERATING IN ICING CONDITIONS.

(a) No pilot may take off an airplane that has—

(1) Frost, snow, or ice adhering to any propeller, windshield, or powerplant installation, or to an airspeed, altimeter, rate of climb, or flight attitude instrument system;

(2) Snow or ice adhering to the wings, or stabilizing or control surfaces; or

(3) Any frost adhering to the wings, or stabilizing or control surfaces, unless that frost has been polished to make it smooth.

(b) Except for an airplane that has ice protection provisions that meet the requirements in section 34 of Special Federal Aviation Regulation No. 23, or those for transport category airplane type certification, no pilot may fly—

(1) Under IFR into known or forecast modeate icing conditions; or

(2) Under VFR into known light or moderate icing conditions; unless the aircraft has functioning de-icing or anti-icing equipment protecting each propeller, windshield, wing, stabilizing or control surface, and each airspeed, altimeter, rate of climb, or flight altitude instrument system.

(c) Except for an airplane that has ice protection provisions that meet the requirements in section 34 of Special Federal Aviation Regulation No. 23, or those for transport category airplane type certification, no pilot may fly an airplane into known or forecast severe icing conditions.

(d) If current weather reports and briefing information relied upon by the pilot in command indicate that the forecast icing conditions that would otherwise prohibit the flight will not be encountered during the flight because of changed weather conditions since the forecast, the restrictions in paragraphs (b) and (c) of this section based on forecast conditions do not apply.

91.211   FLIGHT ENGINEER REQUIREMENTS.

(a) No person may operate the following airplanes without a flight crewmember holding a current flight engineer certificate:

(1) An airplane for which a type certificate was issued before January 2, 1964, having a maximum certificated takeoff weight of more than 80,000 pounds.

(2) An airplane type certificated after January 1, 1964, for which a flight engineer is required by the type certification requirements.

(b) No person may serve as a required flight engineer on an airplane unless, within the preceding 6 calendar months, he has had at least 50 hours of flight time as a flight engineer on that type airplane, or the Administrator has checked him on that type airplane and determined that he is familiar and competent with all essential current information and operating procedures.

91.213   SECOND IN COMMAND REQUIREMENTS.

(a) Except as provided in paragraph (b) of this section, no person may operate the following airplanes without a pilot who is designated as second in command of that airplane:

(1) A large airplane.

(2) A turbojet-powered multiengine airplane for which two pilots are required under the type certification requirements for that airplane.

(b) The Administrator may issue a letter of authorization for the operation of an airplane without compliance with the requirements of paragraph (a) of this section if that airplane is designed for and type certificated with only one pilot station. The authorization contains any conditions that the Administrator finds necessary for safe operation.

(c) No person may designate a pilot to serve as second in command nor may any pilot serve as second in command of an airplane [required under this section to have] two pilots unless that pilot meets the qualifications for second in command prescribed in § 61.55 of this chapter.

91.215   FLIGHT ATTENDANT REQUIREMENTS.

(a) No person may operate an airplane unless at least the following number of flight attendants are on board the airplane:

(1) For airplanes having more than 19 but less than 51 passengers on board—one flight attendant.

(2) For airplanes having more than 50 but less than 101 passengers on board—two flight attendants.

(3) For airplanes having more than 100 passengers on board—two flight attendants plus one additional flight attendant for each unit (or part of a unit) of 50 passengers above 100.

(b) No person may serve as a flight attendant on an airplane when required by paragraph (a) of this section, unless that person has demonstrated to the pilot in command that he is familiar with the necessary functions to be performed in an emergency or a situation requiring emergency evacuation and is capable of using the emergency equipment installed on that airplane for the performance of those functions.

91.217 INSPECTION PROGRAM

(a) No person may operate a large airplane, or a turbojet, or turbopropeller-powered multiengine airplane, unless the replacement times for life-limited parts specified in the aircraft data sheets or other documents approved by the Administrator are complied with, and the airplane, including the airframe, engines, propellers, appliances, survival equipment, and emergency equipment is inspected in accordance with an inspection program selected under the provisions of this section.

(b) The registered owner or operator of each airplane governed by this subpart must select and must use one of the following programs for the inspection of that airplane:

(1) A continuous airworthiness inspection program that is a part of a continuous airworthiness maintenance program currently in use by a person holding an air carrier or commercial operator certificate under Part 121 of this chapter.

(2) An approved aircraft inspection program currently in use by a person holding an ATCO certificate under Part 135 of this chapter.

(3) An approved continuous inspection program currently in use by a person certificated as an Air Travel Club under Part 123 of this chapter.

(4) A current inspection program recommended by the manufacturer.

(5) Any other inspection program established by the registered owner or operator of that airplane and approved by the Administrator under paragraph (e) of this section.

(c) Notice of the inspection program selected shall be sent to the local FAA District Office having jurisdiction over the area in which the airplane is based. The notice must be in writing and include—

(1) Make, model, and serial number of the airplane;

(2) Registration number of the airplane;

(3) The inspection program selected under paragraph (b) of this section; and

(4) The name and address of the person responsible for scheduling the inspections required under the selected inspection program.

(d) The registered owner or operator may not change the inspection program for an airplane unless he has given notice thereof as provided in paragraph (c) of this section and the new program has been approved by the FAA, where appropriate.

(e) Each registered owner or operator of an airplane desiring to establish an approved inspection program under paragraph (b)(5) of this section must submit the program for approval to the local FAA District Office having jurisdiction over the area in which the airplane is based. The program must include the following information:

(1) Instructions and procedures for the conduct of inspections for the particular make and model airplane, including necessary tests and checks.

The instructions and procedures must set forth in detail the parts and areas of the airframe, engines, propellers, and appliances, including emergency equipment required to be inspected.

(2) A schedule for the performance of the inspections that must be performed under the program expressed in terms of the time in service, calendar time, number of system operations, or any combination of these.

91.219 AVAILABILITY OF INSPECTION PROGRAM.

Each owner or operator of an airplane shall make a copy of the inspection program selected under § 91.217 available to—

(a) The person responsible for the scheduling of the inspections;

(b) Any person performing inspections on the airplane; and

(c) Upon request, to the Administrator.

Subpart E—Operating Noise Limits

Part 93

Special Air Traffic Rules and Airport Traffic Patterns

CONTENTS

SUBPART A—GENERAL

SUBPART L—ADDISON (TEXAS) AIRPORT TRAFFIC AREA*

SUBPART M—KETCHIKAN INTERNATIONAL AIRPORT TRAFFIC RULE*

[SUBPART N—SABRE U.S. ARMY HELIPORT (TENN.), AIRPORT TRAFFIC AREA*]

[SUBPART O—JACKSONVILLE, FLA., NAVY AIRPORT TRAFFIC AREA*]

Subpart A – General

[93.1 APPLICABILITY.

(a) This Part prescribes special airport traffic patterns and airport traffic areas. It also prescribes special air traffic rules for operating aircraft in those traffic patterns and traffic areas and in the vicinity of airports described in this Part.

(b) Unless otherwise authorized by ATC (with the exception of § 93.113), each person operating an aircraft shall do so in accordance with the special air traffic rules in this part in addition to other applicable rules in Part 91 of this chapter.

(c) Subpart E prescribes special air traffic rules for operating in the vicinity of Phoenix, Arizona, or Victor Airway No. 16.

(d) Subpart I of this part prescribes the locations at which the special VFR weather minimums do not apply to fixed-wing aircraft.

(e) Subpart K of this part designates high density traffic airports and prescribes air traffic rules and other requirements for operating aircraft to or from those airports.]

Subpart I – Locations At Which Special VFR Weather Minimums Do Not Apply

93.111 APPLICABILITY.

This subpart specifies the control zones in which special VFR weather minimums prescribed in § 91.107 of this chapter do not apply, except for in-flight emergencies.

93.113 CONTROL ZONES WITHIN WHICH SPECIAL VFR WEATHER MINIMUMS ARE NOT AUTHORIZED.

No person may operate a fixed-wing aircraft under the special VFR weather minimums prescribed in 91.107 of this chapter within the following control zones:

1. Atlanta, GA (Atlanta Airport).
2. Baltimore, MD (Baltimore–Washington International Airport).
3. Boston, MA (Logan International Airport).
4. Buffalo, NY (Greater Buffalo International Airport).
5. Chicago, IL (O'Hare International Airport).
6. Cleveland, OH (Cleveland–Hopkins International Airport).
7. Columbus, OH (Port Columbus International Airport).
8. Covington, KY (Greater Cincinnati Airport).
9. Dallas, TX (Love Field, [and Dallas–Ft. Worth Regional Airport).]
10. Denver, CO (Stapleton Municipal Airport).
11. Detroit, MI (Metropolitan Wayne County Airport).
12. Honolulu, HI (Honolulu International Airport).
13. Houston, TX (Intercontinental Airport).
14. Indianapolis, IN (Wier-Cook Municipal Airport).
15. (Reserved.)
16. Los Angeles, CA (Los Angeles International Airport).
17. Louisville, KY (Standiford Field).
18. Memphis, TN (Memphis Metropolitan Airport).
19. Miami, FL (Miami International Airport).
20. Minneapolis, MN (Minneapolis–St. Paul International Airport).
21. Newark, NJ (Newark Airport).
22. New York, NY (John F. Kennedy International Airport).
23. New York, NY (LaGuardia Airport).
24. New Orleans, LA (New Orleans International Airport–Moisant Field).
25. (Reserved.)
26. Philadelphia, PA (Philadelphia International Airport).
27. Pittsburgh, PA (Greater Pittsburgh Airport).
28. Portland, OR (Portland International Airport).
29. San Francisco, CA (San Francisco International Airport).
30. Seattle, WA (Seattle–Tacoma International Airport).
31. St. Louis, MO (Lambert–St. Louis Municipal Airport).
32. Tampa, FL (Tampa International Airport).
33. Washington, DC (Washington National Airport).

Subpart K – High Density Traffic Airports

93.121 APPLICABILITY.

This subpart designates high density traffic airports and prescribes air traffic rules for operating aircraft, other than helicopters, to or from those airports.

93.123 HIGH DENSITY TRAFFIC AIRPORTS.

(a) Each of the following airports is designated as a high density traffic airport and, except as provided in § 93.129 and paragraph (b) of this section, or unless otherwise authorized by ATC, is limited to the hourly number of allocated IFR operations (takeoffs and landings) that may be reserved for the specified classes of users for that airport:

IFR OPERATIONS PER HOUR

Class of user	John F. Kennedy Airport	La Guardia Airport	Newark Airport	O'Hare Airport	Washington National Airport
Air carrier except air taxis	70	48	40	115	40
Scheduled air taxis	5	6	10	10	8
Other	5	6	10	10	12

(b) The following exceptions apply to the allocations of reservations prescribed in paragraph (a) of this section.

(1) The allocations of reservations among the several classes of users do not apply from 12 midnight to 6 a.m. local time, but the total hourly limitation remains applicable.

(2) The allocation of IFR reservations for air carriers except air taxis at the John F. Kennedy Airport is 80 IFR reservations per hour from 5 p.m. to 8 p.m.

(3) The allocation of 40 IFR reservations for air carriers except air taxis at the Washington National Airport does not include charter flights, or other nonscheduled flights of scheduled or supplemental air carriers. These flights may be conducted without regard to the limitation of 40 IFR reservations per hour.

(4) The allocation of IFR reservations for air carriers except air taxis at LaGuardia, Newark, O'Hare, and Washington National Airports does not include extra sections of scheduled air carrier flights. These flights may be conducted without regard to the limitation upon the hourly IFR reservations for air carriers except air taxis at those airports.

(5) Any reservation allocated to, but not taken by, air carrier operations (except air taxis) is available for a scheduled air taxi operation.

(6) Any reservation allocated to, but not taken by, air carrier operations (except air taxis) or scheduled air taxi operations is available for other operations.

93.125   ARRIVAL OR DEPARTURE RESERVATION.

Except between 12 Midnight and 6 a.m. local time, no person may operate an aircraft to or from an airport designated as a high density traffic airport unless he has received, for that operation, an arrival or departure reservation from ATC.

93.129   ADDITIONAL OPERATIONS.

(a) **IFR.** The operator of an aircraft may take off or land the aircraft under IFR at a designated high density traffic airport without regard to the maximum number of operations allocated for that airport if he obtains a departure or arrival reservation, as appropriate, from ATC. The reservation is granted by ATC whenever the aircraft may be accommodated without significant additional delay to the operations allocated for the airport for which the reservation is requested.

(b) **VFR.** The operator of an aircraft may take off or land the aircraft under VFR at a designated high density traffic airport if he obtains a departure or arrival reservation, as appropriate, from ATC. The reservation is granted by ATC whenever the aircraft may be accommodated without significant additional delay to the operations allocated for the airport for which the reservation is requested and the ceiling reported at the airport is at least 1,000 feet and the ground visibility reported at the airport is at least 3 miles.

93.130 SUSPENSION OF ALLOCATIONS.

The Administrator may suspend the effectiveness of any allocation prescribed in § 93.123 and the reservation requirements prescribed in § 93.125 if he finds such action to be consistent with the efficient use of the airspace. Such suspension may be terminated whenever the Administrator determines that such action is necessary for the efficient use of the airspace.

93.133 EXCEPTIONS.

Except as provided in § 93.130, the provisions of §§ 93.123 and 93.125 do not apply to—

(a) The Newark Airport, Newark, NJ; and

(b) The Kennedy International Airport, New York, NY, and the O'Hare International Airport, Chicago, IL, except during the hours from 3 p.m. to 7:59 p.m., local time.

Part 830

Rules Pertaining to the Notification and Reporting of Aircraft Accidents or Incidents and Overdue Aircraft, and Preservation of Aircraft Wreckage, Mail, Cargo, and Records

CONTENTS

SUBPART A—GENERAL

SUBPART B—INITIAL NOTIFICATION OF AIRCRAFT ACCIDENTS, INCIDENTS, AND OVERDUE AIRCRAFT

Subpart A – General

830.1 APPLICABILITY.

This Part contains rules pertaining to:

(a) Providing notice of and reporting, aircraft accidents and incidents and certain other occurrences in the operation of aircraft when they involve civil aircraft of the United States wherever they occur, or foreign civil aircraft when such events occur in the United States, its territories or possessions.

(b) Preservation of aircraft wreckage, mail, cargo, and records involving all civil aircraft in the United States, its territories or possessions.

830.2 DEFINITIONS.

As used in this Part, the following words or phrases are defined as follows:

"Aircraft accident" means an occurrence associated with the operation of an aircraft which takes place between the time any person boards the aircraft with the intention of flight until such time as all such persons have disembarked, in which any person suffers death or serious injury as a result of being in or upon the aircraft or by direct contact with the aircraft or anything attached thereto, or in which the aircraft receives substantial damage.

"Fatal injury" means any injury which results in death within 7 days of the accident.

"Operator" means any person who causes or authorizes the operation of an aircraft, such as the owner, lessee or bailee of an aircraft.

"Serious injury" means any injury which (1) requires hospitalization for more than 48 hours, commencing within 7 days from the date the injury was received; (2) results in a fracture of any bone (except simple fractures of fingers, toes or nose); (3) involves lacerations which cause severe hemorrhages, nerve, muscle or tendon damage; (4) involves injury to any internal organ; or (5) involves second- or third-degree burns, or any burns affecting more than 5 percent of the body surface.

"Substantial damage":

(1) Except as provided in subparagraph (2) of this paragraph, substantial damage means damage or structural failure which adversely affects the structural strength, performance, or flight characteristics of the aircraft, and which would normally require major repair or replacement of the affected component.

(2) Engine failure, damage limited to an engine, bent fairings or cowling, dented skin, small puncture holes in the skin or fabric, ground damage to rotor or propeller blades, damage to landing gear, wheels, tires, flaps, engine accessories, brakes, or wing tips are not considered "substantial damage" for the purpose of this Part.

Subpart B — Initial Notification of Aircraft Accidents, Incidents, and Overdue Aircraft

830.5 IMMEDIATE NOTIFICATION.

The operator of an aircraft shall immediately, and by the most expeditious means available, notify the nearest National Transportation Safety Board (Board), field office[1] when:

(a) An aircraft accident or any of the following listed incidents occur:

(1) Flight control system malfunction or failure;

(2) Inability of any required flight crewmember to perform his normal flight duties as a result of injury or illness;

(3) Turbine engine rotor failures excluding compressor blades and turbine buckets;

(4) Inflight fire; or

(5) Aircraft collide in flight.

(b) An aircraft is overdue and is believed to have been involved in an accident.

830.6 INFORMATION TO BE GIVEN IN NOTIFICATION.

The notification required in § 830.5 shall contain the following information, if available:

(a) Type, nationality, and registration marks of the aircraft;

(b) Name of owner, and operator of the aircraft;

(c) Name of the pilot in command;

(d) Date and time of the accident;

(e) Last point of departure and point of intended landing of the aircraft;

(f) Position of the aircraft with reference to some easily defined geographical point;

(g) Number of persons aboard, number killed, and number seriously injured;

(h) Nature of the accident, the weather and the extent of damage to the aircraft, so far as is known;

(i) A description of any explosives, radioactive materials, or other dangerous articles carried.

[1] The National Transportation Safety Board field offices are listed under U.S. Government in the telephone directories in the following cities: Anchorage, AK; Chicago, IL; Denver, CO; Fort Worth, TX; Kansas City, MO; Los Angeles, CA; Miami, FL; New York, NY; Oakland, CA; Seattle, WA; Washington, DC.

Subpart C — Preservation of Aircraft Wreckage, Mail, Cargo, and Records

830.10 PRESERVATION OF AIRCRAFT WRECKAGE, MAIL, CARGO, AND RECORDS.

(a) The operator of an aircraft is responsible for preserving to the extent possible any aircraft wreckage, cargo, and mail aboard the aircraft, and all records, including tapes of flight recorders and voice recorders, pertaining to the opeation and maintenance of the aircraft and to the airmen involved in an accident or incident for which notification must be given until the Board takes custody thereof or a release is granted pursuant to § 831.17.

(b) Prior to the time the Board or its authorized representative takes custody of the aircraft wreckage, mail, or cargo, such wreckage, mail, or cargo may not be disturbed or moved except to the extent necessary:

(1) To remove persons injured or trapped;

(2) To protect the wreckage from further damage; or

(3) To protect the public from injury.

(c) Where it is necessary to disturb or move aircraft wreckage, mail or cargo, sketches, descriptive notes, and photographs shall be made, if possible, of the accident locale including original position and condition of the wreckage and any significant impact marks.

(d) The operator of an aircraft involved in an accident or incident, as defined in this Part, shall retain all records and reports, including all internal documents and memoranda dealing with the accident or incident, until authorized by the Board to the contrary.

Subpart D — Reporting of Aircraft Accidents, Incidents, and Overdue Aircraft

830.15 REPORTS AND STATEMENTS TO BE FILED.

(a) **Reports.** The operator of an aircraft shall file a report as provided in paragraph (c) of this section on Board Form 6120.1 or Board Form 6120.2 within 10 days after an accident, of after 7 days if an overdue aircraft is still missing. A report on an incident for which notification is required by § 830.5(a) shall be filed only as requested by an authorized representative of the Board.

(b) **Crewmember statement.** Each crewmember, if physically able at the time the report is submitted, shall attach thereto a statement setting forth the facts, conditions, and circumstances relating to the accident or incident as they appear to him to the best of his knowledge and belief. If the crewmember is incapacitated, he shall submit the statement as soon as he is physically able.

(c) **Where to file the reports.** The operator of an aircraft shall file with the Field Office of the Board nearest the accident or incident any report required by this section.

LIST OF FEDERAL AVIATION REGULATIONS

The FAA publishes the Federal Aviation Regulations as individual Parts sold by the Superintendent of Documents.

The more frequently amended Parts are sold on subscription service, while the less active Parts are sold on a single-sale basis.

Changes to single-sale Parts will be sold separately as issued. Information concerning these Changes will be furnished by FAA through its "Status of the Federal Aviation Regulations. AC 00-44." Instructions for ordering this free status list are given in the front of each single-sale Part.

Check or money order made payable to the Superintendent of Documents should be included with each order. Submit orders for single-sales and subscription Parts on different order forms. No COD orders are accepted. All FAR Parts should be ordered from: Superintendent of Documents, U.S. Government Printing Office, Washington, D.C. 20402.

PARTS SOLD ON SINGLE-SALE BASIS

Part	Title	Price [1]
11	General rule-making procedures	$1.30
	Change 1	.45
	Change 2	.40
	Change 3	.40
	Change 4	.80
	Change 5	.85
	[Change 6]	[.90]
	[Change 7]	[1.00]
13	Enforcement procedures	.70
	Change 1	.40
	Change 2	.40
	Change 3	1.10
27	Airworthiness standards: Normal category rotorcraft	2.10
	Change 1	.75
	Change 2	.35
	Change 3	1.30
	Change 4	1.40
	Change 5	1.40
	Change 6	2.10
	[Change 7]	[.90]
	[Change 8]	[1.70]
	[Change 9]	[.70]
29	Airworthiness standards; Transport category rotorcraft	1.70
	Change 1	.70
	Change 2	.35
	Change 3	.40
	Change 4	1.45
	Change 5	1.60
	Change 6	1.40

412

[1] Add 25% for foreign mailing.

[2] Due to their length, complexity, and frequency of issuance, Airworthiness Directives, standard instrument approach procedures, individual airspace designations, airways descriptions, restricted areas, jet route descriptions, and en route IFR altitudes are not included in the publication of these basic Parts.

		Price	
Part	Title	Domestic	Additional for foreign mailing
1	Definitions and abbreviations	$13.00	$3.25
21	Certification procedures for products and parts	18.00	4.50
23	Airworthiness standards: Normal, utility, and acrobatic category airplanes	12.00	3.00
25	Airworthiness standards: Transport category airplanes	22.00	5.50
33	Airworthiness standards: Aircraft engines	10.00	2.50
36	Noise standards: Aircraft type and airworthiness certification	17.00	4.25
37	Technical standard order authorizations	13.00	3.25
63	Certification: Flight crewmembers other than pilots	6.00	1.50
91	General operating and flight rules	26.00	6.50
93	Special air traffic rules and airport traffic patterns	14.00	3.50
[1] 103	(Part revoked as of 7/1/76)	—	—
121	Certification and operations: Domestic, flag, and supplemental air carriers and commercial operators of large aircraft	19.00	4.75
123	Certification and operations: Air travel clubs using large airplanes	10.00	2.50
135	[Air Taxi Operators and Commercial Operators ....]	[14.00]	[3.50]
139	Certification and operations: Land airports serving CAB-certificated scheduled air carriers operating large aircraft (other than helicopters)	10.00	2.50

[1] The regulations for the transportation of hazardous material by air are set forth in Part 175—Carriage by Aircraft, effective July 1, 1976, published in 41 F.R. 16106, 4/15/76. This Part is issued by the Materials Transportation Bureau, Department of Transportation, Washington, DC, 20590.

INDEX